# Osteoporosis
# SOURCEBOOK

## Health Reference Series

*First Edition*

# Osteoporosis
# SOURCEBOOK

*Basic Consumer Health Information about
Primary and Secondary Osteoporosis and
Juvenile Osteoporosis and Related Conditions,
Including Fibrous Dysplasia, Gaucher Disease,
Hyperthyroidism, Hypophosphatasia, Myeloma,
Osteopetrosis, Osteogenesis Imperfecta,
and Paget's Disease*

*Along with Information about Risk Factors,
Treatments, Traditional and Non-Traditional
Pain Management, a Glossary of Related Terms,
and a Directory of Resources*

*Edited by*
**Allan R. Cook**

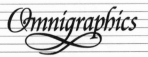

Omnigraphics

615 Griswold Street • Detroit, MI 48226

## Bibliographic Note

Because this page cannot legibly accommodate all the copyright notices, the Bibliographic Note portion of the Preface constitutes an extension of the copyright notice.

Each new volume of the *Health Reference Series* is individually titled and called a "First Edition." Subsequent updates will carry sequential edition numbers. To help avoid confusion and to provide maximum flexibility in our ability to respond to informational needs, the practice of consecutively numbering each volume will be discontinued.

Edited by Allan R. Cook

*Health Reference Series*

Karen Bellenir, *Series Editor*
Peter D. Dresser, *Managing Editor*
Joan Margeson, *Research Associate*
Dawn Matthews, *Verification Assistant*
Maria Franklin, *Permissions Assistant*
Margaret Mary Missar, *Research Coordinator*
Jenifer Swanson, *Research Associate*

EdIndex, Services for Publishers, *Indexers*

Omnigraphics, Inc.

Matthew P. Barbour, *Vice President, Operations*
Laurie Lanzen Harris, *Vice President, Editorial Director*
Kevin Hayes, *Production Coordinator*
Thomas J. Murphy, *Vice President, Finance and Comptroller*
Peter E. Ruffner, *Senior Vice President*
Jane Steele, *Marketing Coordinator*

Frederick G. Ruffner, Jr., Publisher

Library of Congress Cataloging-in-Publication Data

Osteoporosis sourcebook : basic consumer health information about primary and secondary osteoporosis and juvenile osteoporosis and related conditions, including fibrous dysplasia, Gaucher disease, hyperthyroidism, hypophosphatasia, myeloma, osteopetrosis, osteogenesis imperfecta, and Paget's disease; along with information about risk factors, treatments, traditional and nontraditional pain management, a glossary of related terms, and a directory of resources / edited by Allan R. Cook.
    p. cm. -- (Health reference series)
    Includes bibliographical references and index.
    ISBN 0-7808-0239-X
    1. Osteoporosis--Popular works. I. Cook, Allan R. II. Series
    RC931.O73 O777 2001
    616.7'16--dc21
                                                                    00-066907

∞

Printed in the United States

# *Table of Contents*

## Part IV: Related Conditions

## Part V: Osteoporosis Risk Factors and Prevention

## Part VI: Diagnosis, Treatment, and Coping Strategies

## *Part VII: Additional Help and Information*

# *Preface*

## *About This Book*

Many people think of bones as only simple, solid structures that make up the skeletal system. In truth, bones are complex, living tissues that go through a constant process of building up and tearing down. This process, called bone remodeling, rebuilds bones as people age and grow. One of the main components of bone is calcium. In fact, the skeletal system contains 99 percent of the body's calcium. In osteoporosis, which literally means *porous bones*, excessive bone loss results in a depletion of calcium. The gradual weakening of the bones over time makes them more susceptible to fractures and can lead to disfigurement and pain. Most people reach a peak bone mass between the ages of 25 and 35. By age 40, bone loss usually reaches 0.5 percent per year. Postmenopausal women can lose 2 to 3 percent per year and can have lost 50 percent of their bone mass by age 70 or 80.

In osteoporosis, bone loss accelerates. Since the loss occurs over time, the effect may not be noticed until substantial bone loss has occurred, often signaled by an unexpected fracture. Osteoporosis cannot be detected by x-ray until the bone loss has reached 30 to 50 percent of bone mass by which time the calcium depletion cannot be reversed. Because of this, prevention and early diagnosis are critical.

This *Sourcebook* provides information so that the layperson can identify the important risk factors of osteoporosis and the life-style changes needed to offset them. It provides answers to questions about calcium intake and supplements and other dietary needs, hormone replacement therapies, the drugs used to treat osteoporosis, and surgical options. It also suggests coping strategies for those suffering from the disease and provides a glossary of related terms and a directory of resources.

## How to Use This Book

This book is divided into parts and chapters. Parts focus on broad areas of interest. Chapters are devoted to single topics within a part.

*Part I: Introduction: A Quick Overview* contains the March 2000 National Institute of Health Consensus Statement on Osteoporosis prevention, diagnosis, and treatment. The report provides accessible and focused information on the nature and consequences of osteoporosis, the variance of risk factors for different segments of society, factors that affect bone health, treatment and evaluation options, and the direction of current research on osteoporosis. These topics are taken up in greater detail in the following sections.

*Part II: The Nature of Osteoporosis* identifies specific forms of osteoporosis and describes the process of bone "remodeling" the human body uses to maintain strong bones. It highlights the importance of calcium and introduces the concept of the "bone bank": because osteoporosis acts by depleting bones of calcium the effects of the disease can be severely magnified by not "depositing" sufficient calcium early in life. The final chapter in this section distinguishes osteoporosis from arthritis and emphasizes the importance of proper diagnosis. The pain of osteoporosis can be mistaken for arthritis, but some arthritis medicines aggravate bone depletion.

*Part III: Facts and Figures for Osteoporosis* outlines the costs, both monetary and in terms of health effects, for various segments of society. It draws attention to the hidden and unnoticed costs of this "silent disease" that affects more than just older women.

*Part IV: Related Conditions* provides information about diseases and conditions that lead to or aggravate osteoporosis or that have symptoms similar to those produced by osteoporosis. The conditions discussed briefly in this section can be researched more thoroughly in other volumes of the *Health Series*:

- Hyperparathyroidism and hypercalcemia—*Endocrine and Metabolic Diseases and Disorders Sourcebook*

- Osteogenesis imperfecta—*Communications Disorders Sourcebook* and *Skin Disorders Sourcebook*

- Gaucher disease—*Genetic Disorders Sourcebook*

- Hyperphosphatasia—*Kidney and Urinary Tract Diseases and Disorders Sourcebook*

- Myeloma and Paget's disease—*Cancer Sourcebook* and *Cancer Sourcebook for Women*

- Hearing loss—*Communication Disorders Sourcebook*

- Osteopetrosis—*Arthritis Sourcebook* and *Blood and Circulatory Disorders Sourcebook*

- Inflammatory bowel disease—*Gastrointestinal Diseases and Disorders Sourcebook.*

*Part V: Osteoporosis Risk Factors and Prevention* identifies factors that lead to osteoporosis and suggests healthy life-style choices to minimize those factors.

*Part VI: Diagnosis, Treatment, and Coping Strategies* traces the process of diagnosing osteoporosis as early as possible and treating the condition effectively. It reviews the various options in drug and surgical therapies and points out their drawbacks and limitations. The sections ends by discussing ways of treating the pain of osteoporosis both through traditional therapies and alternative methods.

*Part VII: Additional Help and Information* provides a glossary of osteoporosis-related terminology and a list of resources for patients with osteoporosis or related conditions.

## Bibliographic Note

This volume contains documents and excerpts from publications issued by the following U.S. government agencies: Agency for Healthcare Research and Quality (formerly named Agency for Health Care Policy and Research), National Cancer Institute (NCI), National Heart, Lung, and Blood Institute (NHLBI), National Institute on Aging (NIA), National Institute of Arthritis and Musculoskeletal and

Skin Diseases (NIAMS), and National Institutes of Health Consensus Development Program, and the U.S. Food and Drug Administration (FDA).

In addition, this volume contains copyrighted documents from the following organizations and publications: Advanstar Communications; the American College of Physicians—American Society of Internal Medicine; American Council on Science and Health; Aerobics and Fitness Association of America—*American Fitness;* American Medical Association; Lippincott Williams & Wilkins—*The Back Letter;* BMJ Publishing Group—*British Medical Journal;* Cybermedical; Harvard University—*Harvard Health Letter;* Medletter Associated—*Johns Hopkins Medical Letter;* American School Health Association—*Journal of School Health; The Lancet;* Magic Foundation; Mayo Foundation for Medical Education and Research; National Osteoporosis Foundation; Springhouse Corporation—*The Nurse Practitioner;* Osteogenesis Imperfecta Foundation; Osteoporosis and Related Bone Diseases—National Resource Center; Opus Communications Group—*The Brown University Long-Term Care Quality Letter;* Medical Economics—*Patient Care, Pediatrics for Parents,* and *Science News;* St. Jude Children's Research Hospital; *Tuft's University Health & Nutrition Letter; U.S. News and World Report;* Edward White—Miles Health Care; and Women's Health Advocate.

## *Acknowledgements*

In addition to the many organizations and agencies who contributed the material that is included in this book, thanks go to Margaret Mary Missar for her tireless efforts in tracking down documents, Jenifer Swanson for her researching and Internet expertise, Dawn Matthews for her verification assistance, and Maria Franklin for her patient negotiation of reprint permissions. And, of course, Bruce the Scanman for his OCR artistry.

## *Note from the Editor*

This book is part of Omnigraphics' *Health Reference Series.* The series provides basic information about a broad range of medical concerns. It is not intended to serve as a tool for diagnosing illness, in prescribing treatments, or as a substitute for the physician/patient relationship. All persons concerned about medical symptoms or the possibility of disease are encouraged to seek professional care from an appropriate health care provider.

## Our Advisory Board

The *Health Reference Series* is reviewed by an Advisory Board comprised of librarians from public, academic, and medical libraries. We would like to thank the following board members for providing guidance to the development of this series:

Dr. Lynda Baker,
Associate Professor of Library and Information Science
Wayne State University, Detroit, MI

Nancy Bulgarelli,
William Beaumont Hospital Library
Royal Oak, MI

Karen Imarasio,
Bloomfield Township Public Library
Bloomfield Township, MI

Karen Morgan,
Mardigian Library, University of Michigan-Dearborn
Dearborn, MI

Rosemary Orlando,
St. Clair Shores Public Library
St. Clair Shores, MI

## *Health Reference Series* Update Policy

The inaugural book in the *Health Reference Series* was the first edition of *Cancer Sourcebook* published in 1992. Since then, the *Series* has been enthusiastically received by librarians and in the medical community. In order to maintain the standard of providing high-quality health information for the lay person, the editorial staff at Omnigraphics felt it was necessary to implement a policy of updating volumes when warranted.

Medical researchers have been making tremendous strides, and it is the purpose of the *Health Reference Series* to stay current with the most recent advances. Each decision to update a volume will be made on an individual basis. Some of the considerations will include how much new information is available and the feedback we receive from people who use the books. If there is a topic you would like to see added to the update list, or an area of medical concern you feel has not been adequately addressed, please write to:

Editor
*Health Reference Series*
Omnigraphics, Inc.
615 Griswold Street
Detroit, MI 48226

The commitment to providing on-going coverage of important medical developments has also led to some format changes in the *Health Reference Series*. Each new volume on a topic is individually titled and called a "First Edition." Subsequent updates will carry sequential edition numbers. To help avoid confusion and to provide maximum flexibility in our ability to respond to informational needs, the practice of consecutively numbering each volume has been discontinued.

# Part One

# Introduction:
# A Quick Overview

# Chapter 1

# *Osteoporosis Prevention, Diagnosis, and Therapy Consensus Statement*

## *Introduction*

The National Institutes of Health (NIH) sponsored a Consensus Development Conference on Osteoporosis Prevention, Diagnosis, and Therapy on March 27-29, 2000.

Osteoporosis is a major threat to Americans. In the United States today, 10 million individuals already have osteoporosis, and 18 million more have low bone mass, placing them at increased risk for this disorder.

Osteoporosis, once thought to be a natural part of aging among women, is no longer considered age or gender-dependent. It is largely preventable due to the remarkable progress in the scientific understanding of its causes, diagnosis, and treatment. Optimization of bone health is a process that must occur throughout the lifespan in both

National Institutes of Health (NIH) Publication Consensus Development Conference Statement Online 2000, *Osteoporosis Prevention, Diagnosis, and Therapy*, 17(2):1-36, March 27-29, 2000, accessed 08/12/2000. Available at http://odp.od.nih.gov/consensus/cons/111/111_statement.htm. NIH Consensus Statements are prepared by a non-advocate, non-Federal panel of experts, based on (1) presentations by investigators working in areas relevant to the consensus questions during a 2-day public session; (2) questions and statements from conference attendees during open discussion periods that are part of the public session; and (3) closed deliberations by the panel during the remainder of the second day and morning of the third. This statement is an independent report of the panel and is not a policy statement of the NIH or the Federal Government.

males and females. Factors that influence bone health at all ages are essential to prevent osteoporosis and its devastating consequences.

To clarify the factors associated with prevention, diagnosis, and treatment, and to present the latest information about osteoporosis, the NIH organized this conference. After 1 ½ days of presentations and audience discussion addressing the latest in osteoporosis research, an independent, non-Federal consensus development panel weighed the scientific evidence and wrote this draft statement that was presented to the audience on the third day. The consensus development panel's statement addressed the following key questions:

1. What is osteoporosis and what are its consequences?
2. How do risks vary among different segments of the population?
3. What factors are involved in building and maintaining skeletal health throughout life?
4. What is the optimal evaluation and treatment of osteoporosis and fractures?
5. What are the directions for future research?

The primary sponsors of this meeting were the National Institute of Arthritis and Musculoskeletal and Skin Diseases and the NIH Office of Medical Applications of Research. The conference was cosponsored by the National Institute on Aging; National Institute of Diabetes and Digestive and Kidney Diseases; National Institute of Dental and Craniofacial Research; National Institute of Child Health and Human Development; National Institute of Nursing Research; National Institute of Environmental Health Sciences; National Heart, Lung, and Blood Institute; NIH Office of Research on Women's Health; and Agency for Healthcare Research and Quality (formerly the Agency for Health Care Policy and Research).

## What Is Osteoporosis and What Are Its Consequences?

Osteoporosis is defined as a skeletal disorder characterized by compromised bone strength predisposing to an increased risk of fracture. Bone strength reflects the integration of two main features: bone density and bone quality. Bone density is expressed as grams of mineral per area or volume and in any given individual is determined by peak bone mass and amount of bone loss. Bone quality refers to architecture, turnover, damage accumulation (e.g., microfractures) and mineralization. A fracture occurs when a failure-inducing force (e.g., trauma) is applied to osteoporotic bone. Thus, osteoporosis is a significant risk factor for fracture, and a distinction between risk factors that affect bone metabolism and risk factors for fracture must be made.

It is important to acknowledge a common misperception that osteoporosis is always the result of bone loss. Bone loss commonly occurs as men and women age; however, an individual who does not reach optimal (i.e., peak) bone mass during childhood and adolescence may develop osteoporosis without the occurrence of accelerated bone loss. Hence sub-optimal bone growth in childhood and adolescence is as important as bone loss to the development of osteoporosis.

Currently there is no accurate measure of overall bone strength. Bone mineral density (BMD) is frequently used as a proxy measure and accounts for approximately 70 percent of bone strength. The World Health Organization (WHO) operationally defines osteoporosis as bone density 2.5 standard deviations below the mean for young white adult women. It is not clear how to apply this diagnostic criterion to men, children, and across ethnic groups. Because of the difficulty in accurate measurement and standardization between instruments and sites, controversy exists among experts regarding the continued use of this diagnostic criterion.

Osteoporosis can be further characterized as either primary or secondary. Primary osteoporosis can occur in both genders at all ages but often follows menopause in women and occurs later in life in men. In contrast, secondary osteoporosis is a result of medications, other conditions, or diseases. Examples include glucocorticoid-induced osteoporosis, hypogonadism, and celiac disease.

The consequences of osteoporosis include the financial, physical, and psychosocial, which significantly affect the individual as well as the family and community. An osteoporotic fracture is a tragic outcome of a traumatic event in the presence of compromised bone strength, and its incidence is increased by various other risk factors. Traumatic events can range from high-impact falls to normal lifting and bending. The incidence of fracture is high in individuals with osteoporosis and increases with age. The probability that a 50-year-old will have a hip fracture during his or her lifetime is 14 percent for a white female and 5 to 6 percent for a white male. The risk for African Americans is much lower at 6 percent and 3 percent for 50-year-old women and men, respectively. Osteoporotic fractures, particularly vertebral fractures, can be associated with chronic disabling pain. Nearly one-third of patients with hip fractures are discharged to nursing homes within the year following a fracture. Notably, one in five patients is no longer living 1 year after sustaining an osteoporotic hip fracture. Hip and vertebral fractures are a problem for women in their late 70s and 80s, wrist fractures are a problem in the late 50s to early 70s, and all other fractures (e.g., pelvic and rib) are a problem throughout postmenopausal years. The impact of osteoporosis on other body systems, such as gastrointestinal, respiratory, genitourinary, and craniofacial, is acknowledged, but reliable prevalence rates are unknown.

Hip fracture has a profound impact on quality of life, as evidenced by findings that 80 percent of women older than 75 years preferred death to a bad hip fracture resulting in nursing home placement. However, little data exist on the relationship between fractures and psychological and social well-being. Other quality-of-life issues include adverse effects on physical health (impact of skeletal deformity) and financial resources. An osteoporotic fracture is associated with increased difficulty in activities of daily life, as only one-third of fracture patients regain pre-fracture level of function and one-third require nursing home placement. Fear, anxiety, and depression are frequently reported in women with established osteoporosis and such consequences are likely under-addressed when considering the overall impact of this condition.

Direct financial expenditures for treatment of osteoporotic fracture are estimated at $10 to $15 billion annually. A majority of these estimated costs are due to in-patient care but do not include the costs of treatment for individuals without a history of fractures, nor do they include the indirect costs of lost wages or productivity of either the individual or the caregiver. More needs to be learned about these indirect costs, which are considerable. Consequently, these figures significantly underestimate the true costs of osteoporosis.

## How Do Risks Vary among Different Segments of the Population?

### Gender / Ethnicity

The prevalence of osteoporosis, and incidence of fracture, vary by gender and race/ethnicity. White postmenopausal women experience almost three-quarters of hip fractures and have the highest age-adjusted fracture incidence. Most of the information regarding diagnosis and treatment is derived from research on this population. However, women of other age, racial, and ethnic groups, and men and children, are also affected. Much of the difference in fracture rates among these groups appears to be explained by differences in peak bone mass and rate of bone loss; however, differences in bone geometry, frequency of falls, and prevalence of other risk factors appear to play a role as well.

Both men and women experience an age-related decline in BMD starting in midlife. Women experience more rapid bone loss in the early years following menopause, which places them at earlier risk for fractures. In men, hypogonadism is also an important risk factor. Men and perimenopausal women with osteoporosis more commonly have secondary causes for the bone loss than do postmenopausal women.

African American women have higher bone mineral density than white non-Hispanic women throughout life, and experience lower hip fracture rates. Some Japanese women have lower peak BMD than white non-Hispanic women, but have a lower hip fracture rate; the reasons for which are not fully understood. Mexican American women have bone densities intermediate between those of white non-Hispanic women and African American women. Limited available information on Native American women suggests they have lower BMD than white non-Hispanic women.

## *Risk Factors*

Risks associated with low bone density are supported by good evidence, including large prospective studies. Predictors of low bone mass include female gender, increased age, estrogen deficiency, white race, low weight and body mass index (BMI), family history of osteoporosis, smoking, and history of prior fracture. Use of alcohol and caffeine-containing beverages is inconsistently associated with decreased bone mass. In contrast, some measures of physical function and activity have been associated with increased bone mass, including grip strength and current exercise. Levels of exercise in childhood and adolescence have an inconsistent relationship to BMD later in life. Late menarche, early menopause, and low endogenous estrogen levels are also associated with low BMD in several studies.

Although low BMD has been established as an important predictor of future fracture risk, the results of many studies indicate that clinical risk factors related to risk of fall also serve as important predictors of fracture. Fracture risk has been consistently associated with a history of falls, low physical function such as slow gait speed and decreased quadriceps strength, impaired cognition, impaired vision, and the presence of environmental hazards (e.g., throw rugs). Increased risk of a fracture with a fall includes a fall to the side and attributes of bone geometry, such as tallness, hip axis, and femur length. Some risks for fracture, such as age, a low BMI, and low levels of physical activity, probably affect fracture incidence through their effects on both bone density and propensity to fall and inability to absorb impact.

Results of studies of persons with osteoporotic fractures have led to the development of models of risk prediction, which incorporate clinical risk factors along with BMD measurements. Results from the Study of Osteoporotic Fractures (SOF), a large longitudinal study of postmenopausal, white non-Hispanic women, suggest that clinical risk factors can contribute greatly to fracture risk assessment. In this study, 14 clinical risk factors predictive of fracture were identified. The presence of five or more of these factors increased the rate of hip fracture for women in the highest tertile of BMD from 1.1 per 1,000 woman-years to 9.9 per 1,000 woman-years. Women in the lowest tertile of BMD with no other risk factors had a hip fracture rate of 2.6 per 1,000 woman-years as compared with 27.3 per 1,000 woman-years with five or more risk factors present. A second model, derived from the Rotterdam study, predicted hip fractures using a smaller number of variables, including gender, age, height, weight, use of a walking aid, and current smoking. However, these models have not been validated in a population different from that in which they were derived.

*Secondary Osteoporosis*

A large number of medical disorders are associated with osteoporosis and increased fracture risk. These can be organized into several categories: genetic disorders, hypogonadal states, endocrine disorders, gastrointestinal diseases, hematologic disorders, connective tissue disease, nutritional deficiencies, drugs, and a variety of other common serious chronic systemic disorders, such as congestive heart failure, end-stage renal disease, and alcoholism.

The distribution of the most common causes appears to differ by demographic group. Among men, 30 to 60 percent of osteoporosis is associated with secondary causes; with hypogonadism, glucocorticoids, and alcoholism the most common. In perimenopausal women, more than 50 percent is associated with secondary causes, and the most common causes are hypoestrogenemia, glucocorticoids, thyroid hormone excess, and anticonvulsant therapy. In postmenopausal women, the prevalence of secondary conditions is thought to be much lower, but the actual proportion is not known. In one study, hypercalciuria, hyperparathyroidism, and malabsorption were identified in a group of white postmenopausal osteoporotic women who had no history of conditions that cause bone loss. These data suggest that additional testing of white postmenopausal women with osteoporosis may be indicated, but an appropriate or cost-effective evaluation strategy has not been determined.

Glucocorticoid use is the most common form of drug-related osteoporosis, and its long-term administration for disorders such as rheumatoid arthritis and chronic obstructive pulmonary disease is associated with a high rate of fracture. For example, in one study, a group of patients treated with 10 mg of prednisone for 20 weeks experienced an 8 percent loss of BMD in the spine. Some experts suggest that any patient who receives orally administered glucocorticoids (such as Prednisone) in a dose of 5 mg or more for longer than 2 months is at high risk for excessive bone loss.

People who have undergone organ transplant are at high risk for osteoporosis due to a variety of factors, including pre-transplant organ failure and use of glucocorticoids after transplantation.

Hyperthyroidism is a well-described risk factor for osteoporosis. In addition, some studies have suggested that women taking thyroid replacement may also be at increased risk for excess bone loss, suggesting that careful regulation of thyroid replacement is important.

## *Children and Adolescents*

Several groups of children and adolescents may be at risk for compromised bone health. Premature and low birth weight infants have lower-than-expected bone mass in the first few months of life, but the long-term implications are unknown.

Glucocorticoids are now commonly used for the treatment of a variety of common childhood inflammatory diseases, and the bone effects of this treatment need to be considered when steroid use is required chronically. The long-term effects on bone health of intermittent courses of systemic steroids or the chronic use of inhaled steroids, as are often used in asthma, are not well described.

Cystic fibrosis, celiac disease, and inflammatory bowel disease are examples of conditions associated with malabsorption and resultant osteopenia in some individuals. The osteoporosis of cystic fibrosis is also related to the frequent need for corticosteroids as well as to other undefined factors.

Hypogonadal states, characterized clinically by delayed menarche, oligomenorrhea, or amenorrhea, are relatively common in adolescent girls and young women. Settings in which these occur include strenuous athletic training, emotional stress, and low body weight. Failure to achieve peak bone mass, bone loss, and increased fracture rates have been shown in this group. Anorexia nervosa deserves special mention. Although hypogonadism is an important feature of the clinical picture, the profound undernutrition and nutrition-related factors are also critical. This latter point is evidenced, in part, by the failure of estrogen replacement to correct the bone loss.

*Residents of Long-term Care Facilities*

Residents of nursing homes and other long-term care facilities are at particularly high risk of fracture. Most have low BMD and a high prevalence of other risk factors for fracture, including advanced age, poor physical function, low muscle strength, decreased cognition and high rates of dementia, poor nutrition, and, often, use of multiple medications.

## What Factors Are Involved in Building and Maintaining Skeletal Health Throughout Life?

Growth in bone size and strength occurs during childhood, but bone accumulation is not completed until the third decade of life, after the cessation of linear growth. The bone mass attained early in life is perhaps the most important determinant of life-long skeletal health. Individuals with the highest peak bone mass after adolescence have the greatest protective advantage when the inexorable declines in bone density associated with increasing age, illness, and diminished sex-steroid production take their toll. Bone mass may be related not only to osteoporosis and fragility later in life but also to fractures in childhood and adolescence. Genetic factors exert a strong and perhaps predominant influence on peak bone mass, but physiological, environmental, and modifiable lifestyle factors can also play a significant role. Among these are adequate nutrition and body weight, exposure to sex hormones at puberty, and physical activity. Thus, maximizing bone mass early in life presents a critical opportunity to reduce the impact of bone loss related to aging. Childhood is also a critical time for the development of lifestyle habits conducive to maintaining good bone health throughout life. Cigarette smoking, which usually starts in adolescence, may have a deleterious effect on achieving bone mass.

*Nutrition*

Good nutrition is essential for normal growth. A balanced diet, adequate calories, and appropriate nutrients are the foundation for development of all tissues, including bone. Adequate and appropriate nutrition is important for all individuals, but not all follow a diet that is optimal for bone health. Supplementation of calcium and vitamin D may be necessary. In particular, excessive pursuit of thinness may affect adequate nutrition and bone health.

Calcium is the specific nutrient most important for attaining peak bone mass and for preventing and treating osteoporosis. Sufficient data exist to recommend specific dietary calcium intakes at various stages of life. Although the Institute of Medicine recommends calcium intakes of 800 mg/day for children ages 3 to 8 and 1,300 mg/day for children and adolescents ages 9 to 17, only about 25 percent of boys and 10 percent of girls ages 9 to 17 are estimated to meet these recommendations. Factors contributing to low calcium intakes are restriction of dairy products, a generally low level of fruit and vegetable consumption, and a high intake of low calcium beverages such as sodas. For older adults, calcium intake should be maintained at 1,000 to 1,500 mg/day, yet only about 50 to 60 percent of this population meets this recommendation.

Vitamin D is required for optimal calcium absorption and thus is also important for bone health. Most infants and young children in the United States have adequate vitamin D intake because of supplementation and fortification of milk. During adolescence, when consumption of dairy products decreases, vitamin D intake is less likely to be adequate, and this may adversely affect calcium absorption. A recommended vitamin D intake of 400 to 600 IU/day has been established for adults.

Other nutrients have been evaluated for their relation to bone health. High dietary protein, caffeine, phosphorus, and sodium can adversely affect calcium balance, but their effects appear not to be important in individuals with adequate calcium intakes.

*Exercise*

Regular physical activity has numerous health benefits for individuals of all ages. The specific effects of physical activity on bone health have been investigated in randomized clinical trials and observational studies. There is strong evidence that physical activity early in life contributes to higher peak bone mass. Some evidence indicates that resistance and high impact exercise are likely the most beneficial. Exercise during the middle years of life has numerous health benefits, but there are few studies on the effects of exercise on BMD. Exercise during the later years, in the presence of adequate calcium and vitamin D intake, probably has a modest effect on slowing the decline in BMD. It is clear that exercise late in life, even beyond 90 years of age, can increase muscle mass and strength twofold or more in frail individuals. There is convincing evidence that exercise in elderly persons also improves function and delays loss of independence and thus contributes to quality of life. Randomized clinical trials of exercise have been shown to reduce the risk of falls by approximately 25 percent, but there is no experimental evidence that exercise affects fracture rates. It also is possible that regular exercisers might fall differently and thereby reduce the risk of fracture due to falls, but this hypothesis requires testing.

*Gonadal Steroids*

Sex steroids secreted during puberty substantially increase BMD and peak bone mass. Gonadal steroids influence skeletal health throughout life in both women and men. In adolescents and young women, sustained production of estrogens is essential for the maintenance of bone mass. Reduction in estrogen production with menopause is the major cause of loss of BMD during later life. Timing of menarche, absent or infrequent menstrual cycles, and the timing of menopause influence both the attainment of peak bone mass and the preservation of BMD. Testosterone production in adolescent boys and men is similarly important in achieving and maintaining maximal bone mass. Estrogens have also been implicated in the growth and maturation of the male skeleton. Pathologic delay in the onset of puberty is a risk factor for diminished bone mass in men. Disorders that result in hypogonadism in adult men result in osteoporosis.

*Growth Hormone and Body Composition*

Growth hormone and insulin-like growth factor-I, which are maximally secreted during puberty, continue to play a role in the acquisition and maintenance of bone mass and the determination of body composition into adulthood. Growth hormone deficiency is associated with a decrease in BMD. Children and youth with low BMI are likely to attain lower-than-average peak bone mass. Although there is a direct association between BMI and bone mass throughout the adult years, it is not known whether the association between body composition and bone mass is due to hormones, nutritional factors, higher impact during weight-bearing activities, or other factors. There are several observational studies of fractures in older persons that show an inverse relationship between fracture rates and BMI.

## What Is the Optimal Evaluation and Treatment of Osteoporosis and Fractures?

The goals for the evaluation of patients at risk for osteoporosis are to establish the diagnosis of osteoporosis on the basis of assessment of bone mass, to establish the fracture risk, and to make decisions regarding the needs for instituting therapy. A history and physical examination are essential in evaluating fracture risks and should include assessment for loss of height and change in posture. Laboratory evaluation for secondary causes of osteoporosis should be considered when osteoporosis is diagnosed. The most commonly used measurement to diagnose osteoporosis and predict fracture risk is based on assessment of BMD which is principally determined by the mineral content of bone. BMD measurements have been shown to correlate strongly with load-bearing capacity of the hip and spine and with the risk of fracture. Several different techniques have been developed to assess BMD at multiple skeletal sites including the peripheral skeleton, hip, and spine. The World Health Organization (WHO) has selected BMD measurements to establish criteria for the diagnosis of osteoporosis. A T-score is defined as the number of standard deviations (SD) above or below the average BMD value for young healthy white women. This should be distinguished from a Z-score, which is defined as the number of SD above or below the average BMD for age- and gender-matched controls. According to the WHO definition, osteoporosis is present when the T-score is at least minus 2.5 SD. Although T-scores were based originally on assessment of BMD at the hip by dual-energy X-ray absorptiometry (DXA), they have been applied to define diagnostic thresholds at other skeletal sites and for other technologies. Experts have expressed concern that this approach may not produce comparable data between sites and techniques. Of the various sampling sites, measurements of BMD made at the hip predict hip fracture better than measurements made at other sites while BMD measurement at the spine predicts spine fracture better than measures at other sites.

Newer measures of bone strength, such as ultrasound, have been introduced. Recent prospective studies using quantitative ultrasound (QUS) of the heel have predicted hip fracture and all nonvertebral fractures nearly as well as DXA at the femoral neck. QUS and DXA at the femoral neck provide independent information about fracture risk, and both of these tests predict hip fracture risk better than DXA at the lumbar spine. In general, clinical trials of pharmacologic therapies have utilized DXA, rather than QUS, for entry criterion for studies, and there is uncertainty regarding whether the results of these trials can be generalized to patients identified by QUS to have high risk of fracture.

Over the past year, several professional organizations have been working on establishing a standard of comparability of different devices and sites for assessing fracture risk. With this approach, measurements derived from any device or site could be standardized to predict hip fracture risk. However, the values obtained from different instruments cannot be used to predict comparable levels in bone mass. Limitations in precision and low correlation among different techniques will require appropriate validation before this approach can be applied to different skeletal sites and to different age groups.

It has been suggested that the diagnosis and treatment of osteoporosis should depend on risk-based assessment rather than solely on the assessment of a T-score. Consideration of risk factors in conjunction with BMD will likely improve the ability to predict fracture risk. This approach needs to be validated in prospective studies and tested in appropriate randomized clinical trials.

In addition to the effects of bone mass, bone micro architecture, and macrogeometry, bone strength is also affected by the rate of bone remodeling. Bone remodeling can be assessed by the measurement of surrogate markers of bone turnover in the blood or urine. These markers include bone-specific alkaline phosphatase and Osteocalcin, which are indices of bone formation, and the urinary levels of pyridinolines and deoxypyridinolines and serum and urine levels of type I collagen telopeptides (CTX and NTX), which are indices of bone resorption. The level of these markers may identify changes in bone remodeling within a relatively short time interval (several days to months) before changes in BMD can be detected. However, according to available data, marker levels do not predict bone mass or fracture risk and are only weakly associated with changes in bone mass. Therefore, they are of limited utility in the clinical evaluation of individual patients. Despite these limitations, markers have been shown in research studies to correlate with changes in indices of bone remodeling and may provide insights into mechanisms of bone loss.

*Who Should Be Evaluated?*

The value of bone density in predicting fracture risk is established, and there is general consensus that bone density measurement should be considered in patients receiving glucocorticoid therapy for 2 months or more and patients with other conditions that place them at high risk for osteoporotic fracture. However, the value of universal screening, especially in perimenopausal women, has not been established. There are several unknown factors with this approach.

First, the number of women evaluated and treated would need to be high in order to prevent a single fracture. For example, in white women aged 50-59, an estimated 750 BMD tests would be required to prevent just one hip or vertebral fracture over a 5-year period of treatment. Second, the value has not been established for the common practice of beginning preventive drug therapy in the perimenopausal period for the purpose of preventing fractures later in life.

Until there is good evidence to support the cost-effectiveness of routine screening, or the efficacy of early initiation of preventive drugs, an individualized approach is recommended. A bone density measurement should be considered when it will help the patient decide whether to institute treatment to prevent osteoporotic fracture. In the future, a combination of risk factor evaluation and bone density measurements may increase the ability to predict fracture risk and help with treatment decisions. Until assessment by randomized clinical trials is conducted, individual decisions regarding screening could be informed by the preliminary evidence that the risk for fracture increases with age, and with an increased number of additional risk factors.

## *What Are the Effective Medical Treatments?*

In the past 30 years, major strides have been made in the treatment of osteoporosis. Evidence-based reports systematically reviewing the data from randomized clinical trials, including meta-analyses for each of the major treatments, are available and permit conclusions regarding the role of each modality of osteoporosis therapy.

Calcium and vitamin D intake modulates age-related increases in parathyroid hormone (PTH) levels and bone resorption. Randomized clinical trials have demonstrated that adequate calcium intake from diet or supplements increase spine BMD and reduce vertebral and nonvertebral fractures. Low levels of 25-OH vitamin D are common in the aging population, and significant reductions in hip and other nonvertebral fractures have been observed in patients receiving calcium and vitamin D3 in prospective trials. The maximal effective dose of vitamin D is uncertain, but thought to be 400 to 1,000 IU/day. There is consensus that adequate vitamin D and calcium intakes are required for bone health. The therapeutic effects of most of the clinical trials of various drug therapies for osteoporosis have been achieved in the presence of calcium and vitamin D supplementation among control and intervention groups. Optimal treatment of osteoporosis with any drug therapy also requires calcium and vitamin D intake meeting recommended levels. The preferred source of calcium is dietary. Calcium supplements need to be absorbable and should have USP (United States Pharmacopeia) designation.

Physical activity is necessary for bone acquisition and maintenance through adulthood. Complete bed rest and microgravity have devastating effects on bone. Trials of exercise intervention show most of the effect during skeletal growth and in very inactive adults. Effects beyond those directly on bone, such as improved muscular strength and balance, may be very significant in fracture-risk reduction. Trials in older adults have successfully used various forms of exercise to reduce falls. High-impact exercise (weight training) stimulates accrual of bone mineral content in the skeleton. Lower impact exercises, such as walking, have beneficial effects on other aspects of health and function, although their effects on BMD have been minimal.

Randomized placebo-controlled trials (RCTs) of cyclic etidronate, alendronate, and Risedronate analyzed by a systematic review and meta-analysis have revealed that all of these bisphosphonates increase BMD at the spine and hip in a dose-dependent manner. They consistently reduce the risk of vertebral fractures by 30 to 50 percent. Alendronate and Risedronate reduce the risk of subsequent nonvertebral fractures in women with osteoporosis and adults with glucocorticoid-induced osteoporosis. There is uncertainty about the effect of anti-resorptive therapy in reducing nonvertebral fracture in women without osteoporosis. In RCTs, the relative risk of discontinuing medication due to an adverse event with each of the three bisphosphonates was not statistically significant. The safety and efficacy of this therapy in children and young adults has not been evaluated. Since subjects in clinical trials may not always be representative of the community-based population, an individual approach to treatment is warranted.

Hormone replacement therapy (HRT) is an established approach for osteoporosis treatment and prevention. Many short-term studies and some longer term studies with BMD as the primary outcome have shown significant efficacy. Observational studies have indicated a significant hip fracture reduction in cohorts of women who maintain HRT therapy; still there is a paucity of trials with fractures as the endpoint. HRT trials have shown decreased risk of vertebral fractures, but there have been no trials of estrogen with hip fracture as the primary outcome.

The development of selective estrogen receptor modulators (SERMs) has been an important new thrust in osteoporosis research. The goal of these agents is to maximize the beneficial effect of estrogen on bone and to minimize or antagonize the deleterious effects on the breast and endometrium. Raloxifene, a SERM approved by the FDA for the treatment and prevention of osteoporosis, has been shown to reduce the risks of vertebral fracture by 36 percent in large clinical trials. Tamoxifen, used in the treatment and prevention of breast cancer, can maintain bone mass in postmenopausal women. However, effects on fracture are unclear.

There is a great deal of public interest in natural estrogens, particularly plant-derived phytoestrogens. These compounds have weak estrogen-like effects, and although some animal studies are promising, no effects on fracture reduction in humans have been shown. Salmon calcitonin has demonstrated positive effects on BMD at the lumbar spine, but this effect is less clear at the hip. Other than a recently completed randomized controlled trial of nasal calcitonin, no analysis of fracture risk is available. The PROOF study revealed a significant reduction in vertebral fracture risk at the 200 IU dose but not at the 100 IU or 400 IU dose. The absence of dose response, a 60 percent dropout rate, and the lack of strong supporting data from BMD and markers decrease confidence in the fracture risk data from this trial. Non-pharmacologic interventions directed at preventing falls and reducing their effect on fractures have been promising. These include studies to improve strength and balance in the elderly, as well as using hip protectors to absorb or deflect the impact of a fall.

Multifactorial approaches to preventing falls, as well as improving bone mass through combinations of interventions, suggest promising new directions.

*Should the Response to Treatment Be Monitored?*

Several approaches have been introduced for the monitoring of patients receiving therapies for osteoporosis. The goals of monitoring are to increase adherence to treatment regimens and determine treatment responses. Many individuals do not continue prescribed therapy or do not adhere to a treatment protocol, even when enrolled in formal clinical trials. Monitoring by densitometry or measurements of bone markers have not been shown to be effective in improving compliance, and more research is needed about how to improve adherence to treatment protocols.

17

The best tests for monitoring treatment response would reflect the largest changes with the least error, and these assessment tools are not readily available. The Fracture Intervention Trial (FIT) reveals an additional problem with monitoring, the statistical phenomenon of regression to the mean. In this study, the larger the bone loss in the first year, the greater the gain the next year, for both the placebo and active treatment groups. Therefore, physicians should not stop or change therapies with demonstrated efficacy solely because of modest loss of bone density or adverse trends in markers of bone turnover.

*Orthopaedic Management of Osteoporotic Fractures*

While proximal femur (hip) fractures comprise nearly 20 percent of all osteoporotic fractures, this injury is among the most devastating of all the osteoporotic fractures and is responsible for the greatest expenditure of health care resources. The 1-year mortality rate following hip fracture is about 1 in 5. As many as two-thirds of hip fracture patients never regain their preoperative activity status. Early surgical management of hip fractures is associated with improved outcomes and decreased perioperative morbidity.

The adverse health, functional and quality of life effects of vertebral (spine) fractures are commonly underestimated, and such fractures are associated with increased mortality. The occurrence of a single vertebral fracture substantially increases the likelihood of future fractures and progressive kyphotic deformity. Due to the challenges of reconstruction of osteoporotic bone, open surgical management is reserved only for those rare cases that involve neurologic deficits or an unstable spine. Recently, there has been a burgeoning interest in two "minimally invasive" procedures for management of acute vertebral fractures, vertebroplasty and kyphoplasty, which involve the injection of polymethylmethacrylate bone cement into the fractured vertebra. Anecdotal reports with both techniques claim frequent acute pain relief; however, neither technique has been subjected to a controlled trial to demonstrate the benefits over traditional medical management. Furthermore, the long-term effect of one or more reinforced rigid vertebrae on the risk of fracture of adjacent vertebrae is unknown for both of these procedures.

Several issues are critically important to the orthopaedic management of acute osteoporotic fractures. It is most important to avoid the misconception that the only treatment required of an osteoporotic fracture is management of the acute fracture itself. Management

18

during the perifracture period must consider blood clot prevention (mechanical or pharmacologic) in patients who will have delayed ambulation, the avoidance of substances that may inhibit fracture repair (nicotine, corticosteroids), and the frequent need for supplemental caloric intake. Finally, since less than 5 percent of patients with osteoporotic fractures are referred for medical evaluation and treatment, more aggressive diagnostic and therapeutic intervention of this population represents an opportunity to prevent subsequent fractures. Physicians treating the acute fracture should initiate an outpatient evaluation of the patient for osteoporosis and a treatment program, if indicated, or refer the patient for an osteoporosis assessment.

## *What Are the Directions for Future Research?*

The following questions, issues, and concerns should be addressed:

- Peak bone mass is an important factor in determining long-term fracture risk. Strategies to maximize peak bone mass in girls and boys are essential, including how to identify and intervene in disorders that can impede the achievement of peak bone mass in ethnically diverse populations, and, to determine how long these interventions should last. More research regarding the risks for fracture in chronic diseases affecting children is needed. What is the impact of calcium deficiency and vitamin D deficiency in childhood, and can it be reversed? How does gonadal steroid insufficiency, pubertal delay, or undernourishment impact bone mass? What is known about the use of bisphosphonates or other agents in the treatment of children with osteoporosis?

- Genetic factors leading to osteoporosis are being identified. These factors may relate to bone mass acquisition, bone remodeling, or bone structure. Pharmacogenetic approaches for identifying and targeting specific genetic factors predisposing to osteoporosis need to be developed.

- Glucocorticoid use is a common cause of secondary osteoporosis and associated fractures. What is the impact of glucocorticoid-induced osteoporosis in adults and children? What are the mechanisms of disease? What novel approaches can be taken to stimulate bone formation in this condition? Development of glucocorticoids that avoid effects on the skeleton are needed.

- Secondary causes of osteoporosis are prevalent. A number of risk factors have been identified, including specific disease states and medication use. How should patients be identified for diagnosis and treatment of osteoporosis? What is known about the use of bisphosphonates or other agents in young adults with secondary osteoporosis? What is known about the causes of osteoporosis in perimenopausal women? How should they be monitored for treatment response? Are therapies for improving bone mass in postmenopausal women effective in secondary causes?

- There is a need for prospective studies of gender, age, and ethnically diverse individuals to provide data that will permit more accurate fracture risk identification in these populations. Fracture risk is a combination of bone-dependent and bone-independent factors. Bone-independent factors include muscle function and cognition, which also contribute to falls leading to fractures. A comprehensive assessment of bone-dependent and bone-independent factors should be included. There is a need for a comprehensive assessment of a validated risk assessment tool. What is the best way to identify patients in need of treatment for osteoporosis? An algorithm should be constructed that incorporates risk factors for fracture in addition to assessment of bone density. What is the best use of surrogate markers of bone turnover to determine osteoporosis, and how does this impact on fracture risks?

- Quality of life is significantly impaired by osteoporosis. Future research should characterize and validate quality-of-life tools in patients across gender, age, and race or ethnicity. It will be important to identify effects of fracture risk and intervention on quality of life. Quality of life should be incorporated as an outcome in clinical trials evaluating fracture risk and therapy. In addition, the psychosocial and financial effects of osteoporosis on caregivers and family dynamics should be considered.

- There are no available data to suggest which asymptomatic patients should have screening bone-density tests done or when screening is justified. Information regarding screening guidelines is important to obtain.

- Neuropsychiatric disorders may cause or be the result of osteoporosis. Specific psychiatric disorders, including depression and anorexia nervosa, are associated with osteoporosis or clinical fractures. Medications used to treat psychiatric or neurologic disorders may cause osteoporosis, and the diagnosis of osteoporosis may have psychological implications. Research efforts into the relationship between neuropsychiatric disorders and fracture risk should be strongly encouraged.

- There is an urgent need for randomized clinical trials of combination therapy, which includes pharmacologic, dietary supplement, and lifestyle interventions (including muscle strengthening, balance, and management of multiple drug use, smoking cessation, psychological counseling, and dietary interventions). Primary outcomes would be fractures, and secondary outcomes would include quality of life and functional capability. Cost-effectiveness evaluation should be considered in such a trial.

- What is the optimal evaluation and management of fractures? What diagnostic and management paradigm should be employed? What are the long-term consequences of osteoporosis and clinical fractures on non-skeletal body systems? What measures can be taken to prevent subsequent fractures?

- Anabolic agents that stimulate bone formation, such as PTH and fluoride, have been evaluated. Meta-analysis of fluoride therapy revealed no protective effects on fracture risk. PTH peptides are the most promising but are still in clinical trials. Other factors, including growth hormones, are under investigation. There is a critical need to develop and assess anabolic agents that stimulate bone formation.

- Assure accessibility to treatment for people regardless of income and geography.

- There is a need to determine the most effective method of educating the public and health care professionals about the prevention, diagnosis and treatment of osteoporosis.

- There is a need to improve the reporting of BMD and fracture risk so it is understandable to medical specialists and can be explained to patients.

- Study is needed to determine the efficacy and safety of long-term administration of various drug interventions in maintaining BMD and preventing fractures.

- Trials of dietary supplements are needed.

- Study is needed to understand the influence of nutrition on micronutrients and non-patentable medical interventions.

- Study is needed to understand cost-effectiveness and effectiveness of programs encouraging bone health.

- Study of interventions examining the long-term effects of fractures on health, function and quality of life is needed.

## Conclusions

### Question 1:
### What Is Osteoporosis and What Are Its Consequences?

Osteoporosis occurs in all populations and at all ages. Though more prevalent in white postmenopausal females, it often goes unrecognized in other populations.

Osteoporosis is a devastating disorder with significant physical, psychosocial, and financial consequences.

### Question 2:
### How Do Risks Vary among Different Segments of the Population?

The risks for osteoporosis, as reflected by low bone density, and the risks for fracture overlap but are not identical.

More attention should be paid to skeletal health in persons with conditions known to be associated with secondary osteoporosis.

Clinical risk factors have an important, but as yet poorly validated, role in determining who should have BMD measurement, in assessing risk of fracture, and in determining who should be treated.

### Question 3:
### What Factors Are Involved in Building and Maintaining Skeletal Health Throughout Life?

Adequate calcium and vitamin D intake are crucial to develop optimal peak bone mass and to preserve bone mass throughout life. Supplementation of these two components in bioavailable forms may be necessary in individuals who do not achieve recommended intake from dietary sources.

Gonadal steroids are important determinants of peak and lifetime bone mass in men, women, and children.

Regular exercise, especially resistance and high-impact activities, contributes to development of high peak bone mass and may reduce the risk of falls in older individuals.

## *Question 4:*
## *What Is the Optimal Evaluation and Treatment of Osteoporosis and Fractures?*

Assessment of bone mass, identification of fracture risk, and determination of who should be treated are the optimal goals when evaluating patients for osteoporosis.

Fracture prevention is the primary goal in the treatment of patients with osteoporosis.

Several treatments have been shown to reduce the risk of osteoporotic fractures. These include therapies that enhance bone mass and reduce risk or consequences of falls.

Adults with vertebral, rib, hip, or distal forearm fractures should be evaluated for the presence of osteoporosis and given appropriate therapy.

# Part Two


# The Nature of Osteoporosis

# Chapter 2

# *Osteoporosis*

Osteoporosis is a condition characterized by substantial bone loss. When the extent of bone loss reaches a critical point, fractures may occur as a result of very minor stress. Osteoporosis affects the entire skeleton, but fractures occur most notably in the vertebrae, hips and wrists. The bones become so weak that normal workloads overcome their capacity. A simple fall can result in a broken hip. Spinal vertebrae can collapse and in extreme cases cause a "dowager's hump."

Gradual weakening or thinning of bones occurs normally with age. The longer we live, the less bone mass we have and the more prone we are to fractures.

Scientists do not know what causes osteoporosis. They do know a lot about factors which can worsen or lessen the extent of bone loss. Osteoporosis is a very complex disease where many different factors influence the rate of bone loss. Advanced age and being a postmenopausal white female are the predominant risk factors. Other risk factors include hormonal imbalance, nutrient deficiencies (particularly calcium) and immobility.

The role of dietary calcium in the prevention or treatment of osteoporosis is not clear. Calcium may ameliorate or prevent only bone loss directly related to calcium deficiency, but not bone loss due to other causes. Calcium deficiency, however, is common in women. Most bone loss is influenced by hormonal deficiencies.

---

Evidence suggests that exercise helps reduce bone loss. However, too much exercise can be counterproductive for women, because it may lower estrogen levels.

At this time, the most effective treatment of osteoporosis is prevention. The stronger the bones are when people are young, the less likely they are to fracture easily later in life. An effective preventive treatment in postmenopausal women is estrogen replacement therapy (ERT). Other treatments, such as calcitonin therapy, may help if estrogen replacement is not advisable for health reasons.

In some persons, osteoporosis cannot be prevented, but steps can be taken to slow bone loss as much as possible.

Once osteoporosis has proceeded to a very advanced stage, involving fractures, it is difficult to treat. Many of the more promising treatments are still experimental. Advanced osteoporosis interferes with a person's ability to lead a normal life. A simple fall, a wrong movement or even minor stress on the bones can make the difference between an independent or a dependent lifestyle.

As the population ages, the relative percentage and absolute number of elderly will increase, leading to an increase in all diseases associated with aging, including osteoporosis. In 1991, osteoporosis resulted in over 1.5 million fractures, costing over $10 billion in health care. These numbers are expected to increase.

## Types of Osteoporosis

Osteoporosis is traditionally divided into primary and secondary osteoporosis. Both types can occur simultaneously in the same person. The cause of primary osteoporosis is not fully understood. Primary osteoporosis is divided into postmenopausal (type I) and senile (type II) osteoporosis. Secondary osteoporosis is less common and defined as bone loss occurring as a result of other diseases, such as Cushing's syndrome or malignancy.

**(Type I) Accelerated or postmenopausal osteoporosis.** Bone loss is accelerated in women for five to ten years after menopause due to reduced production of the female sex hormone, estrogen. Ten or more years after menopause, accelerated bone loss slows down and approaches the rate of decline observed in older men. In five to ten percent of postmenopausal women, bone loss is severe and leads to fractures before age 75. Postmenopausal osteoporosis most often results in collapsed vertebrae, which may lead to the dowager's hump.

Other bones, such as wrist bones, are also affected. Type I bone loss occurs in women over six times as frequently as in men.

**(Type II) Age-related osteoporosis.** Age-related osteoporosis occurs in both sexes, in women over age 70 and men over age 80.

There is very good evidence that the incidence of fractures increases with the lowering of bone mineral density. Type II bone loss typically results in hip fractures, although fractures occur in other types of bone as well. Elderly men are very susceptible to bone loss, but women get hip fractures about twice as often. It is not clear whether the bone loss is simply an expression of old age which affects some people to a larger extent than others. An underlying disease, a hormonal imbalance or nutrient deficiency may accelerate age-related bone loss.

In general, women have less dense bones than men (usually 30 percent less), and they suffer more bone loss after menopause. This puts women at a disadvantage when age-related bone loss occurs. Women live longer than men, and thus may be more likely to develop fractures. Osteoporosis is rare in young adults and middle-aged men.

**Secondary osteoporosis.** In some instances, osteoporosis is a side effect of another health condition. For example, overproduction of the hormone, cortisone, as in Cushing Syndrome, can lead to osteoporosis. Abnormally low production of sex hormones, as in hypogonadism, castration or "total hysterectomy" can lead to bone loss; certain malignancies, particularly myeloma (a bone marrow cancer); hyperthyroidism and hyperparathyroidism can also result in bone loss. Digestive, kidney, or liver disorders may lead to bone loss (Table 2.1).

**Osteopenia and Osteomalacia.** Osteoporosis is a form of osteopenia. Osteopenia literally means "little bone." In osteoporosis bone mass is lost. However, the composition of the remaining bone is similar to healthy bone, although not as dense.

To diagnose osteoporosis correctly, other bone disorders should be excluded. In osteomalacia, bone tissue is not adequately mineralized, and bone quality is softer than healthy bone. Osteomalacia is primarily due to severe vitamin D deficiency and is an adult form of rickets.

## Bone Is an Active Tissue

Perhaps, because skeletons greatly outlast human life, we get the impression that bones are hard and inert. However, bone is a very active tissue metabolically, and it changes constantly.

The skeleton is soft in the early embryonic state. The fetus starts out with a cartilaginous skeleton, which is gradually replaced by bone. As the embryo grows, mineral salts, deposited into the protein matrix, eventually harden the bones. After birth, bone density increases. By the time an infant is one year old, the skeleton is firm enough to support first attempts at walking. The bones continue to grow in length and mass until adulthood. After longitudinal bone growth is complete, the bones continue to increase in mass and density.

Peak bone density is reached between ages 20 and 35. Thereafter, the process reverses. The bones begin to lose density. At age 40, bones lose less than 0.5 percent of their mass per year. Postmenopausal women can lose up to 2 to 3 percent or more bone mass per year. If accelerated loss is not stopped, a susceptible woman can lose 50 percent of peak bone mass by the time she reaches 70 or 80 years of age.

## *Mechanisms of Bone Formation and Destruction*

Bones are in a continuous state of dissolution and reformation. Two opposing forces occur within the bones to determine their hardness:

- bone resorption: destruction of old bone tissue,
- bone formation: production of new bone tissue.

These two forces occur in sequence and are coupled. Old bone is dissolved and new bone is formed so that the size and shape of bone

**TABLE 2.1.** Causes of Secondary Osteoporosis

| | |
|---|---|
| Steroid therapy and Cushing's syndrome | Amenorrhea |
| Anorexia nervosa | Myeloma |
| Hyperprolactinemia | Skeletal metastases |
| Diabetes mellitus | Gastric surgery |
| Alcoholism | Anticonvulsant therapy |
| Immobilization | Thyrotoxicosis |
| Osteogenesis imperfecta | Male hypogonadism |
| Homocystinuria | |

*(From Francis, R.M., editor, Osteoporosis, Pathogenesis & Management, Kluwer Academic Publishers, 1990.)*

can adapt to the changing shape of the body. Bone resorption initiates the bone remodeling cycle and new bone formation concludes the cycle. However, to maintain bone strength, bone formation must keep up with bone resorption. If bone formation lags behind, bone loss is inevitable. This seems to be what happens in osteoporosis.

Bone loss results either from excessive resorption or from inadequate formation.

- During growth bone formation is greater than bone resorption.

- During adulthood bone formation and bone resorption are in balance.

- During aging, bone resorption begins to exceed bone formation.

High turnover osteoporosis occurs when the bone remodeling cycle performs at high speed; both excess resorption and excess formation takes place. Bone formation, however, rarely keeps up with excess bone resorption, so a high turnover of bone remodeling often results in rapid bone loss. High turnover osteoporosis occurs primarily in younger people and comprises about 10 percent of all osteoporosis cases. Low turnover osteoporosis occurs primarily in the elderly where the remodeling cycle has slowed. Bone resorption is still fairly normal, but formation of new bone is slowed significantly. Postmenopausal women usually have normal bone turnover, but bone resorption rates exceed bone formation rates.

## Bone Composition

Like other tissues, bones are made up of cells. In contrast to soft tissues, however, bone cells lie on the surface of bone, or are enclosed by calcified bone tissue. The enclosed cells, which remain active, are connected to the general circulation through tiny tunnels.

There are three types of bone cells which play different roles in bone maintenance:

1. osteoclasts are responsible for bone resorption and initiation of the bone remodeling cycle.

2. osteoblasts are responsible for bone formation and completion of the bone remodeling cycle.

3. osteocytes are responsible for maintenance work within bone tissue.

Osteoclasts destroy bone tissue by dissolving minerals. Other cells, macrophages, then digest the protein matrix. Osteoblasts form new bone by secreting protein fibers into the cavities produced by the osteoclasts. Calcium salts harden these protein deposits, a process also controlled by osteoblasts. Osteocytes, former osteoblasts trapped by calcified tissue, perform maintenance work within the bone tissue and control local mineral exchange.

The basic framework of bones is a protein, collagen mesh or matrix. Bone becomes hard because mineral salts are incorporated into the protein mesh. The predominant mineral salt is a calcium phosphate salt, called hydroxyapatite. Magnesium, sodium and potassium salts and small amounts of fluoride and chloride also contribute to the inorganic matter in bone. Bone also contains trace amounts of heavy metals, such as lead and strontium.

Calcium is the major mineral in bone. Bone tissue is constantly dissolved and replaced. Therefore, bone calcium is constantly removed and replaced.

Our body contains roughly 1,200 grams (about 2.5 pounds) of calcium. Most of the body's calcium (over 99 percent) is located in the bones. The bones incorporate calcium for hardness while serving as a calcium bank for the rest of the body. Soft tissues require calcium in very small amounts. It is important that these tissues are adequately supplied with calcium by the blood. It is also critical that blood concentrations remain stable at approximately ten milligrams per deciliter. A slight drop or rise in blood calcium concentrations will immediately set off hormonal events that will return blood calcium to normal concentrations.

Bones play an important part in maintaining stable blood calcium concentrations at the expense of their own calcium stores.

Most calcium in the bone is combined with phosphate. About 80 to 85 percent of body phosphate is located in the skeleton. The ratio of calcium to phosphate in the bone is two to one.

## *Calcium Stores Are Determined by Diet and Hormones*

Most calcium is excreted via the urine, sweat and feces. This calcium must be replaced by dietary calcium. The intestine can adjust the absorption of dietary calcium to meet the body's needs.

During growth more calcium is absorbed than in later years. If the amount of dietary calcium intake is low, the intestine compensates (to a degree) by absorbing more calcium. On the other hand, if we consume more calcium than we need, relatively less will be absorbed.

This protects the body from absorbing too much. We depend on vitamin D for this adaptive ability.

The absorptive ability of the intestine diminishes with age. This may be one reason why we lose bone. Therefore, older people may need more calcium than younger people to maintain calcium balance. Very young individuals can absorb up to 75 percent of dietary calcium. Healthy adults can absorb between 30 and 40 percent, while older adults may absorb even less.

The blood delivers calcium to bone tissue. In turn, either dietary sources or the bones deliver needed calcium to the blood. The body deals with bone calcium as being more dispensable than blood calcium. In the long run, therefore, low dietary calcium intake can lead to weakening of the bones.

Several hormones influence blood and bone calcium concentrations, thus affecting bone density and stable blood calcium concentrations.

Blood calcium concentrations can be manipulated by:

- increasing or reducing calcium absorption in the intestine,

- increasing or reducing calcium secretion in the kidney,

- depositing or withdrawing calcium into or from bone tissues.

A small decrease in blood calcium concentrations results in increased output of parathyroid hormone (PTH) and vitamin D (a vitamin which acts as a hormone). Both hormones interact to stimulate bone resorption and calcium absorption in the intestine and to reduce calcium excretion in the kidneys. This results in increased blood concentrations. The two hormones influence each other. For example, adequate blood concentrations of vitamin D depend on the presence of PTH.

When blood calcium concentrations are too high, the hormone calcitonin is released. Calcitonin acts opposite to PTH and vitamin D. It reduces calcium absorption in the intestine, increases calcium deposition in the bone and increases calcium excretion in the kidney. All these events occur just long enough to maintain blood calcium at normal concentrations. Even small reductions in blood calcium concentrations set off bone resorption via PTH. In this way, low dietary calcium can lead to bone loss.

### *The Three Major Calcium Regulators*

1.  Parathyroid Hormone (PTH) is secreted by the parathyroid glands, which are located on the thyroid gland, in response to

low blood calcium concentrations. Its job is to increase blood calcium concentrations. To do this, PTH stimulates bone resorption, reduces calcium excretion in the kidneys, and increases vitamin D conversion in the kidneys, which facilitates greater calcium absorption in the intestine. Too little PTH, by causing low blood calcium concentrations, leads to tetany. Too much PTH leads to weak bones and high blood calcium concentrations. Low blood calcium can lead to secondary hyperparathyroidism.

2.  Vitamin D (cholecalciferol) is absorbed from food or through ultraviolet light conversion in the skin. Vitamin D from either source must be converted into active form by the liver and by the kidney. The activated vitamin D then travels to the intestinal cells. There it affects the cell membranes in such a way that more calcium is absorbed into the body. Vitamin D is technically a hormone. If we get sufficient sunlight, we can make enough vitamin D in our body. However, conditions may be less than ideal, so that we often depend on food to receive the required amount. Severe vitamin D deficiency leads to osteomalacia, inadequate bone mineralization. Mild vitamin D deficiency can lead to secondary hyperparathyroidism, which can contribute to osteoporosis. Excess supplementary vitamin D (over $45\mu$g/day) leads to calcification of soft tissues as well as to loss of calcium from bone. Vitamin D keeps blood calcium levels adequate, either by increasing intestinal absorption or by increasing bone resorption.

3.  Calcitonin is a hormone secreted by a section of the thyroid gland in response to high blood calcium concentrations It reduces blood calcium concentrations by increasing calcium secretion in the kidney, inhibiting calcium absorption inhibiting bone resorption (osteoclasts) and increasing calcium deposition into bone tissues.

## *Other Hormones and Biological Substances Influence Bone Density*

Other hormones affect bone tissue. How they affect bone density is not understood. It is possible that other hormones modulate the calcium regulating hormones or influence the production of other biological substances that act on bone.

Anabolic steroids such as testosterone, estrogen and progesterone prevent bone loss. A sudden lack of estrogen in women or androgens in men leads to bone loss.

These sex hormones may counterbalance PTH and thus control the extent of bone resorption caused by this hormone. Some recent evidence suggests that estrogen has a direct effect on bone cells. The role of progesterone in women is less well established but some evidence suggests that it may increase bone density.

Other hormones, such as corticosteroids, can lead to bone loss, if present in excess. For example, Cushing's Syndrome, where too much cortisone is produced, leads to secondary osteoporosis.

Medications also affect bone strength (Table 2.2). People receiving cortisone as part of arthritis treatment may be losing bone mass. Cortisone reduces the formation of the protein matrix of the bone and also the absorption of calcium in the intestine. Hyperthyroidism also leads to bone loss. Treatment with excess thyroxine increases the risk for osteoporosis. This is of particular concern for women approaching menopause, who are already in danger of losing bone.

Recent research suggests that some cells secrete biochemicals that either stimulate bone resorption or enhance bone formation. For example, macrophages (one type of white blood cell) can produce

**Table 2.2.** Effect of Medication on Bone Strength

Drugs may exacerbate or prevent bone loss.

| Drugs that may worsen bone loss | Drugs that may prevent bone loss |
| --- | --- |
| Thyroxine | Anabolic hormones, such as estrogen |
| Cortisone | Thiazides (calcium sparing diuretic) |
| Some antibiotics | Tamoxifen*: antiestrogen, used to |
| Aluminum antacids | treat breast cancer |
| Chemotherapeutic drugs | |
| Anticonvulsants | |
| Heparin | |

*The paradox as to why an estrogen blocker prevents bone loss is not understood.

interleukin-I which stimulates bone resorption. Certain bone cells may produce prostaglandin E-2, which can also induce bone resorption. It is possible that estrogen blocks the activity of some of these biological agents, which may partly explain why estrogen deficiency results in bone loss.

Some local (produced in the vicinity of the bone) growth factors such as somatomedin C or insulin-like growth factor (IGF) increase bone density. The presence and activity of these local factors are regulated by hormones. For example, human growth hormone (HGH) stimulates the production of local growth factors. Insulin also promotes bone growth by stimulating osteoblast activity. However, lack of insulin has not been shown to play a significant role in osteoporosis. Tumor cells may also produce biological substances that activate osteoclasts, which leads to bone loss.

# Chapter 3

# *Juvenile Osteoporosis*

Osteoporosis literally means "porous bone." It is a disease characterized by too little bone formation or excessive bone loss and an increase in the risk of fractures. Osteoporosis is called a silent disease because it progresses without any symptoms until a fracture occurs. It usually affects people later in life, and is most common in women after menopause.

Osteoporosis is rare among children and adolescents. When it occurs, it is usually caused by an underlying medical disorder or by medications used to treat such disorders. This is called secondary osteoporosis. It may also be the result of a genetic disorder such as osteogenesis imperfecta. Sometimes there is no identifiable cause of juvenile osteoporosis. This is known as idiopathic juvenile osteoporosis (IJO).

No matter what causes it, juvenile osteoporosis can be a significant problem, as it occurs during the prime bone-building years. From birth through young adulthood, up to about 30 years of age, bone formation predominates, resulting in a steady accumulation of bone mass. Most bone mass, in fact, is accumulated by early adulthood (Matkovic, 1994; Teegarden, 1995). After the mid-thirties, bone mass typically begins to decline slowly, speeding up in women after menopause. Both genetic and lifestyle factors (e.g., diet and physical activity)

© 1997. Reprinted with permission of Osteoporosis and Related Bone Diseases-National Resource Center, 1150 17th St., NW, Suite 500, Washington, D.C. 20036 202-223-0344 or 800-624-BONE TTY (202) 466-4315. Available at http://www.osteo.org/juvost.htm.

influence the development of peak bone mass and the rate at which bone is lost.

## Secondary Osteoporosis

Secondary osteoporosis can affect both adults and children, and results from an underlying (primary) disorder or therapeutic activity. Juvenile arthritis (JA) provides a good illustration of the possible causes of secondary osteoporosis.

In some cases, the disease process itself can cause osteoporosis. For example, some studies have found that children with JA have bone mass that is lower than expected, especially near the arthritic joints. Sometimes, medication used to treat the primary disorder may reduce bone mass. For example, certain drugs such as prednisone (glucocorticoids) used to treat JA may affect bone mass. Finally, some behaviors associated with the primary disorder may lead to bone loss or a reduction in bone formation. For example, a child with JA may avoid physical activity (which is necessary for building and maintaining bone mass) because it may aggravate his or her condition or cause pain.

In cases of secondary osteoporosis, the best course of action is to identify and treat the underlying disorder. In the case of medication-induced juvenile osteoporosis, it is best to treat the primary disorder with the lowest effective dose of the osteoporosis-inducing medication.

**Table 3.1.** Disorders, Medications and Behaviors That May Affect Bone Mass

| Primary Disorders | Medications | Behaviors |
|---|---|---|
| • Juvenile arthritis | • Anti-convulsants (e.g., for epilepsy) | • Prolonged inactivity or immobility |
| • Diabetes mellitus | | |
| • Osteogenesis imperfecta | • Corticosteroids (e.g., for rheumatoid arthritis, asthma) | • Inadequate nutrition (especially calcium, vitamin D) |
| • Hyperthyroidism | | |
| • Cushing's Syndrome | • Immunosuppressive agents (e.g., for cancer) | • Excessive exercise leading to amenorrhea |
| • Malabsorption syndromes | | |
| • Anorexia nervosa | • Hyperparathyroidism | • Smoking, Alcohol abuse |
| • Kidney disease | | |

If an alternative medication is available and effective, the child's doctor may also consider prescribing it.

## Idiopathic Juvenile Osteoporosis

Idiopathic juvenile osteoporosis (IJO) is diagnosed after excluding other causes of juvenile osteoporosis (i.e., primary diseases or medical therapies known to cause bone loss, as discussed above). IJO was first identified in the medical literature in 1965 (Dent and Friedman). Since then, fewer than 100 cases have been reported.

This rare form of osteoporosis typically occurs in previously healthy children just before the onset of puberty. The average age of onset is between 8 and 14 years, but it may also occur in younger children during periods of rapid growth. The most notable feature of IJO is that it can remit within two to four years.

**Clinical features.** The first sign of IJO is usually pain in the lower back, hips, and feet, often accompanied by difficulty walking. There may also be knee and ankle pain, and fractures of the lower extremities. Physical deformities may be present, such as kyphosis (abnormal curvature of the thoracic spine), loss of height, a sunken-chest, or a limp. These physical abnormalities are sometimes reversible after the IJO has run its course.

X-rays of children with IJO often show low bone density, fractures of the weight-bearing bones, and collapsed or misshapen vertebrae. However, conventional X-rays may not be able to detect osteoporosis until significant bone mass has already been lost. Newer methods such as dual energy x-ray absorptiometry (DXA), dual photon absorptiometry (DPA) and quantitative computed tomography ("CAT scans") allow for earlier and more accurate diagnosis of low bone mass.

**Treatment.** Early diagnosis of IJO is important, although there is no established medical or surgical therapy for the disease. In fact, there may be no need for treatment, as IJO usually resolves spontaneously. The basic strategy of treatment is to protect the spine and other bones from fracture until remission occurs. This is accomplished through supportive care, which may include physical therapy, use of crutches, and/or avoidance of unsafe weight-bearing activities. Some medications that are used to treat osteoporosis in adults have also been given children with IJO. Examples include bisphosphonates and calcitriol. The physician may try a medical therapy if the problem is severe and not resolving spontaneously.

**Prognosis.** As mentioned above, patients with IJO can experience a complete recovery within two to four years. Growth may be somewhat impaired during the acute phase of the disorder, but normal growth resumes—and catch-up growth often occurs—thereafter. In some cases, IJO can result in permanent disability such as kyphoscoliosis or even collapse of the rib cage.

## Distinguishing IJO from Osteogenesis Imperfecta

Osteogenesis imperfecta (OI) is a genetic disorder characterized by bones that break easily, often from little or no apparent cause. Most forms of OI are caused by imperfectly formed bone collagen, the result of a genetic defect. There are at least four distinct forms of the disorder, representing extreme variation in severity from one person to another. For example, a person may have as few as ten or as many as several hundred fractures in a lifetime. While the prevalence of OI in the United States is not known, the best estimate suggests that about 20,000 people are affected by this disorder.

The clinical features of OI vary greatly from person to person; there is also great variation in their severity. The most common features of OI include:

- bones that fracture easily
- family history usually present
- small stature common
- blue sclera ("whites" of the eyes) common
- possible hearing loss
- possible dental problems

The features that most often distinguish OI and IJO are the family history and blue sclera commonly found in cases of OI. There are also radiographic differences: patients with OI often have Wormian bones (irregular bone patterns in the skull).

## The Bottom Line

- Secondary osteoporosis is best addressed by treating the primary disorder and/or using the lowest effective dose of an osteoporosis-inducing medication.

- Idiopathic juvenile osteoporosis is quite rare. It is often suspected after a series of fractures not caused by serious trauma.

The condition usually resolves itself within two to four years, and permanent disability is uncommon.

* Juvenile osteoporosis can be most easily distinguished from osteogenesis imperfecta by the lack of family history and the absence of blue sclera.

For more information about weight-bearing exercise and other ways to prevent osteoporosis, contact the Osteoporosis and Related Bone Diseases-National Resource Center.

## References

Dent, C. and Friedman, M. (1965). Idiopathic juvenile osteoporosis. *Quarterly Journal of Medicine, New Series* XXXIV(134). 177-210.

Khosla, S. and Melton, L.J. (1995). Secondary osteoporosis. In Riggs, B.L., Melton, L.J. (eds) *Osteoporosis: Etiology, Diagnosis and Management*, Second Edition. Lippincott-Raven: Philadelphia.183-204.

Khosla, S., Riggs, B.L., and Melton, L.J. (1995). Clinical spectrum. In Riggs, B.L., Melton, L.J. (eds) *Osteoporosis: Etiology, Diagnosis and Management*, Second Edition. Lippincott-Raven:Philadelphia. 205-223.

Matkovic, V., Jelic, T.,Wardlaw, G., Ilich, J., Goel, P., Wright, J., Andon, M., Smith, K., and Heaney, R. (1994). Timing of peak bone mass in Causasian females and its implication for the prevention of osteoporosis. *Journal of Clinical Investigation*, 93,799-808.

Norman, M. (1996). Juvenile osteoporosis. In Favus, M.J. (ed) *Primer on the metabolic bone diseases and disorders of mineral metabolism*. Third edition. Lippincott-Raven: Philadelphia. 275-278.

Smith, R. (1996). Osteoporosis in young people. *Osteoporosis Review: Journal of the National Osteoporosis Society*, 4(2).

Teegarden, D., Proulx, W., Martin, B., Zhao, J., McCabe, G., Lyle, R., Peacock, M., Slemenda, C., Johnston, C. and Weaver, C.

(1995). Peak bone mass in young women. *Journal of Bone and Mineral Research*, 10(5), 711-715.

ORBD-NRC is supported by the National Institute of Arthritis and Musculoskeletal and Skin Diseases, National Institutes of Health

# Chapter 4

# *Bone Basics*

## *Bone Basics for Kids*

### *Be a Bone Builder*

Have you ever thought about your bones? Your bones are the frame that your body is built on. You need healthy bones to help you grow taller and stronger. That's why being a bone builder is so important. You can build bones now that will last for the rest of your life. There are lots of things you can to do to make sure your bones grow bigger and stronger.

### *Drink Your Milk*

You may have heard it a million times, but your parents really know what they're talking about. Milk, as well as other dairy foods, has a lot of calcium. Calcium is the mineral that makes bones strong.

Kids age 10 and under need 800-1,200 milligrams (mg) of calcium each day, and those over 10 need about 1,200-1,500 mg a day. How much calcium do you get each day? You can find out how much calcium different foods have by reading the label or looking it up at the

---

This chapter includes the following publications: "Bone Basics for Kids," © 1997 National Osteoporosis Foundation (NOF), "Bone Basics for Teens," © 1997 NOF; "Bone Basics for Young Women," © 1998 NOF; "Bone Basics for Midlife Women," © 1997 NOF; "Bone Basics for Men of All Ages," © 1997 NOF; "Bone Basics for Older Women and Men," © 1995 NOF. Reprinted with permission from the National Osteoporosis Foundation, Washington, DC 20037.

library. If you're not getting enough calcium, here are some ways to add more calcium to your daily diet:

Drink three to five glasses of low-fat or skim milk every day or substitute a milk shake, or make chocolate milk.

Eat more low-fat yogurt and have frozen yogurt once in a while. Have cheese on hamburgers. Sprinkle cheese on popcorn and salads. Make brownies with low-fat or skim milk instead of water. Eat calcium-rich dark green vegetables like broccoli and collard greens. Eat a balanced diet including fruits and green vegetables everyday. Calcium isn't just found in dairy foods.

Can you think of some more ways to get more calcium in your diet?

### Don't Be a Lazy Bones

You can walk, run, hike, skateboard, jump rope, dance, or ski, but do something! Being active and getting plenty of exercise is good for your bones. Don't be a couch potato! Your bones need exercise to grow big and strong just as your muscles do.

One way to become more active is to play sports or take dance lessons regularly. Just find something you like and do it!

## Bone Basics for Teens

### How to Look and Feel Good, Inside and out

Have you ever thought about your bones? They are the framework your body is built on.

One way to look and feel your best is to have strong, healthy bones. Think about it this way: Your favorite clothes look their best on a healthy body, and your body looks its best on a set of strong, healthy bones.

Now is the perfect time for you to build strong bones to last a lifetime.

### The Bone Bank Account

Bones are not lifeless structures, they're living tissue. Bone is made of proteins and minerals, especially the mineral calcium. Bone is constantly changing, with bits of old bone being removed to be replaced by new bone. In fact, you can think of bone as a bank account, where you make "deposits" and "withdrawals" of bone tissue.

During your teenage years, hormones (estrogen in girls and testosterone in boys) help bones grow in size and strength. You deposit much more bone than you withdraw until around age 30, when your bones reach their maximum strength and density.

You'll need a large bank account of bone tissue to draw from when you're older. At menopause (generally around age 50), women's bodies change in a way that has a big effect on their bones: they produce less of the female hormone estrogen. Estrogen helps slow down bone loss—so, with less estrogen in women's systems, they lose a great deal of bone tissue in the years after menopause. While men do not stop producing the male hormone testosterone, they also experience bone loss as they age, but at a far slower rate than women.

The teen years are your best chance to build up your bone bank account, so take advantage of it! This way, you will have plenty of bone tissue to "withdraw" when the time comes.

## What Is Osteoporosis?

Have you noticed that some older women and men have a stooped posture? They were once as straight and as strong as you are, but now they suffer from osteoporosis. Fractures cause stooped posture.

Osteoporosis is a disease where bones become fragile and break easily. When a person has osteoporosis, it means their bank account of bone tissue has been withdrawn to such a low level that even a sneezing or bending over to tie a shoe can cause a bone in the spine to break. Hips, ribs, and wrist bones also break easily. Osteoporosis is painful and disfiguring, and there is no cure.

The way to prevent osteoporosis from happening to you when you get older is to build strong bones NOW with a balanced diet including calcium and an active lifestyle.

## The Balancing Act

To build healthy bones, you need to eat a balanced diet rich in calcium. You should be getting 1,200-1,500 mg of calcium everyday. If you're like most people, you're not getting enough calcium to build strong bones—maybe because you're on a diet. But you can boost your calcium intake and not gain weight. Sometimes, you get more calcium from low-fat foods than from "fat" foods—for example, a cup of skim milk gives you a little more calcium than a cup of whole milk.

Here are some easy ways to get more calcium each day:

- Ask for cheese on your burgers, extra cheese on pizza, or add cheese to salads.

- Have low-fat yogurt, frozen yogurt, or ice milk for dessert.

- Snack on broccoli with low-fat dip, it's a lot less fattening than chips!

- Drink milk or milkshakes instead of soft drinks.

You should know that starving yourself or purging to lose weight (disorders called anorexia nervosa and bulimia) can be so harmful that you can develop osteoporosis by the time you're in your 20s. Starvation and fad diets can be extremely dangerous. Instead, make sure you eat a balanced diet which, in combination with proper exercise, should keep you at your proper weight and make you feel and look good. If you are concerned about losing weight, talk to your doctor about a safe diet and exercise program that is right for you.

### Get a Bone Workout

Don't be a couch potato! Bones are living tissue and they need exercise to grow and stay healthy just as your muscles do. An active lifestyle that includes weight-bearing exercise is an important element in building strong bones. Weight-bearing exercise causes muscles to work against gravity.

Weight-bearing exercises are such activities as jogging, skating, weight-lifting, soccer, skiing, tennis, volleyball, basketball, dancing, and even walking. See if you and your friends can organize some regular activities that include weight-bearing exercise! There are plenty of easy ways to be more active throughout the day:

- Walk to school and other places instead of driving or riding with someone.

- Take the stairs instead of the elevator.

- Join a team sport at school, or take dance classes.

- Surprise your parents—do house or yardwork! Physical work is great for building bones.

Remember, physical activity of any kind is good for your bones! In addition, exercise burns calories, so by working out on a regular basis you can eat the foods you need to stay healthy and keep your weight under control.

*Healthy Habits Make Healthy Bones*

Certain substances are toxic to bones. For example, smoking and drinking alcohol are both harmful to your bones. They can slow bone growth, and damage bone tissue. Remember, your bones provide the support your body depends on.

## Bone Basics for Young Women

*Simple Health Tips for Your Busy Life*

You're leading a busy, active life, packing as much as you can into each day. But remember to build time into your schedule for your health, especially to take care of your bones. Having healthy bones will have benefits for you today and in the future.

The best way to build strong bones is through a balanced diet rich in calcium and regular exercise. The immediate benefits are a strong body, more energy, and a terrific, healthy look. The biggest benefit you'll enjoy in your later years is prevention of osteoporosis, a painful and disfiguring bone disease that occurs in one in two women. By taking a few simple steps every day, you'll build strong bones that will last you for the rest of your life.

*Now Is the Time to Build Strong Bones*

Contrary to popular belief, bones are not lifeless structures, but are, in fact, living tissue. Bone changes constantly, with bits of old bone, being removed to be replaced by new bone. Think of bone as a bank account, where you make "deposits" and "withdrawals" of bone tissue.

During childhood and adolescence, much more bone is deposited than withdrawn, so that the skeleton grows both in size and density. The amount of bone tissue in the skeleton known as bone mass can continue to increase until you're around 30. At this point, the amount of bone typically begins to decline slowly, as withdrawals exceed deposits of new bone. That is why it is so important to build as much bone as you can now!

Around the time of menopause, the ovaries produce less estrogen. Estrogen is a hormone that has been proven to have a protective effect on bone. After menopause, the loss of estrogen greatly accelerates bone loss in most women.

## *What Is Osteoporosis?*

The most important reason to take care of your bones now is to prevent osteoporosis, an exaggerated loss of bone tissue that makes bones weak and more likely to fracture.

With osteoporosis, simply bending over to tie your shoe can put you at risk of a serious fracture. Osteoporosis can cause painful fractures, deformity, and disability.

Although there is no cure for osteoporosis, it can be prevented. But you must work on building strong bones now, while you're young. During your young adult years, you should take advantage of your opportunity to build up your bone bank account, so you'll have plenty of bone mass to "withdraw" when the time comes. If you didn't get enough calcium as a teen, it's not too late to start now. With proper diet and exercise, you can reduce your risk of developing osteoporosis later in life.

## *Quick and Easy Ways to Add Calcium to Your Daily Diet*

To prevent osteoporosis, you need to eat a balanced diet rich in calcium. Young adult women need 1,200 mg. of calcium per day, which is equal to four 8 oz. glasses of milk. If you're like most American women, you're taking in only one-third to one-half of the calcium you need for healthy bones. If you're worried about the calories, you should know that calcium-rich foods don't have to be fattening. For example, a cup of skim milk actually gives you somewhat more calcium than a cup of whole milk and has fewer calories, and no fat.

Even when your busy schedule only allows you to grab a quick meal, you can easily add calcium to your diet. For example:

- Add a dairy product to every meal. Grate cheese over your salad, add slices of low-fat cheese to your sandwich, or drink milk instead of other beverages.

- Drink calcium-fortified fruit juices.

- Try low-fat yogurt, frozen yogurt, or ice milk for dessert or snacks.

- Enjoy high calcium foods like broccoli and tofu.

Some people have difficulty digesting milk products; this is a condition known as lactose intolerance. People who are lactose intolerant can satisfy their daily calcium requirements in a number of ways by incorporating non-dairy, calcium rich foods into the diet, taking calcium supplements, and using lactase pills or drops which make the milk products digestible.

### Exercise for Strong Bones

Bones are living tissue and they need exercise to grow and remain strong. Regular weight-bearing exercise, which causes muscles to work against gravity, is the most effective type of exercise to build bone mass. Some examples of weight-bearing exercises are jogging, tennis, stair climbing, weight-lifting, walking, and dancing. Experts believe that other forms of exercise, like swimming, bicycling, and rowing, while not weight-bearing, may have other benefits. The bottom line is that keeping active allows you to eat more without gaining weight, making it easier to maintain an adequate intake of calcium and other nutrients. Adopt an active lifestyle. Walk short distances instead of driving. Do housework and yardwork that involves walking and carrying. If you spend a lot of time at a desk in your office, it's especially important that you exercise. Use the stairs instead of the elevator and whenever possible, walk to appointments.

### Healthy Habits Make Healthy Bones

Certain substances such as nicotine and alcohol are toxic to bones. They can interfere with proper nutrition and taking extra calcium cannot make up for the damage. To help protect your bones, avoid smoking and practice moderation with alcoholic beverages.

### Pregnancy and Motherhood

If you are pregnant or nursing an infant, you need even more calcium in your diet, both for yourself and your child's early bone development. Your baby's calcium needs will be satisfied by taking calcium from your bones. If you're pregnant or nursing under age 24, you need 1,500 mg. of calcium per day. If you are over 24, you need 1,200 mg. per day.

Getting enough calcium during pregnancy is a great way to start bone healthy habits for both you and your child.

### Estrogen Replacement Therapy

Estrogen, a hormone produced naturally by the ovaries, has been proven to slow or stop bone loss after menopause, lowering the chances that osteoporosis will develop.

Estrogen replacement therapy (ERT) has been used to help prevent osteoporosis in women who no longer produce estrogen because of menopause or surgical removal of the ovaries.

ERT can help—but it also has risks. If you are interested in learning more, you should discuss ERT with your doctor

## Bone Basics for Midlife Women

### Bone Health to Last a Lifetime

Midlife is a critical time for women to be concerned about their bone health. You might be surprised to know that 8 million American women have osteoporosis and another 14 million are at high risk with low bone mass.

Following menopause, the amount of estrogen produced by the ovaries sharply declines. Estrogen is a female hormone that affects the skeleton. This decline causes a period of rapid bone loss that lasts five to ten years after menopause. In fact, it is this postmenopausal bone loss that accounts for the high proportion of women with osteoporosis.

You might be wondering how you can lose bone. Contrary to popular belief, bones are not lifeless structures, but are, in fact, living tissue. Bone changes constantly, with bits of old bone being removed to be replaced by new bone. Think of bone as a bank account, where you make "deposits" and "withdrawals" of bone tissue.

During childhood and adolescence, much more bone is deposited than withdrawn, so that the skeleton grows both in size and density. The amount of bone tissue in the skeleton, known as bone mass, can continue to increase until you're around 30. At this point the amount of bone typically begins to decline slowly as withdrawals exceed deposits of new bone. Osteoporosis occurs when deposits are too low or when withdrawals are excessive.

Around the time of menopause, when estrogen production diminishes, rapid bone loss begins, which increases a woman's risk of developing osteoporosis.

Osteoporosis is an exaggerated loss of bone tissue, a painful and disabling disease that develops in older person—usually women—who do not have enough bone density. Osteoporosis makes bones more susceptible to fracture, most often of the hip, spine or wrist. Spinal fractures cause stooped posture, loss of height, and chronic back pain. Hip fracture, the most serious consequence of osteoporosis, threatens one's independence and life. Once you reach midlife, you need to take action to protect your bones. There are several steps you can take to maintain the strength of your bones. You can start by finding out what your bone density is by having a bone density test.

## *Risk Factors*

- Being female
- Thin and small frame
- Advanced age
- A family history of osteoporosis
- Postmenopause, including early or surgically induced menopause
- Abnormal absence of menstrual periods (amenorrhea)
- Anorexia nervosa or bulimia
- A diet low in calcium
- Use of certain medications, such as corticosteroids and anticonvulsants
- Low testosterone levels in men
- An inactive lifestyle
- Excessive use of alcohol
- Being Caucasian or Asian, although African Americans and Hispanic Americans are at significant risk as well.

## *Bone Density Testing*

Once bone mass has been lost, it can't be replaced. That's why the best "treatment" for osteoporosis is preventing it in the first place! Since osteoporosis can develop silently for decades until a fracture occurs, early detection of low bone mass is essential so that therapy to prevent further bone loss will be most effective.

Assessing your risk for osteoporosis and finding out the density of your bones (your bone mass) is necessary to determine whether you need medication to help maintain your bone mass.

Safe, accurate, and non-invasive tests are available for measuring bone mass. Use of these techniques is the only accurate way to measure bone mass and to assess the risk of fracture. If you would like to learn more about bone density testing, ask your doctor.

### Prevention and Treatment of Osteoporosis

Estrogen replacement therapy (ERT) is medication that replaces or supplements the body's falling level of estrogen which results from menopause. ERT helps keep calcium in the bones and maintains bone density, thereby preventing osteoporosis. Recent research findings indicate that ERT also may protect against heart disease.

Estrogen usually is given with another hormone called progesterone, to prevent an increased risk of endometrial cancer. This does not apply to women who have had their uterus removed.

Experts believe that ERT is most effective in reducing bone loss during the five to ten years following menopause, when bone loss is at its greatest. But if you are older, there may still be benefits in starting ERT to prevent further bone loss. While ERT can be beneficial, it also has risks and should be undertaken only after a careful discussion with your doctor.

Raloxifene is a drug that was recently approved for the prevention of osteoporosis. It is from a new class of drugs called "Selective Estrogen Receptor Modulators" (SERMS) that appears to prevent bone loss throughout the body.

Alendronate is another medication used to treat and prevent osteoporosis. It is from a class of drugs called bisphosphonates, which inhibit bone breakdown. Alendronate has been shown to increase bone density and prevent fractures.

Calcitonin is another treatment option for postmenopausal women. Calcitonin is a hormone produced in the thyroid gland that is involved in calcium regulation and bone metabolism. This hormone has been shown to slow bone loss. It is available in nasal spray form or can be administered by injection.

Other medications currently being studied are other bisphosphonates, selective estrogen receptor modulators, sodium fluoride, parathyroid hormone and vitamin D metabolites.

### Calcium: A Necessity at Every Age

Children aren't the only ones who need calcium. Because bone tissue is constantly building up and breaking down, calcium is important for people of all ages. To prevent osteoporosis, you need to eat a balanced diet rich in calcium throughout your lifetime.

- Postmenopausal women on ERT need 1,000 mg of calcium daily.
- Postmenopausal women not on ERT need 1,500 mg of calcium daily.

52

Adding more calcium to your daily diet is easy. Add a dairy product to every meal by grating cheese over your salad or adding low-fat cheese to your sandwich. Try low-fat yogurt or frozen yogurt for dessert. Enjoy other high calcium foods like broccoli or calcium-fortified fruit juices.

Some people have difficulty digesting milk products, a condition known as lactose intolerance. People who are lactose intolerant can satisfy daily calcium requirements by incorporating non-dairy, calcium-rich foods into the diet, taking calcium supplements, and using lactase pills or drops that make the milk products digestible.

### Exercise for Strong Bones

Regular weight-bearing exercise, which causes muscles to work against gravity, helps to build and maintain bone mass. Walking is an excellent weight-bearing exercise, as are jogging, tennis, aerobics, and dancing. Experts believe that other forms of exercise like swimming and bicycling, while not weight-bearing, have important cardiovascular benefits. Remember, keeping active allows you to eat more without gaining weight, making it easier to maintain an adequate intake of calcium and other nutrients.

Adopt an active lifestyle. Walk short distances instead of driving, use the stairs instead of the elevator, and do house or yardwork. If you spend a lot of time sitting, it's especially important that you exercise.

REMEMBER: Before embarking on an exercise program, be sure to consult your physician.

### Healthy Habits Make Healthy Bones

Certain substances are toxic to bones, such as nicotine and alcohol. Smoking is toxic to bone cells, and extra calcium can't make up for the damage. Alcohol is also harmful. Not only is it directly toxic to bones, but it also interferes with proper nutrition. To help protect your bone density, avoid smoking and practice moderation with alcoholic beverages.

## Bone Basics for Men of All Ages

### Understanding Osteoporosis in Men

You might be surprised to learn that more than 2 million American men have osteoporosis and another 3 million men are at risk for developing the disease. In fact, osteoporosis affects nearly half of all people—women and men—over the age of 75. Although this disease has been studied more often in women, there are steps that can be taken to prevent and treat osteoporosis in men.

### Understanding Your Bones

Bones are not lifeless structures, but are, in fact, living tissue. Bone constantly changes, with bits of old bone being removed to be replaced by new bone. During childhood, more bone is produced than removed, so the skeleton grows in both size and strength. The amount of tissue or bone mass in the skeleton reaches its maximum amount by age 30. At this point, the amount of bone in the skeleton typically begins to decline slowly as removal exceeds deposits of new bone.

While women lose bone mass rapidly in the years after menopause, by age 65 or 70 women and men lose bone mass at the same rate, and calcium absorption decreases in both sexes. When bone loss is excessive, bone can become fragile and break. Once bone is lost, it cannot, as yet, be replaced.

### What Is Osteoporosis?

Osteoporosis is a painful and disabling disease that weakens bones and makes them more likely to fracture. Osteoporosis occurs because of inadequate bone formation, excessive bone removal or both. Fractures resulting from osteoporosis typically occur in the hip, spine, and wrist and can be permanently disabling.

### Risk Factors for Men

There are several risk factors that have been linked to osteoporosis in men.

- Prolonged exposure to certain medications, such as steroids used to treat asthma, arthritis, or other diseases, anticonvulsants, certain cancer treatments, and aluminum-containing antacids.
- Chronic diseases that affect the kidneys, lungs, stomach, and intestines, or that alter hormone levels.
- Undiagnosed low levels of the sex hormone testosterone.
- Unhealthy lifestyle habits (e.g., smoking, excessive alcohol use, low calcium intake, inadequate physical exercise).
- Age: The older you are, the greater your risk.

* Heredity

* Race: Caucasian men appear to be at greater risk, but all men can develop this disease.

In the absence of research findings, there may be other risk factors that have not yet been identified. Men who develop osteoporosis often do not have any of the above risk factors.

### Calcium: A Necessity at Any Age

To prevent osteoporosis, you need to eat a balanced diet rich in calcium throughout your lifetime. Adult men need 1,000 mg of calcium per day and those over 65 need 1,500 mg per day. It's easy to add calcium to your diet. Try having a dairy product at every meal. Grate cheese over your salad, drink skim milk, or add a slice of low-fat cheese to your sandwich. Try low-fat yogurt, frozen yogurt, or ice milk for dessert or snacks. Enjoy high calcium foods like broccoli, tofu, and calcium-fortified fruit juice.

Some people have difficulty digesting milk products, a condition known as lactose intolerance. People who are lactose intolerant can satisfy their daily calcium requirements in a number of ways: by incorporating non-dairy, calcium-rich foods into the diet, by taking calcium supplements, and by using lactase pills or drops that make milk products digestible.

### Exercise for Strong Bones

Regular weight-bearing exercise, which causes muscles to work against gravity, can help build bone density. Jogging is an excellent weight-bearing exercise, as are walking, tennis, and dancing. Experts believe that other forms of exercise, like swimming, bicycling, and rowing, while they are not weight-bearing, have cardiovascular benefits. And keeping active allows you to eat more without gaining weight, making it easier to maintain an adequate intake of calcium and other nutrients.

Adopt an active lifestyle. Walk short distances instead of driving. Do housework and yardwork. If you spend a lot of time at a desk in your office, it's especially important that you exercise. Use the stairs instead of the elevator and, whenever possible, walk to appointments. If you are older and have not been exercising regularly, check with your doctor before embarking on an exercise program.

## *Healthy Habits Make Healthy Bones*

Adequate calcium and vitamin D intake, proper exercise, and good health habits are essential throughout life to ensure that the body has enough bone tissue to draw from in later years.

Certain substances, such as nicotine and alcohol, are toxic to bones. Smoking is toxic to bone cells, and extra calcium can't make up for the damage. Alcohol abuse is also harmful. Not only is it directly toxic to bones, but it also interferes with proper nutrition. To help protect your bone density, avoid smoking and practice moderation with alcoholic beverages.

## *Bone Density Testing*

You cannot feel your bones becoming weak and fragile. Because of this, you can have osteoporosis and not even know it—until a bone breaks. The key to preventing osteoporosis is to find out how weak or strong your bones are before a bone breaks. The sooner you know this, the sooner you can take action to prevent the disease.

The best way to find out how strong or weak your bones are is to have a bone density test. This safe, painless, and non-invasive test can determine your bone density, which is a measure of bone strength, and can predict your chances of sustaining a fracture in the future. It uses very low amounts of radiation and is much more sensitive than standard x-rays.

Risk factors help identify some of the people who will develop osteoporosis, but not all. Only a bone density test can detect low bone density and diagnose osteoporosis. If you are interested in learning more about bone density testing, your doctor can explain the test further and refer you to an exam site.

## *Living with Osteoporosis*

If you have osteoporosis, you can live actively and comfortably if you seek proper medical care and make some lifestyle adjustments. Your doctor may prescribe a treatment program that includes calcium, exercise, or medication. There are several osteoporosis medications approved by the Food and Drug Administration (FDA) for women that are often prescribed for men with osteoporosis, such as alendronate or calcitonin. If low levels of testosterone (hypogonadism) is determined to be a cause of your osteoporosis, your doctor may prescribe testosterone replacement therapy as a treatment.

## *Bone Basics for Older Women and Men*

### *Prevention is Ageless*

Typically, when most people think about health, they don't think about their bones. But keeping your bones healthy by preventing osteoporosis is particularly important with age.

Bones are not lifeless structures, but are, in fact, living tissue. Bone changes constantly, with bits of old bone being removed and replaced with new bone. Think of bone as a bank account, where you make "deposits" and "withdrawals" of bone tissue. During childhood, more bone is produced than removed, so that the skeleton grows both in size and density. The amount of tissue or bone mass in the skeleton reaches its maximum amount by age 30. At this point, the amount of bone tissue in the skeleton typically begins to decline slowly as withdrawals exceed deposits of new bone.

Women are at greater risk for developing osteoporosis. Not only do women have smaller, thinner skeletons, but around the time of menopause, the ovaries' production of estrogen diminishes. The female hormone estrogen is protective of bone. This decrease in estrogen production greatly accelerates the loss of bone in most women. It is the five-to ten-year period of rapid postmenopausal bone loss that probably accounts for the high proportion of women with osteoporosis.

Men also develop osteoporosis, but generally later than women. By age 65 or 70, women and men lose bone mass at the same rate, and dietary calcium absorption decreases for both sexes. Nearly half of all people over the age of 75 are affected by this disease.

### *Risk Factors*

- Being female
- Thin and small frame
- Advanced age
- A family history of osteoporosis
- Postmenopause, including early or surgically induced menopause
- Abnormal absence of menstrual periods (amenorrhea)
- Anorexia nervosa or bulimia
- A diet low in calcium

- Use of certain medications, such as corticosteroids and anticonvulsants

- Low testosterone levels in men

- An inactive lifestyle

- Excessive use of alcohol

- Being Caucasian or Asian, although African Americans and Hispanic Americans are at significant risk as well.

### What Is Osteoporosis?

Osteoporosis is a painful and disfiguring disease that weakens bones and makes them more susceptible to fracture. Osteoporosis occurs when bone formation is inadequate, bone removal is excessive, or both. Fractures occur most often in the hip, spine, wrist, and ribs. Spinal fractures cause a stooped posture, loss of height, and chronic back pain. Hip fracture, the most serious consequence of osteoporosis, threatens one's independence and life.

Fortunately, in your older years, you can still take steps to protect your bones. You'll need a balanced diet rich in calcium and vitamin D, a regular program of exercise, and, in some cases, medication. These steps can help you slow bone loss. In addition, you'll want to learn how to fall-proof your home and alter your lifestyle to avoid fracturing fragile bones.

### Calcium: A Necessity at Any Age

Calcium is not just important for growing children—it is needed to help maintain healthy, strong bones throughout life. To make sure that a lack of calcium is not weakening your bones, be sure to eat a balanced diet rich in calcium.

Women on estrogen replacement therapy (ERT) and men need 1,000 mg of calcium every day. Women not on ERT need 1,500 mg. However, once over age 65, both women and men need 1,500 mg of calcium daily.

To add calcium to your diet, have a dairy product at every meal. Grate cheese over your salad, or add a slice of low-fat cheese to your sandwich. Try low-fat or frozen yogurt for dessert or snacks. Enjoy high calcium foods like broccoli, tofu, canned salmon with bones, and calcium-fortified fruit juice. If you cannot get enough calcium in your diet, you may want to consider taking calcium supplements.

Some people have difficulty digesting milk products. This is known as lactose intolerance. People who are lactose intolerant can satisfy their daily calcium requirements in a number of ways: by taking dairy products in small amounts spread out over the day; by including more non-dairy, calcium-rich foods into the diet; by taking calcium supplements; and by using lactase pills or drops that make milk products more digestible.

## *Exercise*

It Is essential to consult a physician before embarking on any exercise program. If you have osteoporosis, you will want to follow carefully the activity program set up by your physician and a physical therapist in order to decrease your chances of fracturing.

In general, weight-bearing exercises, which cause muscles to work against gravity, can help maintain bone strength. Walking is an excellent weight-bearing exercise: it strengthens the legs, hips, and lower back, improves heart function, helps control weight, and, when done with friends, can be a source of social enjoyment.

Other forms of exercise, like tennis, gardening, swimming, and bicycling, are beneficial as well. Keeping active allows you to eat more without gaining weight, making it easier to maintain an adequate intake of calcium and other nutrients. Regular exercise will also help you increase your flexibility and improve your balance.

## *Bone Density Testing*

Since osteoporosis can develop undetected for decades until a fracture occurs, early diagnosis is important. Assessing your risk for osteoporosis and finding out the density of your bones (your bone mass) is necessary to determine whether you need medication to help maintain your bone mass. Safe, accurate, and non-invasive tests are available for measuring bone mass. These tests are the only accurate way to measure bone mass and to assess the risk of fracture. With the results of a bone mass measurement, physicians can identify areas in the body with low bone mass and determine the type of therapy that should be used to prevent further bone loss. To learn more about bone mass measurements, ask your doctor.

## *Living with Osteoporosis*

If you have osteoporosis, you can live actively and comfortably. Be sure to seek proper medical care and make some lifestyle adjustments, including making your environment safe so you can avoid falls.

Your doctor may prescribe a regimen that includes calcium and vitamin D, exercise, and medication. For men with hypogonadism, testosterone may be prescribed. A woman might consider estrogen replacement therapy (ERT). Experts believe that ERT is most effective in reducing bone loss during the five to ten years following menopause, when bone loss is at its peak, but studies show that starting ERT later in life can still be beneficial.

Raloxifene is a drug that was recently approved for the prevention of osteoporosis. It is from a new class of drugs called "Selective Estrogen Receptor Modulators" (SERMS). Ralixofene appears to prevent bone loss throughout the body.

Other treatment options include alendronate and calcitonin. Alendronate has been approved for the treatment and prevention of postmenopausal osteoporosis. It is from a class of drugs called bisphosphonates that inhibit bone breakdown. Alendronate has been shown to increase bone density and prevent fractures.

Calcitonin is another treatment option. Calcitonin is a hormone produced in the thyroid gland that is involved in calcium regulation and bone metabolism. This hormone has been shown to slow bone loss. Calcitonin has few side effects and is safe. It is available in nasal spray form or can be administered by injection.

Other investigational medications currently being studied include other bisphosphonates, other selective estrogen receptor modulators, sodium fluoride, parathyroid hormone and vitamin D metabolites.

# Chapter 5

# *Boning Up*

## *Turning on Cells That Build Bone and Turning off Ones That Destroy It*

Construction and demolition crews working side by side. It sounds insane, but that's how the human skeleton grows and maintains itself. Each of its 206 bones harbors cells that continually deposit a rigid protein matrix that becomes mineralized. Each bone also contains cells that can break that structure down.

The bone builders keep ahead of the bone destroyers as a child grows, but the balance can shift as a person gets older. Bones weaken when osteoclasts, the matrix-resorbing cells, outpace osteoblasts, the matrix-making cells. A wide variety of conditions—most notably osteoporosis, but also rheumatoid arthritis, leukemia, and HIV infection—shift the cellular tug of war in favor of the bone destroyers. The weak bones that result can suffer debilitating, even deadly, fractures.

Scientific advances on two complementary fronts now offer new hope in the body's battle against bone loss. In one of the most exciting stories in bone research in many years, scientists have unearthed a fundamental mechanism by which osteoblasts communicate with osteoclasts. Medical researchers are already testing a new drug that exploits this knowledge to stop bone deterioration.

---

Travis, John, "Boning Up," in *Science News*, January 15, 2000, Vol. 157, Issue 4, p. 41. Reprinted with permission from *Science News*, the weekly newsmagazine of science, copyright 2000 by Science Service, Inc.

61

In a more surprising development, popular cholesterol-lowering drugs known as statins seem to stimulate growth of new bone. Statins have thickened the bones of mice in laboratory experiments, and test-tube studies suggest a mechanism for this action. However, it's not clear yet whether statin drugs will jump-start bone growth in people.

The excitement began in 1996 when X rays of some genetically engineered mice revealed something unusual about their skeletons. "We found that [the animals] had extraordinarily dense bones," recalls Colin R. Dunstan of Amgen, a biotech firm in Thousand Oaks, Calif.

He and his colleagues at the company had been puzzling over the role of a protein encoded by a gene that they had recently discovered. As part of their investigation into the protein's function, the investigators created mice with extra copies of the gene. The animals synthesized abnormally large amounts of the protein, which somehow led to the thicker-than-normal bones.

The puzzling protein—dubbed osteoprotegerin (OPG) by Amgen because it seemed to protect the integrity of bones—turned out to be a key part of the molecular conversation between osteoblasts and osteoclasts. While the goals of these two cell types appear at odds, scientists have long known that the cells cooperate.

"The cells that make the bone also control its removal or resorption," says Dunstan.

How the two types of cells communicate had been a mystery until studies in the past few years revealed that OPG binds to a protein called OPG-ligand. This attachment prevents OPG-ligand from rousing osteoclasts into action.

"OPG-ligand is like the accelerator of your car. If you step on OPG-ligand, you lose bone. OPG is the brake of the system. If you step on OPG, then you have more bone. The balance between the two determines how much bone we have," says Josef M. Penninger of the University of Toronto.

Osteoblasts make both OPG and OPG-ligand, scientists have learned. OPG-ligand binds to surface proteins on osteoclasts, triggering proliferation of these cells and increasing their bone degradation. OPG secreted in the bone matrix serves as a decoy, sequestering OPG-ligand and preventing it from triggering bone resorption.

Since many proteins in the body stimulate osteoclast activity, investigators wanted to confirm the importance of OPG-ligand by creating mice lacking its gene. In the Jan. 28, 1999 *Nature*, Amgen scientists and Penninger's team reported that like the mice producing excess OPG, mice without OPG-ligand develop unusually thick bones. The latter mice have no osteoclasts at all.

"OPG-ligand is the essential molecule for osteoclast development," says Penninger. By controlling the balance between OPG and OPG-ligand, he speculates, "you can treat hundreds of diseases that have associated bone loss."

These molecules do seem to make up "a key and previously unrecognized system in the regulation of osteoclast genesis," agrees William J. Sharrock of the National Institute of Arthritis and Musculoskeletal and Skin Diseases in Bethesda, Md.

A variety of natural body chemicals and drugs leads to bone loss when administered to animals or people. Scientists are now finding that almost all of those substances slash production of OPG, boost creation of OPG-ligand, or do both.

Consider the glucocorticoids, a class of steroids that includes prednisone. Prescribed for a variety of medical reasons, these drugs sometimes set off quick and dramatic bone loss. Treating laboratory-grown osteoblasts with such steroids inhibits their synthesis of OPG and heightens their OPG-ligand production, Dunstan and other researchers from Amgen and the Mayo Clinic in Rochester, Minn., reported in the October 1999 *Endocrinology*.

In the September 1999 *Endocrinology*, some of the same scientists showed that applying estrogen to human osteoblasts stimulates activity of the gene for OPG. This may explain why an aging female's diminishing estrogen production leads to bone loss and may account for the bone-protecting effects of hormone-replacement therapy. "Now, we have the molecular explanation for postmenopausal osteoporosis," says Penninger.

The interplay of OPG and OPG-ligand may resolve another medical mystery. Rheumatoid arthritis, diabetes, multiple sclerosis, lupus, hepatitis, lymphomas, AIDS, and many seemingly unrelated diseases can produce osteoporosis along with their other symptoms. "Kids with leukemia are growth retarded because of bone loss," adds Penninger.

The only thing the diseases seem to have in common is that they involve a class of immune cells called activated T cells. How do T cells, which normally fight infections, interact with bone?

The first glimpse of an explanation came in 1997 from the Seattle biotech firm Immunex. Scientists there described a protein made by activated T cells. That protein turned out to be OPG-ligand. The unanticipated connection between OPG-ligand and T cells grew stronger in 1998 when Penninger found that his mice lacking the gene for OPG-ligand had no lymph nodes, one of the tissues where T cells mature.

Scientists have since found that almost anything that stirs quiescent T cells into action also triggers their synthesis of OPG-ligand.

Although no one can explain why the immune cells react this way, this link suggests that chronic infections, autoimmune disorders, and T cell cancers can all make osteoclasts go wild.

"Every time you turn on T cells, they make OPG-ligand, and this leads to bone loss," says Penninger. "This explains hundreds of clinical studies."

To buttress that argument, he and his colleagues recently tested whether OPG could slow the progression of an artificially induced rodent condition similar to rheumatoid arthritis. In patients with this autoimmune disorder, joint inflammation is followed by the destruction of surrounding bone and cartilage. Rheumatoid arthritis afflicts more than a million people in the United States, crippling many of them.

When signs of inflammation appeared in mice treated to develop arthritis, the investigators started giving the animals daily injections of OPG. The inflammation persisted, but the shots prevented bone and cartilage destruction, Penninger and his colleagues report in the Nov. 18, 1999 *Nature*.

They were pleasantly surprised that OPG blocked cartilage as well as bone damage, particularly since scientists aren't sure how rheumatoid arthritis destroys the cartilage in people.

"The simplest explanation is the cartilage breakdown has been a matter of the underlying bone deteriorating," notes Sharrock. An alternative explanation is that OPG-ligand may stimulate osteoclasts to degrade cartilage as well as bone, says Sharrock, or it may incite other cells to destroy the cartilage.

Moving biological advances from the laboratory bench to the doctor's office can take years and frequently fails, but Amgen has already begun the long trek with OPG. The company's first step was to modify the protein so that it circulates in the blood much longer than the natural version does.

Last September, at the American Society for Bone and Mineral Research meeting in St. Louis, Dunstan and his colleagues announced results of initial safety tests. Forty women who had just gone through menopause received a single shot, in varying doses, of the modified OPG. Physicians documented no side effects other than some minor irritation at the injection site.

While the researchers didn't design this initial trial to test the drug's efficacy, they did monitor daily the rate of bone resorption in the women by measuring a bone-breakdown product in their urine. At the highest dose, the single shot of modified OPG reduced a woman's normal bone resorption rate by as much as 85 percent. The drug's effect lasted for up to a month, says Dunstan.

Amgen now plans larger trials of the drug with postmenopausal women, as well as with people suffering localized bone destruction due to metastatic bone cancer. As for rheumatoid arthritis, specialists on the topic warn that the rat condition studied by Penninger and his colleagues doesn't perfectly model the human disease.

"It has a lot of shortcomings," cautions Gary S. Firestein of the University of California, San Diego. He adds that other T cell-based strategies have failed to help people with rheumatoid arthritis. Still, he believes that testing OPG on people with the autoimmune disorder is warranted. Indeed, Amgen may begin such a trial this year.

Penninger admits that he can barely contain his enthusiasm about using OPG to stop bone loss in osteoporosis and T cell disorders. He compares its potential significance to the realization that giving insulin to diabetics prevents the most serious consequences of the disease.

"I think it's the insulin for the bone," says Penninger. "I've never been as confident in my whole scientific life."

Stopping bone loss is one thing. Tricking the body into growing new bone is quite another. Physicians desperately need such a technique because they often don't diagnose osteoporosis until bones have already become irrevocably weakened.

"The Holy Grail of osteoporosis research is a drug that will restore or rebuild bone that is lost," notes Gregory Mundy, a researcher at the University of Texas Health Science Center and founder of the biotech firm OsteoScreen, both in San Antonio.

"We need something for the little old lady who has already lost 40 percent [of her bone mass]," agrees C. Conrad Johnston Jr. of Indiana University School of Medicine in Indianapolis, who is president of the National Osteoporosis Foundation.

The widely used statins may provide the answer to Johnston's request. In the Dec. 3, 1999 *Science*, Mundy and his colleagues report that statins stimulate bone formation in test-tube studies and in experiments with rodents. Since physicians have prescribed statins for more than a decade and the drugs have a well-documented safety record, the unexpected results tantalize bone researchers.

The initial hint that statins have bone-building properties came when the scientists began looking for small molecules that trigger the maturation of osteoblasts. The researchers used automated machines to screen more than 30,000 natural compounds for their ability to activate a gene encoding a molecule—bone morphogenetic protein-2, or BMP-2—that promotes local bone formation.

Mundy's team found just one molecule, lovastatin, that turned on the gene for BMP-2. Startled by this unanticipated result, the researchers quickly tested whether other statins, not among the compounds they originally screened, would also stimulate BMP-2 production. All but one did so.

The investigators next examined whether statins can influence bone creation. By adding the drugs to laboratory dishes in which pieces of mouse skulls were growing, they showed that statins could double or triple the amount of new bone formation. The statins seem to stimulate activity, proliferation, and maturation of osteoblasts.

Mundy and his colleagues then began testing statins on animals, initially injecting the drugs three times a day into tissue above the upper part of the skull of mice just a few weeks old. Five days of such injections produced 50 percent more bone than normal.

Since part of the appeal of the statins is that people can take them as pills rather than as injections, the scientists also administered oral doses of the drugs to female rats. In rodents that have had their ovaries removed, osteoporosis normally occurs quickly. When the researchers examined such rats after they had taken statins for a month, those on the highest doses had double the bone-formation rate of untreated rats, Mundy and his colleagues report.

Hans Oxlund of the University of Aarhus in Denmark and his colleagues have confirmed the bone-building properties of statins in rodents. Compared with adult female rats receiving a saline solution, those getting statin had twice as much bone formation over three months, Oxlund reported at the St. Louis meeting of the American Society for Bone and Mineral Research. This extra bone has normal properties, Oxlund told *Science News*.

Statins slash cholesterol production in the body by inhibiting an enzyme that creates a cholesterol precursor. Laboratory results suggest that the drugs also increase bone production by inhibiting that same enzyme. Pharmaceutical firms may ultimately need to develop statin-related drugs that increase bone formation while allowing the body to continue making the cholesterol that all animal cells need, Mundy notes.

Yet companies probably won't go to such lengths until they're certain that statins build bone in people. Since human and rodent bone metabolisms differ significantly, the jury is still out on that question.

In an attempt to address the issue, Mundy, along with Steven R. Cummings of the University of California, San Francisco, recently analyzed bone density and hip-fracture data from about 600 women over the age of 55 who had participated in trials of statins' effects on cholesterol. They were compared with similarly aged women taking other cholesterol-lowering agents.

The results were not conclusive, says Mundy, who calls upon the makers of statins to launch clinical trials specifically designed to test the bone-forming abilities of their drugs.

Even such trials may not resolve the issue. Drug developers selected the current statins for their ability to move quickly from the bloodstream to the liver, the primary site of cholesterol synthesis, rather than to the skeleton. Statins that target bone may be needed, but such drugs could lose the benefit of the current statins' enviable record. "You might have to start all over again on safety and toxicity," says Sharrock.

While physicians don't yet have mastery over the skeleton's cellular construction and demolition crews, bone researchers are finally providing them with the commands they need to instruct their skilled workers.

*—John Travis*

# Chapter 6

# *Peak Bone Mass in Women*

Bone mass in adults is based on the maximum amount achieved during skeletal growth, known as peak bone mass, and the subsequent degree of bone loss. Until recently, much of the effort in osteoporosis prevention has been devoted to minimizing bone loss following the attainment of peak levels. However, given the knowledge that increased peak bone density reduces osteoporosis risk later in life, increased attention is being paid to those factors that affect peak bone mass. Such a shift in emphasis has resulted in prevention efforts directed at children and adolescents.

## *Skeletal Growth and Maturation*

The majority of bone mass is achieved during the first two decades of life. Rapid skeletal growth occurs *in utero* and infancy, while children tend to experience steady but slow growth until puberty. During the adolescent growth spurt, young people achieve up to 60 percent of their total bone mass.

© July 1999. Reprinted with permission of the Osteoporosis and Related Bone Diseases—National Resource Center. The National Resource Center is supported by the National Institute of Arthritis and Musculoskeletal and Skin Diseases with contributions from the National Institute of Child Health and Human Development, National Institute of Dental and Craniofacial Research, National Institute of Environmental Health Sciences, NIH Office of Research on Women's Health, Office of Women's Health, PHS, and the National Institute on Aging. The Resource Center is operated by the National Osteoporosis Foundation, in collaboration with The Paget Foundation and the Osteogenesis Imperfecta Foundation. Web link: http://www.osteo.org/peak.html

By age 18, skeletal growth is nearly complete, with minor accumulations in bone density occurring until around the age of 30. In women, between the ages of 30 and menopause, there tends to be minimal change in total bone mass. But in the first few years after menopause, most women experience rapid bone loss that slows but persists throughout the postmenopausal years.

## Factors Affecting Peak Bone Mass

Peak bone mass is influenced by a variety of genetic and environmental factors. It has been suggested that genetic factors may account for up to 60-80 percent of bone mass, while environmental factors account for the remaining 20-40 percent.

*Gender.* Peak bone mass tends to be higher in men than in women. Before puberty, bone mass is acquired at similar rates among boys and girls. After puberty, however, males tend to acquire greater bone mass than their female counterparts.

*Race.* For reasons still being investigated, African-American females tend to achieve higher peak bone mass than Caucasian females. These differences in bone density are apparent even during youth.

*Hormonal factors.* Estrogen is an important determinant of peak bone mass. Early menarche and use of oral contraceptives, for example, have been positively correlated with high bone mineral density. Young women who become amenorrheic experience significant deficits in bone density, that may not be recovered even after menses returns.

*Nutritional status.* Calcium is an essential nutrient for bone health. It has been suggested that calcium deficiencies in the young can account for a 5-10 percent difference in peak bone mass and can significantly increase the risk for hip fracture in later life. Surveys indicate that adolescent females in the United States are less likely than their male counterparts to consume their recommended levels of calcium. In fact, less than 25 percent of adolescent females are actually getting the calcium they need each day. Calcium is shown to positively impact peak bone mass when given up to the threshold dose of 1000 milligrams per day.

*Physical Activity.* Studies suggest that physical activity is a strong determinant of peak bone mass. The benefits of activity are most pronounced in those areas of the skeleton under mechanical loads.

# Chapter 7

# *Calcium and Vitamin D: Important at Every Age*

The foods we eat contain a variety of vitamins, minerals, and other important nutrients that help keep our bodies healthy. Two nutrients in particular—calcium and vitamin D—are needed for strong bones. It is also needed for our heart, muscles, and nerves to function properly, and for blood to clot normally

## *Vitamin D*

Vitamin D is needed for the body to absorb calcium. Without enough vitamin D, we can't form enough of the hormone "calcitriol (known as the "active vitamin D") causing insufficient calcium adsorption from the diet. In this situation, the body must take its calcium from its stores in the skeleton, which weakens bone already there and prevents the formation of strong, new bone.

You can get vitamin D safely in two ways: through the skin and from the diet. Vitamin D is formed naturally in the body after exposure to sunlight. Fifteen minutes in the sun each day is plenty of time to manufacture and store all the Vitamin D you need. Experts recommend a daily intake of between 400 and 800 IU of vitamin D which also can be obtained through the diet, from supplements, or vitamin D fortified dairy products, egg yolks, saltwater fish, and liver. Do not take more than 800 IU per day unless prescribed by your doctor, since massive doses of vitamin D may be harmful.

## The Role of Calcium

Calcium is needed for our heart, muscles, and nerves to function properly, and for blood to clot. Inadequate calcium is thought to significantly contribute to the development of osteoporosis. Many published studies show that low calcium intakes throughout life are associated with low bone mass and high fracture rates. National nutrition surveys have shown that many women and young girls consume less than half the amount of calcium recommended to grow and maintain healthy bones. To find out how much calcium you need, see Table 7.1.

Remember, calcium is not a substitute for medication that may be needed to curb excessive bone loss.

## Calcium Culprits

High levels of protein and sodium in the diet are thought to increase calcium excretion through the kidneys. Excessive amounts of

**Table 7.1.** Recommended Calcium Intakes*

| Ages | Amount mg/day |
|------|---------------|
| Birth-6 months | 210 |
| 6 months-1 year | 270 |
| 1-3 | 500 |
| 4-8 | 800 |
| 9-13 | 1300 |
| 14-18 | 1300 |
| 19-30 | 1000 |
| 31-50 | 1000 |
| 51-70 | 1200 |
| 70 or older | 1200 |
| | |
| Pregnant or Lactating | 1000 |
| 14-18 | 1300 |
| 19-50 | 1000 |

*Source: National Academy of Sciences (NAS), Recommended Calcium Intake, 1997.*

these substances should be avoided especially in those who have low calcium intakes.

Lactose intolerance can lead to inadequate calcium intake. Those who are lactose intolerant have insufficient amounts of the enzyme lactase that is needed to break down the lactose found in dairy products. In order to include dairy products in the diet, dairy foods can be taken in very small quantities, treated with lactase drops, or lactase can be taken as pills. There are even some milk products on the market that have already been treated with lactase.

## Calcium Supplements

If you have trouble getting enough calcium in your diet, you may need to take a calcium supplement. The amount of calcium you will need from a supplement depends on how much calcium you obtain from food sources. There are several different calcium compounds from which to choose, such as calcium carbonate and calcium citrate among others.

**Table 7.2.** Good Sources of Calcium. The items listed below are examples of foods containing calcium. This is not a complete list.

- Most foods in the milk group: milk and dishes made with milk, such as puddings and soups made with milk; cheeses such as Mozzarella, Cheddar, Swiss, and Parmesan; and yogurt (Some foods in this group are high in fat, cholesterol, or both. Choose lower fat, lower cholesterol foods most often. Read the labels.)

- Canned fish with soft bones such as sardines, anchovies, and salmon

- Dark-green leafy vegetables, such as kale, mustard greens, and turnip greens, and pak-choi

- Tofu, if processed with calcium sulfate. Read the labels.

- Tortillas made from lime-processed com. Read the labels.

*Source: From* Nutrition and Your Health: Dietary Guidelines for Americans, Fourth Edition, *U.S. Department of Agriculture (USDA) and U.S. Department of Health and Human Services (DHHS), 1995.*

It is necessary for the calcium tablet to disintegrate in order to be absorbed by the body. If you are unsure whether a tablet will break down, you can test how well it disintegrates by placing it in 6 ounces of vinegar or warm water, stirring occasionally for 30 minutes. If the tablet has not almost completely disintegrated at this time, it probably will not do so in your stomach.

All calcium supplements are better absorbed when taken in small doses several times throughout the day. In many individuals, calcium supplements are better absorbed when taken with food.

## A Complete Osteoporosis Program

Remember, a calcium-rich diet is only one part of an osteoporosis prevention or treatment program. Like exercise, getting enough calcium is a strategy that helps strengthen bones at any age. But these approaches may not be enough to stop bone loss caused by lifestyle, medical conditions, or menopause. It is important to speak to your doctor about the need for medication in addition to diet and exercise.

# Chapter 8

# *Osteoporosis and Arthritis: Two Common but Different Conditions*

"Osteoarthritis is a disease of the joints, while osteoporosis is a disease of fragile bones. At least $50 billion a year are spent on medical costs and lost wages due to these two conditions." That's what Dr. Joan McGowan, Chief of the Musculoskeletal Diseases Branch and Director of the Bone Diseases Program at NIAMS, told the standing-room-only crowd attending the Arthritis and Osteoporosis Seminar that was held at the NIH on March 6, 1997. The seminar, sponsored by the Office of Research on Women's Health (ORWH), is one of several held each year. "These seminars are designed to inform the community about common health issues that affect many women in their middle and later years," said Dr. Vivian Pinn, Director of ORWH. The March 6 seminar was coordinated by Dr. McGowan and Dr. Nancy Cummings, Associate Director for Research and Assessment at NIDDK, members of the ORWH's Women's Health Seminar Committee.

"There are many institutes at the NIH that are interested in arthritis and osteoporosis. It is through these collaborative efforts that we get the research done. As caretakers and scientists these diseases affect us all," said Dr. Stephen I. Katz, Director of NIAMS.

Dr. Rosemarie Hirsch, an NIAMS rheumatologist currently assigned to the Epidemiology, Demography, and Biometry Program at the National Institute on Aging, said that more than 37 million Americans have some form of arthritis. "By the year 2020, 60 million

---

"Arthritis and Osteoporosis: Women's Health Seminar," National Institute of Arthritis and Musculoskeletal and Skin Diseases, March 2, 1997.

Americans are projected to have arthritis." She said that arthritis literally means joint inflammation but is often used to refer to more than 100 different rheumatic diseases that can affect children and adults. Her discussion focused on three diseases that affect women more than men: osteoarthritis, rheumatoid arthritis, and lupus.

"Osteoarthritis is the most common form of arthritis," said Hirsch. The disease ranges from mild to severe and may cause pain, stiffness and tenderness around the joint. It most often affects the hands, feet, knees, and hips. Contributory factors include age, injury, obesity, and genetics. Hirsch said that therapies for osteoarthritis include weight reduction, exercise, and rehabilitation; simple pain-killing medications, such as acetaminophen or topical capsaicin cream; short courses of nonsteroidal anti-inflammatory drugs (NSAIDs), such as ibuprofen, for more severe symptoms; corticosteroid injections into affected joints for temporary pain relief; and surgery, such as surgical replacement of the joints, as a treatment option in severe cases.

Hirsch said that rheumatoid arthritis is less common than osteoarthritis, but not rare. In the joint with rheumatoid arthritis, the synovium (joint lining) becomes inflamed, leading to destruction of joint tissue (synovium and cartilage), which can result in chronic pain and deformity. The disease may cause pain and stiffness, weight loss, decreased appetite, and tender swollen joints, especially in the hand, wrist, shoulder, hip, knees, and feet. Possible causes of rheumatoid arthritis may include a genetic susceptibility combined with environmental factors, such as bacteria or viruses. Treatment of RA may include NSAIDs to relieve pain and reduce inflammation; disease-modifying drugs, such as oral or injected gold salts, sulfasalazine, and methotrexate; and low-dose corticosteroids. Other therapies may include splinting of the hands to prevent further joint problems and decrease pain. Joint replacement may also be used in severe cases to decrease pain and increase function.

"Lupus is less common than either osteoarthritis or rheumatoid arthritis. It tends to occur in women in their reproductive years, but can affect older individuals. Its frequency is higher in Blacks and Hispanics," said Hirsch. In lupus, the immune system attacks the body's healthy cells and tissues. The disease may range from mild to severe and is characterized by periods of flares and remissions. Lupus may cause weight loss, fever, fatigue, aching, and weakness and may involve different organ systems such as the central nervous system, the heart, lungs, kidneys, muscles, and joints. Treatment for the disease, depending on its severity and on the organ systems involved, can include NSAIDs, corticosteroids (which may cause osteoporosis), and immunosuppressants such as cyclophosphamide.

Hirsch discussed some recent discoveries. In osteoarthritis, defective collagen genes have been identified in some families. In rheumatoid arthritis, a group of genes with the same amino acid sequence have been identified as susceptibility markers. In lupus, a gene on chromosome 1 has been linked with susceptibility to lupus in Caucasians, Asians, and African Americans. In the area of cartilage research, Hirsch said that medications that counteract cartilage-destroying enzymes have been identified and that improved implants for replacing areas of worn cartilage and better artificial joints for longer lasting joint replacements are being investigated. Finally Hirsch discussed the area of biologics (messenger molecules that allow communication in or between cells). She said that one example of the use of biologics is their use as drugs to enhance or interfere with immune system activity in arthritis inflammation.

Dr. Ethel S. Siris, Madeline C. Stabile Professor of Clinical Medicine at Columbia University College of Physicians and Surgeons in New York City, and Director of the Toni Stabile Center for the Prevention and Treatment of Osteoporosis at the Columbia-Presbyterian Medical Center in the same city, discussed diagnosis and treatment options for osteoporosis. She said that low bone mass is the single most predictable factor for osteoporosis, a disease that affects more than 25 million Americans. Other factors include postmenopausal status, early menopause (before age 45), being white or Asian, being thin, having a small build, having a family history of osteoporosis, and taking certain drugs such as corticosteroids and thyroid medications over a long period. She added that bone is a living, dynamic tissue. Peak bone mass is achieved at 20-30 years and then declines with age. At menopause, with diminished levels of estrogens, there is rapid bone loss.

Siris said that osteoporosis causes 1.3 million fractures of the wrist, vertebrae, and hips a year. "About half the people who break their hips end up in nursing homes, and in the year following the fracture, 20 percent will die. The lifetime risk of death due to hip fracture is comparable to the risk of death from breast cancer," she said. Siris then discussed vertebral fracture, which can lead to deformity of the spine, chronic back pain, and a loss of height. She said that osteoporosis is a silent disease, and she recommends that people at risk for the disease have a non-invasive test called dual x-ray absorptiometry that will scan the spine, hip, and arm, in order to measure bone density.

Prevention and treatment of osteoporosis may include calcium (1,000 milligrams per day at 25-50 years of age, 1,500 milligrams per day after age 50) and vitamin D. For the menopausal woman, Siris said that therapies may include estrogen, calcitonin, bisphosphonates, and fluoride. "Every woman at menopause should consider taking estrogen since it is highly effective against osteoporosis and heart disease, and may protect the brain from Alzheimer's disease. Women who take estrogen can reduce their fracture risk by 50 percent." She added that osteoporosis is not an inevitable part of aging. It is a highly diagnosable and treatable disease.

Dr. Kate Lorig, Associate Professor (research) at Stanford University School of Medicine Division of Rheumatology and Immunology, and Director of the Stanford Patient Education Research Center in Palo Alto, California, discussed self-management and how to break the pain cycle. Lorig said when you have a chronic disease you need to learn how to manage it. Three things are important: (1) take medicine, exercise, go to the doctor, (2) learn how to get on with your life, and (3) learn how to deal with your emotions. Lorig said that with a chronic disease, your future is altered. "In arthritis, the biggest problem is pain. If you make a small change in the amount of pain, you may be able to lessen the disability." She said that not all pain comes from the disease. Other things such as tense and deconditioned muscles, depression, fatigue, and stress all may contribute. Lorig discussed several ways to break the pain cycle and get relief. These include exercise, distraction, and self-talk. She said that exercise is very important for people with arthritis, and recommended that it be done in gradually increasing amounts 4-5 times a week. Another technique is to substitute distraction for pain. Keep your mind occupied, think of something else. Finally she mentioned self-talk as a way to deal with depression. Lorig said that we constantly talk to ourselves and our emotions are ruled by what we say. "You should pay attention to the messages that you give yourself, and make an effort to change your mental messages, "she said. "Management of your pain is up to you."

*—by Barbara Weldon*

# Part Three

# Facts and Figures for Osteoporosis

# Chapter 9

# *The Importance and Impact of Osteoporosis*

Osteoporosis is a brittle bone disorder that affects over 20 million American women.[1,2] Osteoporosis deforms the skeletal structure. In its severest form, spontaneous fractures occur in the bones of the back, and at the wrist, elbow, shoulder, hip, knee and ankle. It is painful and disabling.

Osteoporosis in women is more common than heart attack or breast cancer. Osteoporosis in women of all ages occurs nearly double the incidence of heart attack in women 29 and older,[1,3] and occurs more than five times the incidence of new cases of breast cancer in women of all ages.[4] The World Health Organization recently placed osteoporosis on the priority list of the non-transmissible diseases for which preventive programs have to be implemented throughout the world.

Osteoporosis occurs primarily in women as they move into their elder years, but it can occur in younger females and men as well. Typically, the disease is caused by hormonal changes associated with aging. The prevention of age related osteoporosis begins in youth with lifelong habits of exercise, proper nutrition and abstinence from tobacco. The most severely affected group of patients, those who are genetically predestined to osteoporosis, can be taught early intervention measures to help resist the consequences of the disease.

---

© 1998 The Osteoporosis Initiative, Miles Memorial Hospital, Edward R. White. M.D. Reprinted by permission of the author. Available at http://lincoln.midcoast.com/~ewhite/OSTEOIMPACT.html.

## The Gap between Research Knowledge and Public Knowledge

Partly because osteoporosis has only recently attracted research attention and resources, awareness and treatment are at an early stage. According to a 1991 survey of 750 American women, 80 percent did not associate osteoporosis with disabling hip fractures, and 90 percent did not know death was a potential outcome. In addition, 60 percent of these women could not identify potential osteoporosis risk factors, such as family history. Most women at risk for osteoporosis have not discussed it with their physician.[5] A white woman over the age of 50 has a 40 percent risk of osteoporotic fracture of her wrist, spine or hip during her lifetime.

## The Economic Cost of Osteoporosis

Osteoporosis costs the nation over $10 billion annually—more than congestive heart failure or asthma. If the population continues to increase at its current rate, the costs of hip fractures alone are estimated to reach $62 billion by the year 2020 (based on 5 percent annual inflation).[6] It is estimated that the next ten years will bring 5.2 million osteoporosis related fractures to white women over the age of 44, costing at least 45 billion dollars.[7]

*—by Edward R. White, M.D.*
RR2 Box 4500
Damariscotta, ME 04543
Phone: (207) 563-1040
FAX: (207) 563-1039
E-Mail: ewhite@lincoln.midcoast.com

## Notes

1. Consensus Development Conference: Diagnosis, prophylaxis, and treatment of osteoporosis, *Am. J. Med.* 94:646-650, June 1993.

2. *Osteoporosis Research, Education and Health Promotion*, National Institute of Arthritis and Musculoskeletal and Skin Diseases, NIH Publication No. 91-3216, September 1991.

3. Heart and Stroke Facts: 1995 Statistical Supplement, American Heart Association.

4.  Cancer Facts & Figures—1995, American Cancer Society, Revised 1/95.

5.  Gallup survey finds women underestimate severity, consequences of osteoporosis, *Menopause Management* 1(3):27, November/December 1992.

6.  Cummings, S.R., Rubin, S.M., and Black, D.: The future of hip fractures in the United States: Numbers, Costs, and potential effects of post menopausal estrogen, *Clin. Orthrop.* 252:163-166, March 1990.

7.  Chrischilles E., Shireman, T., Wallace, R.: Costs and health effects of osteoporotic fractures. *Bone* 15:377-386, 1994.

# Chapter 10

# *Fast Facts on Osteoporosis*

## *Definition*

Osteoporosis, or porous bone, is a disease characterized by low bone mass and deterioration of bone tissue, leading to bone fragility and an increased susceptibility to fractures of the hip, spine, and wrist.

## *Prevalence*

- Osteoporosis is a major public health threat for more than 28 million Americans, 80 percent of whom are women. In the U.S. today 10 million individuals already have disease and 18 million more have low bone mass, placing them at increased risk for osteoporosis.

- 80 percent of those affected by osteoporosis are women.

- 8 million American women and two million men have osteoporosis, and millions more have low bone density.

- One in two women and one in eight men over age 50 will have an osteoporosis-related fracture in their lifetime.

- 10 percent of African-American women over age 50 have osteoporosis; an additional 30 percent have low bone density that puts them at risk of developing osteoporosis.

- Significant risk has been reported in people of all ethnic backgrounds.

- While osteoporosis is often thought of as an older person's disease, it can strike at any age.

- Osteoporosis is responsible for more than 1.5 million fractures annually, including:

  - 300,000 hip fractures; and approximately
  - 700,000 vertebral fractures,
  - 250,000 wrist fractures, and
  - 300,000 fractures at other sites.

## Cost

The estimated national direct expenditures (hospitals and nursing homes) for osteoporotic and associated fractures was $13.8 billion in 1995 ($38 million each day) and the cost is rising.

## Symptoms

Osteoporosis is often called the "silent disease" because bone loss occurs without symptoms. People may not know that they have osteoporosis until their bones become so weak that a sudden strain, bump, or fall causes a fracture or a vertebra to collapse.

Collapsed vertebrae may initially be felt or seen in the form of severe back pain, loss of height, or spinal deformities such as kyphosis or stooped posture.

## Risk Factors

Certain people are more likely to develop osteoporosis than others. Factors that increase the likelihood of developing osteoporosis are called "risk factors." The following risk factors have been identified:

- Being female
- Thin and/or small frame
- Advanced age
- A family history of osteoporosis
- Postmenopause, including early or surgically induced menopause

- Abnormal absence of menstrual periods (amenorrhea)
- Anorexia nervosa or bulimia
- A diet low in calcium
- Use of certain medications, such as corticosteroids and anticonvulsants
- Low testosterone levels in men
- An inactive lifestyle
- Cigarette smoking
- Excessive use of alcohol
- Being Caucasian or Asian, although African Americans and Hispanic Americans are at significant risk as well

Women can lose up to 20 percent of their bone mass in the 5-7 years following menopause, making them more susceptible to osteoporosis.

## Detection

Specialized tests called bone density tests can measure bone density in various sites of the body. A bone density test can:

- Detect osteoporosis before a fracture occurs
- Predict your chances of fracturing in the future
- Determine your rate of bone loss and/or monitor the effects of treatment if the test is conducted at intervals of a year or more

### Prevention

By about age 20, the average woman has acquired 98 percent of her skeletal mass. Building strong bones during childhood and adolescence can be the best defense against developing osteoporosis later. A comprehensive program that can help prevent osteoporosis includes:

- A balanced diet rich in calcium and vitamin D
- Weight-bearing exercise
- A healthy lifestyle with no smoking or excessive alcohol use, and
- Bone density testing and medication and when appropriate

## Fractures

The most typical sites of fractures related to osteoporosis are the hip, spine, wrist, and ribs, although the disease can affect any bone in the body.

The rate of hip fractures is two to three times higher in women than men; however the one year mortality following a hip fracture is nearly twice as high for men as for women.

A woman's risk of hip fracture is equal to her combined risk of breast, uterine and ovarian cancer.

In 1991, about 300,000 Americans age 45 and over were admitted to hospitals with hip fractures. Osteoporosis was the underlying cause of most of these injuries.

An average of 24 percent of hip fracture patients age 50 and over die in the year following their fracture.

One-fourth of those who were ambulatory before their hip fracture require long-term care afterward.

White women 65 or older have twice the incidence of fractures as African-American women.

## Medications

Although there is no cure for osteoporosis, the following medications are approved by the FDA for postmenopausal women to either prevent and/or treat osteoporosis:

- Estrogens (brand names such as Premarin®, Estrace®, Ogen®, Prempro®, Estraderm® and Estratab® and others)

- Calcitonin (brand name Miacalcin®)

- Alendronate (brand name Fosamax®)

- Raloxifene (brand name Evista®)

- Risedronate (brand name Actonel®)

- Alendronate and risedronate are approved for use in glucocorticoid-induced osteoporosis in both men and women.

- Treatments under investigation include sodium fluoride; vitamin D metabolites; parathyroid hormone; other bisphosphonates and SERMs.

Medical experts agree that osteoporosis is highly preventable. However, if the toll of osteoporosis is to be reduced, the commitment to osteoporosis research must be significantly increased. It is reasonable to project that with increased research, the future for definitive treatment and prevention of osteoporosis is very bright.

## *About the National Osteoporosis Foundation*

The National Osteoporosis Foundation is the nation's leading resource for patients, healthcare professionals, and organizations seeking up-to-date, medically sound information on the causes, prevention, diagnosis, and treatment of osteoporosis. Please contact us to learn more about NOF, National Osteoporosis Prevention Month, or how to become a member.

National Osteoporosis Foundation
1232 22nd Street N.W.
Washington, DC 20037-1292
(202) 223-2226

# Chapter 11

# *Old Bones in Young Bodies*

Low caloric intake and excessive exercise can often lead to osteoporosis—even in young women.

The bones of some young women, particularly athletes, are sometimes equivalent to the bones of 50- to 60-year-old women—and occasionally 70- or 80-year-old women. In one study, a roentgenogram (an X-ray of internal body structures) showed a young woman with a hip fracture, pelvic fracture and multiple stress fractures in her spine. Another study reported that poor bone formation in young women is "not just in the spine, but every place. These women have significantly lower bone densities throughout their entire bodies." The study, conducted by Barbara L. Drinkwater, Ph.D., a pioneer in osteoporosis research, cited the case of a woman who at 19 had a normal spine, but by age 23 had three vertebral fractures. "She will never have normal posture," she says. "We're not looking at a little old lady of 85. We're looking at a youngster."

Osteoporosis in young women sounds like a contradiction. After all, it is typically a disease found in older, post-menopausal women. Unfortunately, when young women, particularly athletes, maintain a low caloric intake and exercise to excess to keep their weight osteoporosis often results. This is particularly troubling because these are the years when young bodies should be building bone for the future, not losing it.

---

Reprinted with permission from the Aerobics and Fitness Association of America. *American Fitness Magazine*, September 1999. © 1999 AFAA.

# What Is Osteoporosis?

Osteoporosis is a metabolic bone disease in which bones lose density and the spaces within them become enlarged, resulting in increased fragility and chance of breakage. It is a disease which is easier to prevent than treat.

## The Causes of Osteoporosis in Young Women

Osteoporosis in young women usually results from disordered eating, low body weight and amenorrhea—the cessation of menstruation. For athletes, excessive exercise bordering on addiction is a major contributor. In addition, low calcium levels caused by constant dieting and calcium loss through sweating during exercise contribute to osteoporosis in young female athletes.

According to Dr. Mark Timmerman, assistant clinical professor in sports medicine at the University of Wisconsin and doctor of sports and family medicine at the Dean Clinic in Madison, Wisconsin, another problem in young female athletes is that 30 percent to 40 percent of them are anemic. Dr. Timmerman says young women concerned about their weight and athletic performance tend to eat low fat, higher fiber diets deficient in iron. The consequent anemia contributes to amenorrhea.

The focus on achieving or maintaining a specific body weight and shape contributes to osteoporosis. According to Dr. Kimberly K. Yeager, assistant director for Public Health Practice, San Diego State University, "There tends to be an increased incidence of osteoporosis among young women participating in appearance-based and endurance sports." This includes gymnastics, figure skating, ballet and running, where thin, girlish bodies are considered desirable. Women participating in these activities are believed to have higher levels of amenorrhea and osteoporosis than women in sports where weight and body type are not a major issue. Yeager found that "15.4 percent of college female swimmers were affected by eating disorders and amenorrhea, while the figure may be as high as 62 percent among gymnasts."

Dr. Ronald Young, director of the Division of Gynecology at Baylor College in Houston, Texas, says the need for calcium in both boys and girls increases dramatically around the time of puberty. For boys, this coincides with a period of life when food intake—particularly of calcium-rich foods—skyrockets. Girls, however, need calcium when they are beginning to worry about their figures, often trying to imitate the unrealistic bodies of fashion models and Barbie® dolls. Both caloric and calcium intake decline significantly when they should be trying to build bone.

Dr. Young says that between puberty and approximately age 30, young women should be acquiring bone mass. By 30, most women reach their maximum bone density, then level off and begin losing bone by age 35. This process accelerates considerably when estrogen levels decline after menopause. Dr. Young stresses anything that hinders bone development during puberty will hurt later in life. He has seen too many young women with bones "like their grandmothers." Bone damage is cumulative and irreversible.

## Exercise Addictions

In addition to disordered eating, young female athletes may be addicted to exercise. An exercise addiction damages a woman's body because there is no chance for the body to rest and repair itself. It also contributes to low body weight, amenorrhea and osteoporosis. Some of the hallmarks of exercise addiction are feeling angry or depressed when exercise is not possible, missing important events or not spending time with family or friends in favor of exercising, extreme fatigue and exercising even when sick.

## Detection

Because it is a silent disease, there are no reliable statistics on how many young women have osteoporosis. Screening for osteoporosis is not routine in young women and is often not detected until fractures occur, sometimes accompanied by severe pain. According to doctors, however, there are several red flags which should not be ignored. The most important red flag is amenorrhea or other menstrual irregularities. "The cessation of menstruation should be like a smoke alarm going off," says Dr. Carol Otis in the *Journal of the American Medical Association*. "It is a symptom of things going wrong." Abnormal menstruation is a marker of ovarian dysfunction and low estrogen levels.

Young women who do not menstruate regularly should be screened for eating disorders, abnormal amounts of exercise and osteoporosis. Screening for osteoporosis is becoming easier as less expensive tests have been developed.

A second red flag is low body weight and low levels of fat. Young woman with these symptoms are likely to have menstrual disorders.

## Implications

The implications of osteoporosis at a young age are serious. Bone density is extremely low because bone is being lost while its formation and density augmentation is not taking place as it should. The result is permanent bone loss. "Bone that is lost or never formed may not be completely regained," according to Dr. Drinkwater. "Very few athletes have above-average bone densities, which one would expect to find in young physically active women." Even after menses resumes, bone density does not increase at a normal rate. Four years after resuming menses, one group of young women had not reached normal bone mass.

Another implication is that bones may be thin enough to actually fracture—such as in older women. Stress fractures can be painful and contribute to misshapen skeletal structures and long-term disability. When young women with low bone density approach menopause, they are likely to have severe osteoporosis.

## Treatment

Treatment of osteoporosis in young women has to be dealt with on three levels:

1. Determine whether a woman has osteoporosis.

2. The underlying causes must be addressed—disordered eating (often bordering on anorexia and bulimia) and/or excessive exercise. For this type of treatment, professional experts on eating disorders and exercise addiction should be consulted.

3. Osteoporosis should be dealt with before permanent damage to the skeletal structure occurs.

Dr. Robert Haney, professor of medicine at Creighton University in Omaha, Nebraska, emphasizes that young women with low bone densities should take birth control pills to increase their estrogen levels. He also emphasizes that weight gain is essential to restoring normal menstrual function. Young women with osteoporosis also need to boost their calcium intake through calcium-rich foods and calcium supplements.

Young women believe their athletic performance will be improved by low body weight and constant training. In fact, the reverse is true. "Dieting can hurt performance," Dr. Yeager says. "Muscle mass, as well as fat, is lost during extreme dieting. Fatigue, anemia, electrolyte abnormalities and depression can also contribute to poor performance." In addition, stress fractures and skeletal abnormalities can end an athlete's career and contribute to long-term disability.

## Act Now

Annual physicals or pre-participation examinations are opportunities to screen for osteoporosis.

1. A physician should take a complete menstrual history.

2. A physician should screen for disordered eating by obtaining a history of the young woman's eating habits, particularly her caloric intake. She should be asked if she vomits or purges frequently and if, in spite of normal weight, she feels too fat. She should also be asked to keep an eating log for several days.

3. A young woman should be weighed to determine if her weight is appropriate.

4. Young women reporting depression or fatigue should be screened for eating disorders and exercise addiction.

5. Any young woman who has an eating disorder or menstrual irregularities should be tested for osteoporosis.

## Osteoporosis Test

1. A urine test developed by OSTEOMARK can determine whether a woman's body is losing bone density. The test, known as NTx assay, measures a type of protein which the body releases into the urine when bone is being lost. The greater the amount of protein in the urine, the higher the rate of bone loss. According to Dr. Charles H. Chestnut of the University of Washington Medical Center's Osteoporosis Research Center, the test is dynamic and indicates whether a woman is losing or gaining bone. This differs from bone density scans which are static, measuring bone mass at a single point in time. The dynamic test is significant because it is predictive. Women with high levels of the protein in their urine are losing bone mass at a greater-than-normal level and are heading toward

osteoporosis. Knowing this, preventive measures can be implemented.

2.  Bone density tests on wrists, ankles, etc., correlate with full body bone density tests 60 percent to 70 percent of the time and are significantly easier and less expensive to administer.

*—by Christine F. Ridout*

Christine F. Ridout is a freelance writer living outside of Boston, Massachusetts.

# Chapter 12

# *Osteoporosis and African-American Women*

## *What is osteoporosis?*

Osteoporosis is a metabolic bone disease characterized by low bone mass, which makes bones fragile and susceptible to fracture. Osteoporosis is commonly called the "silent disease" because there are no symptoms or pain until fracture occurs. Fractures can result in loss of height, pain, and deformity. While African-American women tend to have higher bone mineral density (BMD) than white women throughout life, they are still at significant risk of developing osteoporosis. Furthermore, as African-American women age, their risk of developing osteoporosis more closely resembles the risk among white women. So, as the number of older African-American women in the United States increases, there will be an increasing number of African-American women with osteoporosis.

## *What are the risk factors for osteoporosis?*

Risk factors for developing osteoporosis include: thinness or small frame; family history of osteoporosis; being postmenopausal or having had early menopause; abnormal absence of menstrual periods; prolonged use of certain medications, such as those used to treat diseases like systemic lupus erythematosus, asthma, thyroid deficiencies, and seizures; low calcium intake; physical inactivity; smoking; and excessive alcohol intake.

---

Recent scientific studies highlight the risk that African-American women face with regard to developing osteoporosis and fracture.

• Approximately 300,000 African-American women currently have osteoporosis.

• Between 80-95 percent of fractures in African-American women over 64 are due to osteoporosis.

• African-American women are more likely than white women to die following a hip fracture.

• As African-American women age, their risk for hip fracture doubles approximately every seven years.

• Diseases more prevalent in the African-American population, such as sickle-cell anemia and systemic lupus erythematosus, are linked to osteoporosis.

### How does nutrition affect African-Americans and their risk of osteoporosis?

Adequate intake of calcium plays a crucial role in building peak bone mass and preventing bone loss. Studies indicate that African-American women consume 50 percent less calcium than the Recommended Dietary Allowance. The recommendations made at the NIH Consensus Development Conference on Optimal Calcium Intake suggest the following intake levels:

• Women ages 11-24 = **1,200 - 1,500 mg/day (4-5 glasses of milk)**

• Women ages 25-49 (premenopausal) = **1000 mg/day ( 3 1/2 glasses of milk)**

• Women over 50 (postmenopausal, on estrogen) = **1000 mg/day (3 1/2 glasses of milk)**

• Women over 50 (postmenopausal, not on estrogen) = **1500 mg/ day (5 glasses of milk)**

Lactose intolerance can also hinder optimal calcium intake. As many as 75 percent of all African-Americans are lactose intolerant. However, a recent study found that many people who are lactose intolerant can actually digest as much as two cups of milk per day, if divided into small servings, without symptoms. Although milk and other dairy products such as cheese and yogurt are the best calcium sources, there are many non-dairy foods that also contain calcium. Turnip greens, mustard greens, and kale are good sources of calcium among green vegetables: however large quantities must be consumed to equal the amount of calcium supplied by dairy products. Sardines and salmon with edible bones and calcium-fortified orange juice are also good sources of calcium.

### How is osteoporosis diagnosed?

Osteoporosis is diagnosed by a bone mineral density (BMD) test, a safe and painless test used to detect low bone mass. Talk to your doctor about a BMD test if you have reached menopause and/or if you have some of the risk factors for osteoporosis listed earlier. With the results of a BMD test, you and your doctor can decide what prevention or treatment steps are right for you.

### How can osteoporosis be prevented?

The prevention of osteoporosis begins in childhood. The recommendations listed below should be followed throughout life to lower your risk of osteoporosis.

- Eat a balanced diet adequate in calcium and vitamin D.
- Exercise regularly, especially weight-bearing activities such as walking, jogging, dancing and weight-lifting.
- Avoid smoking and excessive alcohol intake.

### What treatments are available?

Although there is no cure for osteoporosis, there are treatments available to help stop further bone loss and lower a persons risk of fracture. Talk to your doctor about these medications:

- estrogen
- alendronate (bisphosphonates)
- calcitonin

### What are some special considerations for caring for elderly individuals with osteoporosis?

For people with osteoporosis preventing falls is essential to decrease the risk of fracture. Some basic preventive measures include:

getting regular exercise to increase balance and muscle strength; having regular physical exams, including vision and hearing tests; learning the proper way to use walkers and canes; reviewing with your doctor the medications you are taking; and, removing throw rugs from the house, installing grab bars, stair rails, and applying non-skid tape on the outer edges of stairs are tips that will help avoid potentially dangerous situations in the home. Make sure you consult a doctor before embarking on an exercise program or participating in other physical activities.

## *About the Osteoporosis and Related Bone Diseases– National Resource Center*

ORBD-NRC is supported by the National Institute of Arthritis and Musculoskeletal and Skin Diseases, National Institutes of Health

Osteoporosis and Related Bone Diseases–National Resource Center
1150 17th St., NW, Suite 500
Washington, DC 20036
202-223-0344 or 800-624-BONE
TTY (202) 466-4315
E-Mail: orbdnrc@nof.org

# Chapter 13

# *Asian-American Women and Osteoporosis*

Asian American women are at high risk for developing osteoporosis (porous bones), a disease that is preventable and treatable. Studies that have been conducted on this population group indicate that Asian Americans share many of the risk factors that apply to Caucasian women. As an Asian American woman, it is important that you understand what osteoporosis is and what steps you can take to prevent or treat it.

### *What is osteoporosis?*

Osteoporosis is a debilitating disease characterized by low bone mass and, thus, bones that are susceptible to fracture. If not prevented or if left untreated, osteoporosis can progress painlessly until a bone breaks, typically in the hip, spine, or wrist. A hip fracture can limit mobility and lead to a loss of independence, while a vertebral fracture can result in loss of height and stooped posture.

### *What are the risk factors for osteoporosis?*

There are several factors that increase your chances of developing osteoporosis, including a thin, small-boned frame; previous fracture or family history of osteoporotic fracture; estrogen deficiency resulting from early menopause (before age 45), either naturally or from surgical removal of the ovaries or as a result of prolonged amen-orrhea (abnormal absence of menstruation) in younger women; ad-vanced age; a diet low in calcium; Caucasian and Asian ancestry (African American and Hispanic women are at lower but significant risk); cigarette smoking; excessive use of alcohol; and prolonged use of certain medications.

- Recent studies indicate a number of facts that highlight the risk that Asian American women face with regard to developing os-teoporosis:

- White women and Asian women have osteoporosis more often than black women, due largely to differences in bone mass and density.

- The average calcium intake among Asian women has been ob-served to be about half that of Western population groups. Calcium is essential for building and maintaining a healthy skeleton.

- Asian women generally have lower hip fracture rates than Cau-casian women, although the prevalence of vertebral fractures among Asians seems to be as high as that in Caucasians. In re-cent decades, there has been a sharp increase in hip fracture in-cidence in some parts of the Far East; in fact, it is estimated that about half of the expected 6.3 million hip fractures world-wide in 2050 will occur in Asia.

- Slender women have less bone mass than heavy or obese women and are therefore at greater risk for osteoporotic bone fractures.

### How can osteoporosis be prevented?

Building strong bones, especially before the age of 35, can be the best defense against developing osteoporosis, and a healthy lifestyle can be critically important for keeping bones strong. To help prevent osteoporosis:

- Eat a balanced diet rich in calcium

- Exercise regularly, especially weight-bearing activities

- Don't smoke and limit alcohol intake

- Talk to your doctor if you have a family history of osteoporosis or no longer have the protective benefit of estrogen due to natural or surgically induced menopause. Your doctor may suggest that you have your bone density measured at menopause through a safe and painless test that can help predict your chance of fracturing in the future.

### *What treatments are available?*

Although there is no cure for osteoporosis, there are treatments available to help stop further bone loss and reduce the risk of fractures:

- Studies have shown that estrogen can prevent the loss of bone mass in postmenopausal women.

- Alendronate, a bisphosphonate recently approved by the Food and Drug Administration for treatment of postmenopausal osteoporosis, is an alternative to estrogen for bone protection.

- Calcitonin is another treatment used by women for osteoporosis. This drug has been shown to slow bone breakdown and also may reduce the pain associated with osteoporotic fractures.

- Treatments under investigation include other bisphosphonates, sodium fluoride, para-thyroid hormone, vitamin D metabolites, and selective estrogen receptor modulators.

## Additional Resources

Office of Minority Health Resource Center
P.O. Box 37337
Washington, D.C. 20013-7337
(800) 444-MHRC (6472); FAX 301-589-0884

### *Osteoporosis and Related Bone Diseases– National Resource Center*

ORBD–NRC is supported by the National Institute of Arthritis and Musculoskeletal and Skin Diseases, National Institutes of Health

Osteoporosis and Related Bone Diseases–National Resource Center
1150 17th St., NW, Suite 500
Washington, DC 20036
202-223-0344 or 800-624-BONE
TTY (202) 466-4315
E-Mail: orbdnrc@nof.org

# Chapter 14

# *Latina Women and Osteoporosis*

Osteoporosis is a major public health threat for 28 million Americans, 80 percent of whom are women. It is a disease that causes the skeleton to weaken and bones to break. It can result in loss of height, severe back pain, and deformity; it can impair a person's ability to walk; and it may cause prolonged or permanent disability or even death.

## *What causes osteoporosis?*

Bone is constantly changing—that is, old bone is removed and replaced by new bone. During childhood, more bone is produced than removed, so the skeleton grows in both size and strength. The amount of tissue or bone mass in the skeleton reaches its maximum amount by the mid-thirties. At this point, the amount of bone in the skeleton typically begins to decline slowly as removal of old bone exceeds formation of new bone.

## *What are the risk factors for developing osteoporosis?*

Risk factors for developing osteoporosis include: previous fracture or family history of osteoporotic fracture; estrogen deficiency resulting from early menopause (before age 45, either naturally or from surgical removal of the ovaries; normal menopause or menopause resulting from amenorrhea (abnormal absence of menstruation);

---

© 1996. Reprinted with permission of Osteoporosis and Related Bone Diseases-National Research Center. Available at http://www.osteo.org/hispan.htm.

advanced age; unhealthy lifestyle habits (e.g., smoking, excessive alcohol use, low calcium intake, inadequate physical exercise); and prolonged use of certain medications.

Latina women are at significant risk for developing osteoporosis. Studies have shown that Latina women, along with Caucasian women, consume less calcium than the Recommended Dietary Allowance in all age groups. And, it is estimated that the number of hip fractures worldwide will increase sharply over the next half century, especially in Asia and Latin America. Another area of concern stems from the rapid aging of the population, since the elderly are at greatest risk for developing fractures. The Latino population is growing at a faster rate than the non-Latino: Between 1980 and 1990, it increased by 53 percent, in comparison with only 6.7 percent for non-Hispanics. The Bureau of the Census estimates that the Latino population is expected to almost triple between 1995 and 2050.

According to the National Health and Nutrition Examination Survey (NHANES III) (1988-91), between 36-49 percent of Mexican American women age 50 and older (300-400,000 women) have experienced significant loss of bone density. Among the Mexican American women identified in the NHANES study, 13-16 percent (100,000) already have osteoporosis. Although there are no statistics on the incidence of fracture among Latina women, the likelihood of osteoporotic fracture increases with age and loss of bone density.

### How is osteoporosis diagnosed?

Osteoporosis can be effectively treated if it is detected before significant bone loss has occurred.

A medical workup to diagnose osteoporosis will include a complete medical history, x-rays, and urine and blood tests. The doctor may also order a Bone Mineral Density Test (BMD) or bone mass measurement. A special type of x-ray, the BMD test is accurate, quick, non-invasive, and painless and can detect low bone density, predict risk for future fractures, and diagnose osteoporosis. It is important to inform the doctor about risk factors for developing osteoporosis, loss of height or change in posture, a fracture, or sudden back pain.

### What treatments are available?

Although there is no cure for osteoporosis, the three treatments currently available to help stop further bone loss and reduce the risk of fractures include estrogen, alendronate, and calcitonin.

Talk to your doctor to find out more about these medications.

### *How can osteoporosis be prevented?*

It is important that all people, regardless of race or gender, take the following steps to preserve their bone health:

- Avoid smoking, reduce alcohol intake, and increase level of activity.

- Ensure a daily calcium intake of 1000 mg/day (which equals approximately 3 1/2 glass of milk) to age 65 and 1500 mg/day (approximately 5 glasses of milk) over age 65. Some food sources other than milk that are high in calcium include: corn or flour tortillas, cheese, yogurt, oranges, dark green vegetables, and ice cream.

- Ensure an adequate vitamin D intake. Normally, enough vitamin D is made from exposure to as little as 10 minutes of sunlight a day. If exposure to sunlight is inadequate, dietary vitamin D intake should be at least 400 IU but not more than 800 IU/day, the amount that is found in one cup of fortified milk and most multivitamins.

- Engage in a regular regimen of weight-bearing exercises where bones and muscles work against gravity. This includes walking, jogging, racquet sports, stair climbing, team sports, and lifting weights. A doctor should evaluate the exercise program of anyone already diagnosed with osteoporosis to determine if twisting motions and impact activities, such as those used in housework, basketball, or dancing, need to be curtailed.

- Discuss with your doctor the use of medications, such as steroids, that are known to cause bone loss.

### *Additional Resources:*

Spanish language brochure on osteoporosis available from the National Osteoporosis Foundation
Office of Minority Health Resource Center
P.O. Box 37337
Washington, D.C. 20013-7337
(800) 444-MHRC (6472)

Provides publications in Spanish about nutrition, exercise, alcohol; Spanish-speaking person available to receive calls.

National Institutes of Health
Osteoporosis and Related Bone Diseases–National Resource Center
1150 17th St., NW, Suite 500
Washington, DC 20036
202-223-0344 or 800-624-BONE
Fax (202) 223-2237
TTY (202) 466-4315
E-Mail: orbdnrc@nof.org

The National Resource Center is supported by the National Institute of Arthritis and Musculoskeletal and Skin Diseases, with contributions from the National Institute of Child Health and Human Development, National Institute of Dental and Craniofacial Research, National Institute of Environmental Health Sciences, NIH Office of Research on Women's Health, Office of Women's Health, PHS, and the National Institute on Aging.

# Chapter 15

# *Osteoporosis in Men*

### *How often does osteoporosis occur in men?*

Men are less likely than women to develop osteoporosis, the disease that causes porous bones and leads to fractures. This may be because, on the average, men have a heavier bone structure than women, do not live as long as women, and do not experience a rapid decline in sex hormone production similar to the menopause in women. Men suffer about one-fifth to one-fourth of the hip fractures and one-seventh of the fractures of bones of the back (vertebrae).

### *What are the risk factors and causes of osteoporosis in men?*

The following are the most-often identified risk factors for osteoporosis in men:

- Aging
- Too little calcium intake or absorption
- Possible heredity
- Too little testosterone, the male hormone produced in the testes (see below)

---

NIH Publication No. AR-167, Office of Scientific and Health Communications, National Institute of Arthritis and Musculoskelatal and Skin Diseases, Department of Health and Human Services, June 1994 (ed. 8/95).

The following are other risk factors for osteoporosis in men:

- Lack of physical movement and exercise, including that caused by injury or long-term illness.

- Inadequate amount of vitamin D.

- Diseases of the lung, liver, or certain glands (e.g., adrenal, thyroid, parathyroid or pituitary) or a cancer that destroys bone.

- Medications used to treat certain illnesses (e.g., steroids, chemotherapy used to treat cancer, anticoagulants [blood thinners]), medications to prevent convulsions (seizures), or high doses of thyroid medication.

- Cigarette smoking, which affects calcium absorption, or heavy alcohol intake, which affects calcium, vitamin D, and protein absorption. Both lower the level of testosterone.

Testosterone is as important to the health of the male skeleton as estrogen is to the health of the female skeleton. It is believed to stimulate bone-forming cells and prevent the activity of bone-resorbing cells, which break down bone, through the action of a hormone produced by the thyroid gland called calcitonin. Therefore, an inadequate amount of testosterone, leading to increased bone breakdown and decreased bone formation, is one cause of osteoporosis in men. Determining the function of the gonads (sex glands) is one of the first steps doctors take to evaluate a man for osteoporosis. A low level of testosterone has been found in 20−30 percent of men with crush fractures in the spine due to bone loss. Twenty to thirty years of a low level of testosterone is typical of men with spinal osteoporosis.

Secondary risk factors for osteoporosis play a greater role in men than in women, in whom a decline in estrogen is the primary cause. Osteomalacia, a softening of bones due to lack of vitamin D, has been shown to cause osteoporosis in men. Vitamin D plays a role in the absorption of calcium in the intestine (gut), which is essential for building and maintaining strong, healthy bones. Osteomalacia may result from too little vitamin D in the diet, a lack of exposure to sunlight, gastrointestinal surgery, or other circumstances that interfere with vitamin D absorption from the digestive tract. Osteomalacia may also result from kidney defects or failure that impairs production of vitamin D.

### *How is osteoporosis in men detected?*

A complete blood count and the measurement of levels in the blood of testosterone, gonadotropin (hormone stimulating the testes), certain proteins, and calcium are usual tests. Levels of certain substances in the blood (alkaline phosphatase) and urine (hydroxyproline) indicate bone turnover (formation and resorption). Although they are not specific for osteoporosis, these tests can reveal if there is a high rate of bone resorption, which is associated with the disorder.

The amount of bone loss can be determined by measuring bone mass through dual-energy X-ray absorptiometry (DXA) or quantitative computed tomography (QCT). If no cause of bone loss can be detected, a tiny piece of bone may be removed (biopsy) for examination.

### *How is osteoporosis in men treated?*

Research is being conducted to find treatments that are effective in reducing the fracture rate. In men with a low level of testosterone, treatment with injections of the synthetic hormone may partly reverse the bone loss. (This treatment is not safe for men with prostate cancer and requires particular care in the presence of an enlarged prostate or heart disease.)

The role that calcium plays in men is not fully understood. A panel convened by the National Institutes of Health, in June 1994, recommended that men between 25 and 65 years of age ingest 1,000 mg of calcium per day and men over 65 ingest 1,500 mg per day. Also, some doctors advise men over 70 years to take 400–800 IU of supplemental vitamin D per day. Good nutrition and weight-bearing exercise should be added to enhance the benefit of calcium.

Several treatments for osteoporosis in men are still under investigation to determine their usefulness. Small doses of parathyroid gland hormone with calcitriol (a form of vitamin D) are being tried experimentally in men. Thus far, bone mass has increased for an 18- to 24-month period, but it is unknown whether this increase can be maintained. It is also too soon to determine whether a group of drugs called bisphosphonates (e.g., etidronate), which have been used for many years to treat the bone disorder Paget's disease in men and women, will become an approved treatment for men with osteoporosis. Studies are being conducted to determine if these drugs reduce fractures.

Several treatments have been found to help women with osteoporosis, but their effects in men have not been sufficiently studied. For example, a synthetic calcitonin hormone that is believed to prevent bone resorption has led to an increase in bone mass in women. However, the treatment may not provide the same benefit to men because men already produce a higher level of natural calcitonin in the body than women do. Specially prepared sodium fluoride has been used to treat postmenopausal women with osteoporosis who had suffered fractures. The treatment increased bone minerals and decreased the incidence of new fractures. However, the impact of fluoride in men has not yet been reported in the United States.

## How can osteoporosis be prevented?

- Osteoporosis is best prevented by increasing peak bone mass at the time the skeleton matures, minimizing bone loss thereafter, and preventing falls that cause fractures. The following accomplish these three measures:

- Adequate intake of calcium, beginning early in life

- Adequate level of vitamin D obtained from the diet, exposure to sunlight (a few minutes a day is usually adequate), or both

- Weight-bearing exercise that improves strength and coordination

- Elimination of tobacco and excess alcohol intake

- Early diagnosis and treatment of testosterone deficiency

# Part Four

# Related Conditions

# Chapter 16

# *Hyperparathyroidism*

Primary hyperparathyroidism is a disorder of the parathyroid glands. Most people with this disorder have one or more enlarged, overactive parathyroid glands that secrete too much parathyroid hormone. In secondary hyperparathyroidism, a problem such as kidney failure makes the body resistant to the action of parathyroid hormone. This e-pub focuses on primary hyperparathyroidism.

## *What are the parathyroid glands?*

The parathyroid glands are four pea-sized glands located on the thyroid gland in the neck. Occasionally, a person is born with one or more of the parathyroid glands embedded in the thyroid, the thymus, or elsewhere in the chest. In most such cases, however, the glands function normally.

Though their names are similar, the thyroid and parathyroid glands are entirely separate glands, each producing distinct hormones with specific functions. The parathyroid glands secrete parathyroid hormone (PTH), a substance that helps maintain the correct balance of calcium and phosphorous in the body. PTH regulates release of the calcium from bone, absorption of calcium in the intestine, and excretion of calcium in the urine.

When the amount of calcium in the blood falls too low, the parathyroid glands secrete just enough PTH to restore the balance.

NIH Publication No. 95-3425. February 1995 e-text posted: 12 February 1998: http://www.niddk.nih.gov/health/endo/pubs/hyper/hyper.htm.

115

## *What is hyperparathyroidism?*

If the glands secrete too much hormone, as in hyperparathyroidism, the balance is disrupted: blood calcium rises. This condition of excessive calcium in the blood, called hypercalcemia, is what usually signals the doctor that something may be wrong with the parathyroid glands. In 85 percent of people with this disorder, a benign tumor (adenoma) has formed on one of the parathyroid glands, causing it to become overactive. In most other cases, the excess hormone comes from two or more enlarged parathyroid glands, a condition called hyperplasia. Very rarely, hyperparathyroidism is caused by cancer of a parathyroid gland.

This excess PTH triggers the release of too much calcium into the bloodstream. The bones may lose calcium, and too much calcium may be absorbed from food. The levels of calcium may increase in the urine, causing kidney stones. PTH also acts to lower blood phosphorous levels by increasing excretion of phosphorus in the urine.

## *Why are calcium and phosphorous so important?*

Calcium is essential for good health. It plays an important role in bone and tooth development and in maintaining bone strength. It is also important in nerve transmission and muscle contraction. Phosphorous is found in every body tissue. Combined with calcium, it gives strength and rigidity to your bones and teeth.

## *What causes hyperparathyroidism?*

In most cases doctors don't know the cause. The vast majority of cases occur in people with no family history of the disorder. Only about 3 to 5 percent of cases can be linked to an inherited problem. Familial endocrine neoplasia type I is one rare inherited syndrome that affects the parathyroids as well as the pancreas and the pituitary gland. Another rare genetic disorder, familial hypocalciuric hypercalcemia, is sometimes confused with typical hyperparathyroidism.

## *How common is hyperparathyroidism?*

In the U.S., about 100,000 people develop the disorder each year. Women outnumber men by 2 to 1, and risk increases with age. In women 60 years and older, 2 out of 1,000 will get hyperparathyroidism.

116

## *What are the symptoms of hyperparathyroidism?*

A person with hyperparathyroidism may have severe symptoms, subtle ones, or none at all. Increasingly, routine blood tests that screen for a wide range of conditions including high calcium levels are alerting doctors to people who, though symptom-free, have mild forms of the disorder.

When symptoms do appear, they are often mild and nonspecific, such as a feeling of weakness and fatigue, depression, or aches and pains. With more severe disease, a person may have a loss of appetite, nausea, vomiting, constipation, confusion or impaired thinking and memory, and increased thirst and urination. Patients may have thinning of the bones without symptoms, but with risk of fractures. Increased calcium and phosphorous excretion in the urine may cause kidney stones. Patients with hyperparathyroidism may be more likely to develop peptic ulcers, high blood pressure, and pancreatitis.

## *How is hyperparathyroidism diagnosed?*

Hyperparathyroidism is diagnosed when tests show that blood levels of calcium as well as parathyroid hormone are too high. Other diseases can cause high blood calcium levels, but only in hyperparathyroidism is the elevated calcium the result of too much parathyroid hormone. A blood test that accurately measures the amount of parathyroid hormone has simplified the diagnosis of hyperparathyroidism.

Once the diagnosis is established, other tests may be done to assess complications. Because high PTH levels can cause bones to weaken from calcium loss, a measurement of bone density may be done to assess bone loss and the risk of fractures. Abdominal radiographs may reveal the presence of kidney stones and a 24-hour urine collection may provide information on kidney damage and the risk of stone formation.

## *How is hyperparathyroidism treated?*

Surgery to remove the enlarged gland (or glands) is the only treatment for the disorder and cures it in 95 percent of cases. However, some patients who have mild disease may not need immediate treatment, according to a panel of experts convened by the National Institutes of Health in 1990. Patients who are symptom-free, whose blood calcium is only slightly elevated, and whose kidneys and bones are normal, may wish to talk to their doctor about long-term monitoring.

In the panel's recommendation, monitoring would consist of clinical evaluation and measurement of calcium levels and kidney function every 6 months, annual abdominal x-ray, and bone mass measurement after 1 to 2 years. If the disease shows no signs of worsening after 1 to 3 years, the interval between exams may be lengthened. If the patient and doctor choose long-term follow-up, the patient should try to drink lots of water, get plenty of exercise, and avoid certain diuretics, such as the thiazides. Immobilization and gastrointestinal illness with vomiting or diarrhea can cause calcium levels to rise, and if these conditions develop, patients with hyperparathyroidism should seek medical attention.

### Are there any complications associated with parathyroid surgery?

Surgery for hyperparathyroidism is highly successful with a low complication rate when performed by surgeons experienced with this condition. About 1 percent of patients undergoing surgery have damage to the nerves controlling the vocal cords, which can affect speech. One to five percent of patients develop chronic low calcium levels, which may require treatment with calcium and/or vitamin D. The complication rate is slightly higher for hyperplasia than it is for adenoma since more extensive surgery is needed.

### Are parathyroid imaging tests needed before surgery?

The National Institutes of Health panel recommended against the use of expensive imaging tests to locate benign tumors before initial surgery. Research shows that such tests do not improve the success rate of surgery, which is about 95 percent when performed by experienced surgeons. Localization tests are useful in patients having a second operation for recurrent or persistent hyperparathyroidism.

### Which doctors specialize in treating hyperparathyroidism?

Endocrinologists (doctors who specialize in hormonal problems), nephrologists (doctors who specialize in kidney and mineral disorders), and surgeons who are experienced in endocrine surgery. A listing of medical specialists and members of the American Association of Endocrine Surgeons, the American Society of Clinical Endocrinologists, and the American Society for Bone and Mineral Research is available at a public library.

## Additional Resources

The Paget Foundation for Paget's Disease of Bone and
Related Disorders
120 Wall Street, Suite 1602
New York, NY 10005-4001
201-509-5335

## Further Reading

Bilezikian, John P. et al. *The Parathyroids: Basic and Clinical Concepts*. New York: Raven Press, 1994.

Parisien, May, et al. "Bone Disease in Primary Hyperparathyroidism," *Endocrinology and Metabolism Clinics of North America*. Vol. 19, No. 1, March, 1990.

Potts, John T., Jr. "Management of Asymptomatic Hyperparathyroidism," *Journal of Endocrinology and Metabolism* Vol. 70, No. 6, 1990. 1489-1493.

National Institutes of Health. "Diagnosis and Management of Asymptomatic Primary Hyperparathyroidism: Consensus Development Conference Statement," *Annals of Internal Medicine* Vol. 114, No. 7, April 1, 1991. 593-596. Reprints are also available from the Office of Medical Applications of Research (OMAR) Consensus Program Clearinghouse, P.O. Box 2577, Kensington, MD 20891 1-800-NIH-OMAR.

# Chapter 17

# *Osteogenesis Imperfecta*

## *Facts on Osteogenesis Imperfecta*

### *Definition*

Osteogenesis Imperfecta (OI) is a genetic disorder characterized by bones that break easily, often from little or no apparent cause. There are at least four distinct forms of the disorder, representing extreme variation in severity from one individual to another. For example, a person may have as few as ten or as many as several hundred fractures in a lifetime.

### *Prevalence*

While the number of persons affected with OI in the United States is unknown, the best estimate suggests a minimum of 20,000 and possibly as many as 50,000.

---

This chapter includes text from the following publications of the Osteogenesis Imperfecta Foundation: "Fast Facts on Osteogenesis Imperfecta," © August 1997, "OI Issues: Osteoporosis," © August 1997; "OI Issues: Pain Management," © August 1997; "Rodding Surgery in Children with Osteogenesis Imperfecta," © June 1997; "OI Issues: Psychosocial Needs of the Family," © August 1997; "OI Issues: Child Abuse," © September 19997; and "OI Issues: Education," undated. Reprinted by permission of Osteogenesis Imperfecta Foundation. For more information visit http://www.oif.org.

## *Diagnosis*

Most forms of OI are caused by imperfectly formed bone collagen, the result of a genetic defect. Collagen is the major protein of the body's connective tissue and can be likened to the framework around which a building is constructed. In OI, a person has either less collagen or a poorer quality of collagen.

Collagen testing, which is done through a skin biopsy, is used to determine the amount of collagen present and its structure. While these studies identify the vast majority of people who have OI, approximately 15 percent of individuals with obvious features of OI do not demonstrate a collagen abnormality sufficient enough to be detected by the testing. Because of the complexity of the test, as well as the limited number of laboratories that are qualified to do the testing, it may take 3 to 6 months before test results are known.

## *Clinical Features*

The characteristic features of OI vary greatly from person to person and not all characteristics are evident in each case; however, the general features of OI, which vary in characteristics as well as severity, are:

### Type I OI:

- Most common
- Bones fracture easily
- Can usually be traced through the family
- Near normal stature or slightly shorter
- Blue sclera
- Dental problems
- Hearing loss beginning in the early twenties and thirties
- Most fractures occur before puberty; occasionally women will have fractures after menopause
- Triangular face
- Tendency toward spinal curvatures

### Type II OI:

- Newborns severely affected; frequently lethal
- Usually resulting from a new gene mutation

- Very small stature with extremely small chest and under developed lungs

## Type III OI:

- Tend to be isolated family incidents
- Very small in stature—some only three feet tall
- Fractures at birth very common
- X-ray may reveal healing of *in utero* fractures
- Severe early hearing loss
- Loose joints and poor muscle development in arms and legs
- Barrel-shaped rib cage

## Type IV OI:

- Can frequently be traced through the family
- Bones fracture easily—most before puberty
- Normal or near normal colored sclera
- Problems with teeth—more than type 1
- Spinal curvatures
- Loose joints

### *Inheritance Factors*

OI can be dominantly or recessively inherited and can also occur as a mutation. Therefore, individuals with OI and parents of children with OI are strongly encouraged to seek genetic counseling to determine the likelihood of OI recurring in their families.

### *Treatment*

At present there is no cure for OI. Treatment is directed toward preventing or correcting the symptoms. Care of fractures, extensive surgical and dental procedures, and physical therapy are often recommended for persons with OI. Wheelchairs, braces, and other custom-made equipment are often necessary. Individuals are encouraged to seek out medical centers where all aspects of OI, including biochemical, orthopedic, dental, and hearing problems, can be treated.

An orthopedic procedure called "rodding" is frequently considered for individuals with OI. This treatment involves inserting metal rods through the length of the long bones to strengthen them and prevent deformities.

## *Prognosis*

The prognosis for an individual with OI varies greatly depending on the number of symptoms as well as the severity of the symptoms. Despite numerous fractures, restricted activity, and short stature, many adults and children with OI lead productive and happy lives.

## *Osteoporosis and Osteogenesis Imperfecta*

The information for this section is reprinted from *ORBD–NRC News You Can Use*, "Osteoporosis in Osteogenesis Imperfecta," Osteoporosis and Related Bone Diseases–National Resource Center, Vol. III, No. 9, July 14, 1997.

Osteogenesis imperfecta (OI) is a genetic disorder in which the bones are fragile due to defective collagen. Collagen is an important protein found in the body's connective tissues, such as bone and cartilage. In people with OI, either the quantity or the quality of collagen is abnormal, resulting in bones that are less dense and break easily.

At least four types of OI have been identified. Type I is the most common form of OI. People with this type of the disease tend to fracture easily and exhibit other features, such as blue sclera, hearing loss, a triangular face, spinal curvature, and dental problems. Type II OI, though less common, is a very severe form of the disease. Newborns with Type II often fracture before birth and usually die shortly after birth. Individuals with Type III OI tend to be very small in stature, experience hearing loss at a young age, and have a barrel-shaped rib cage, while those with Type IV tend to fracture easily and often have spinal curvature and significant dental problems.

### *The Osteoporosis Connection*

While the traits of each type of osteogenesis imperfecta can vary greatly from person to person, consistent among all types of OI is the tendency for patients to develop low bone density at some point in their lives. For this reason, osteoporosis is an almost universal consequence of osteogenesis imperfecta. The goal of osteoporosis therapy in patients with OI involves two main concerns: increasing bone density at every age and minimizing bone loss that occurs as a result of aging. Generally, the strategies for prevention and treatment of osteoporosis among patients with OI are the same as those strategies for the rest of the population.

## Minimizing Bone Loss in OI Patients

Immobilization is a critical risk factor for the development of osteoporosis in anyone. However, immobility may be virtually unavoidable for those with serious skeletal deformities or recurrent fractures. When possible, however, activities such as isometric exercise, weight lifting, standing, and walking can help reduce bone loss in people with OI.

Adequate calcium intake is another important factor for bone health. However, urine calcium excretion should be measured before substantially increasing dietary calcium, since urinary calcium excretion may be increased in some patients with OI. Eliminating other risk factors for osteoporosis, such as smoking, excessive alcohol, and prolonged use of certain bone-wasting medications, should also be considered.

Though published data are limited, various therapeutic agents continue to be investigated for their ability to minimize bone loss in people with OI at all ages. Agents currently under investigation include calcium supplements, fluoride, growth hormone, and bisphosphonates such as alendronate and pamidronate. Pamidronate has been associated with significant increases in bone density among children with OI and among adults with Type I OI.

## OI and Menopause

Given the low bone density found in many patients with osteogenesis imperfecta, many women with OI are concerned about the effects of ovarian estrogen loss after menopause. It has been reported that women with OI have an increased fracture rate after menopause, although it is not clear whether the increased rate is due to aging, a lack of estrogen, or both. Despite a lack of research in this area, it is generally recommended that all postmenopausal women with osteogenesis imperfecta consider estrogen replacement therapy.

## The Osteoporosis Diagnosis

Bone density measurements are often recommended for patients with OI. The three sites that are commonly measured include the spine, wrist, and hip. Unfortunately, several factors can interfere with a bone density reading in individuals with OI, such as significant curvature of the spine, past vertebral fractures, or the presence of metal rodding in the wrist or hip. Also, some bone density techniques (such as dual energy absorptiometry and dual energy radioabsorptiometry) may not produce accurate readings on short-statured individuals. In fact, short individuals with normal bone density may be diagnosed with low bone density by these tests. Serial measurements with such techniques can be useful, however, in evaluating changes in bone density in people with OI.

If you would like more information about osteoporosis, its diagnosis and treatment, contact the Osteoporosis and Related Bone Diseases–National Resource Center at (800) 624-BONE.

## Pain Management

This information is adapted from the "Osteoporosis Report," Winter 1996, National Osteoporosis Foundation.

For individuals with osteogenesis imperfecta (OI), the pain associated with multiple fractures can lead to needless suffering and, when untreated, may result in a chronic condition. Since pain may impair a person's ability to lead a productive life, chronic pain is a serious economic as well as a major health problem.

Pain is the body's way of responding to damaged tissue. When a bone breaks, nerves send pain messages through the spinal cord to the brain, where they are interpreted. How a person responds to pain is determined by many factors, including his or her emotional outlook. For example, depression seems to increase a person's perception of pain and to decrease his or her ability to cope with it. Often, treating the depression treats the pain as well. If pain is not adequately treated, the transmission of pain impulses to the brain occurs more readily. Therefore, it is more effective to prevent pain than to treat it after it occurs.

Acute pain is usually characterized by a short duration, normal functioning of both the peripheral and central nervous systems, a predictable course and, in most cases, a good outcome. Chronic pain is pain that lasts beyond the expected time for healing and interferes with normal life. The damaged tissues have healed, but the pain continues. The pain message may be triggered by muscle tension, stiffness, weakness, or spasms. Nonverbal responses to pain include elevated heart rate and blood pressure and immobilization of an injured part in order to avoid pain from movement. Whatever the cause of chronic pain, feelings of frustration, anger, and fear make the pain more intense. Chronic pain can often diminish the quality of a person's life psychologically, socially, and physically. It is also the most frequent cause of suffering and disability in the world today.

With OI, there can be associated conditions of acute and chronic pain resulting from multiple fractures, vertebral collapse, joint deformity, osteoarthritis, contractures, deformity/malalignment of limbs, and recurrent abdominal pain. Pain management for OI, in both adults and children, requires adequate assessment and implementation of a regimen that should address the multifaceted presentation of acute and chronic pain. With the increased longevity of individuals with OI, the incidence of pain syndromes relating to degenerative changes becomes more likely. An interdisciplinary approach to pain management is best.

The following information provides an overview of different options for pain management in OI. Individuals who need help managing the chronic pain associated with OI may wish to discuss the options listed below with a physician.

## Coping Strategies

### Physical Methods of Pain Management

**Heat and Ice.** Heat in the form of warm showers or hot packs can relieve chronic pain or stiff muscles. Cold packs or ice packs provide pain relief by numbing the pain-sensing nerves in the affected area. Cold may also prevent swelling and inflammation. Heat or ice should be applied for 15 to 20 minutes at a time to the painful area, and a towel should be placed between the skin and the source of the cold or heat to protect the skin:

- Warm towels or hot packs in the microwave provide a quick source of heat.

- Frozen juice cans or bags of frozen vegetables make instant cold packs.

- A damp towel that has been completely wrung out and frozen can provide relief from pain.

- Freezing a plastic, resealable bag filled with water makes a good ice bag.

**Transcutaneous Electrical Nerve Stimulation (TENS).** A TENS machine is a small device that sends electrical impulses to

127

certain parts of the body to block pain signals. Two electrodes are placed on the body where the person is experiencing the pain. The electrical current that is produced is very mild, but it can prevent pain messages from being transmitted to the brain. Pain relief can last for several hours. Some people may use a small, portable TENS unit that hooks on a belt for more continuous relief. TENS machines should be used under the supervision of a physician or physical therapist. They can be purchased or rented from hospital supply or surgical supply houses; however, a prescription is necessary for insurance reimbursement.

Other forms of electrical therapy that can be beneficial include high volt, low volt, micro stimulation, bipolar, interferential, and Russian stimulation. Each of these therapies has different properties to control not only pain but to decrease swelling and strengthen weakened muscles. Most of them, however, must be used in the physician's office.

**Exercise or Physical Therapy.** Exercise or physical therapy, under the supervision of a health professional who understands the nature of OI, can be effective in strengthening muscles, improving stamina, and helping an individual have a more positive outlook on life. Because exercise raises the body's level of endorphins (natural painkillers produced by the brain), pain can diminish. It is beneficial for children with OI to begin physical therapy as soon as possible. Physical therapists can teach proper positioning, posture, and exercises to strengthen muscles without injuring bones. Exercise can be as simple as moving a joint through its range of motion. Pool therapy is one of the best exercise techniques to gently improve muscle strength and reduce pain.

**Acupuncture and Acupressure.** Acupuncture involves the use of special needles that are inserted into the body at specific points. These needles are believed to stimulate nerve endings and cause the brain to release endorphins. It may take several acupuncture sessions before the pain is relieved. Acupressure is direct pressure over trigger areas of pain. This technique can be self-administered after training with a certified instructor.

**Massage Therapy.** Massage therapy can be a light, slow, circular motion with the fingertips or a deep and kneading motion that moves from the center of the body outward toward the fingers or toes. Massage relieves pain, relaxes stiff muscles, and smoothes out muscle knots by increasing the blood supply to the affected area and warming it. The person doing the massage uses oils or powder so that his/her hands slide smoothly over the skin. Massage can also include gentle pressure over affected areas or hard pressure over trigger points in muscle knots. Special care must be taken when working on individuals with OI to avoid putting too much pressure on bones that might possibly fracture.

*Psychological Methods of Pain Management*

**Relaxation training.** Relaxation involves concentration and slow, deep breathing to release tension from muscles and to relieve pain. Learning to relax takes a great deal of practice, but relaxation training can focus attention away from pain and release tension from all muscles. Relaxation audiotapes are available to help achieve the desired effects.

**Biofeedback.** Biofeedback is taught by a professional who uses special machines to help a person control certain functions such as heart rate and muscle tension. As the person learns to release muscle tension, the machine immediately indicates success. Biofeedback can be used to reinforce relaxation training. Once the technique is mastered, it can be practiced without the use of the machine.

**Visual imagery or distraction.** Imagery involves concentrating on mental pictures of pleasant scenes or events or mentally repeating positive sayings to reduce pain. Videotapes are also available to help visual imagery. Distraction techniques focus the person's attention away from negative painful images to more positive thoughts. This technique may include watching television or a favorite movie, reading a book or listening to a book on tape, listening to music, or talking to a friend.

**Hypnosis.** Hypnosis can be used in two ways to reduce a person's perception of pain. Some people are hypnotized by a therapist and given a post-hypnotic suggestion that reduces the pain they feel; others are taught self-hypnosis and can hypnotize themselves when pain interrupts their ability to function. Self-hypnosis is a form of relaxation training.

**Individual or family therapy.** A psychologist, psychiatrist, or psychiatric social worker can help people cope with feelings of depression, frustration, and anger that often accompany chronic pain.

*Medications for Pain Management*

To be most effective in alleviating pain, medications should be administered before pain appears and certainly before it worsens. Pain medications should be administered prior to painful procedures or before the performance of an activity that may be painful, such as deep breathing exercises after a spine fusion. As stated earlier, it is easier to prevent pain rather than to attempt to alleviate it. Pain is best prevented or treated by providing pain medication on a continuous or around-the-clock basis rather than as needed. Pain medications should be administered in an acceptable manner that is less uncomfortable than the pain itself. Ideally, they should be administered orally, intravenously, or under the tongue. Medications taken orally are generally the least expensive and most convenient alternative. Intramuscular injections are painful and may be a last resort.

**Over-the-counter pain relievers.** Aspirin, ibuprofen, naprosyn sodium, and acetaminophen can effectively relieve pain. While these medications are relatively safe, they can still cause side effects, such as stomach upset, and may result in complications from excessive dosing or prolonged administration. For this reason, these medications should be taken according to the doctor's or manufacturers' directions. Before increasing the frequency of use or the dosage, the person should first check with the doctor or pharmacist.

**Non-steroidal anti-inflammatory medications (NSAIDs).** NSAIDs may be prescribed to treat mild to severe pain. These preparations block pain and treat inflammation. There are dozens of NSAIDs on the market, and a person may have to try several different brands to find the one that works best.

**Topical pain relievers.** A variety of topical creams may also relieve pain when they are rubbed directly into the painful area. While some of these creams are available by prescription only, others may be purchased over-the-counter.

**Narcotic pain medication.** Narcotics are powerful pain-relieving medications derived from opium or synthetic opium. Narcotics alter a person's perception of pain and can also induce euphoria, mood changes, mental cloudiness, and deep sleep. These drugs may also cause nausea, lethargy, and constipation. People with OI must be especially careful when taking these medications. Narcotics can affect a person's balance and increase the chance of falling. After repeated and prolonged use, some people may become dependent on or addicted to these medications, which are available only by prescription.

There are new medications that appear to relieve pain without the serious side effects of narcotics. There is also a skin patch that releases small amounts of a narcotic into the body through the skin. These medications can only be prescribed by a physician.

**Antidepressant medications.** People who suffer from chronic pain frequently suffer from chronic depression as well. Several studies using antidepressant medications have noted that these medications may not only improve depression but may also relieve or reduce the amount of pain a person feels. Additional research is needed to determine whether antidepressants can treat the chronic pain of OI and which antidepressants produce the best results.

**Nerve block.** In some cases, a physician may perform a nerve block that involves the injection of pain-relieving medications into the tissues around an affected nerve. The block numbs the nerves and surrounding tissues and eliminates the sensation of pain. Pain relief may last for hours or months, depending on the medications used and the person's response to them. All of these methods of pain management, alone and in combination, are used in hospitals and clinics across the country. People who are suffering from unrelieved chronic pain may wish to consult a physician for a referral to a physical therapist or a clinic specializing in pain management.

Pain management for individuals with OI often requires a multidisciplinary approach involving specialists in medicine, psychology, and rehabilitation for adequate treatment. The goal for treatment is effective therapy that will not only reduce or remove the pain but will also achieve mental well-being and an improvement in physiological function.

## *Rodding Surgery in Children with Osteogenesis Imperfecta*

Rodding surgery is usually restricted to children with moderate and severe forms of osteogenesis imperfecta (OI). The treatment, which is tailored to a patient's needs, involves straightening and internal splinting (Rodding) of one or more long bones.

### Purpose of Rodding

Rodding is recommended when a child is having repeated fractures of one or more long bones. In most cases, the long bone is deformed from repeated fractures and bending of the soft bone. A curved long bone is not in itself a reason for Rodding unless it worsens or becomes painful because of stress fractures.

When a child is ready to walk but is not making progress because of repeated fractures, rodding is used to help strengthen and straighten the child's bones. Under these circumstances, straightening of the bone and internally splinting it with a rod corrects the deformities, reduces the fracture rate, and improves the child's well being.

### Timing of Surgery

Babies with severe forms of OI have numerous fractures at birth and repeated fractures over the following months. The fractures are usually treated with splints or casts rather than surgery. Surgery may be needed over the following years if repeated fractures of one or more long bones occur. Children with moderately severe forms of OI also have numerous fractures at birth but few new fractures until they start to stand and walk, which is when repeated fractures of the upper thigh bone (femur) may occur; at this time, surgery may be required.

Rodding is usually undertaken as a scheduled elective procedure after the fracture has healed. However, it can also be undertaken soon after a fracture to avoid a second period in a cast.

### Surgery, Anesthesia, and After-Care

In 1946, Dr. H. Sofield developed the commonly used method of straightening the deformed bone and internally splinting it with a stainless steel rod. This method, which used a non-expanding rod, was refined by Drs. Miller and Williams. Drs. Bailey and Dubow developed a method that used an expanding rod, in which one half of the rod consists of a tube and the other half a spike. Flanges at the end of the rod anchor it to the ends of the bone so that the spike can slide within the tube during growth. A modified version of this rod, the Sheffield expanding rod, was developed by Drs. Sharrard and Bell in Sheffield, U.K.

In the original Sofield procedure, the full length of the deformed long bone is exposed, divided into pieces, and threaded onto a straight, non-expanding rod (like a shish kebab). It requires a long incision in the skin and underlying tissues, and bone healing may be slow. Alternatively, small incisions can be made at the end of each deformed bone, which is corrected with minimal disturbance of the blood supply to the bone, thus encouraging the bone cut to heal rapidly. The rod is introduced through the skin and moved through the bone under x-ray guidance.

Non-expanding rods come in various widths and lengths and can, therefore, be used in almost any OI long bone. They are inserted to support the full length of the long bone. In some cases, the rod is advanced across the growth areas, which are near the ends of the bone, to provide better support. The smooth surface of the rod does not reduce the growth of the bone. The major disadvantage of the non-expanding rod is that it fails to support the bone that grows beyond it. If the unsupported bone gradually bends, the end of the rod may protrude from the bone surface and the bone may fracture. Under these circumstances, the bone is straightened and a new rod inserted. In many children, however, the non-expanding rods are inserted in early childhood, when they are needed most, and may not need to be changed later even though the x-ray may show mild bowing of the unsupported bone beyond the rod.

The expanding rods have the advantage of supporting the bone while it grows. Their use is limited to bones that are sufficiently wide to accommodate the thicker expanding rod, and the bone needs to be sufficiently strong to anchor the flanges at the ends of the rod.

Rodding procedures are most often undertaken in the thigh bone (femur) and shin bone (tibia). Occasionally, the arm bone requires rodding as well. With modem anesthesia, children can be sedated for longer periods of time, thereby enabling several bones to be rodded at one time (e.g., the femur and tibia of one leg).

After the surgery, the limb is often supported by a lightweight cast for about four weeks. An above-the-knee cast is used following tibial surgery.

The knee may be bent so that the child can sit in a wheelchair or stroller. Casting following femoral surgery is more difficult. A hip spica, which extends from the ribs down the affected leg, may be required. However, an above-the knee half cast that does not extend above the hip may be sufficient. Bracing may be used after the removal of the cast to provide added support for standing and walking.

### Summary

There are many considerations in determining whether rodding is necessary and, if so, when and how it should be done. Because OI is so variable, the treatment plan needs to be specific for each child.

Overall, the rodding procedures are successful with a low frequency of complications.

This information was prepared by Dr. William G. Cole, MBBS, PhD, FRACS, FRCSC, who is Head, Division of Orthopedics, Professor of surgery, University of Toronto, Canada. He also is a member of the OIF Medical Advisory Committee.
ORBD-NRC is supported by the National Institute of arthritis and Musculoskeletal and Skin Diseases, National Institutes of Health

## *Psychosocial Needs of the Family*

Most of the information in this section was adapted from "Walking the tightrope: Juggling the psychological needs of the whole family," by Kay Harris Kriegsman, Ph.D., in *Managing Osteogenesis Imperfecta: A Medical Manual Osteogenesis Imperfecta Foundation*, 1996.

Osteogenesis imperfecta (OI) is a complex disorder that affects each individual and family in a unique way. The degree to which differences resulting from OI change lives depends to some extent on the type of OI the person has, the history of the disorder, the extent to which physical appearance is affected, and the personal mobility and presence of other family members who have OI. These factors may influence the way in which these individuals adjust to their community and work environment. It is, therefore, important to understand and appreciate the psychological and social aspects of OI and how they affect the individual and the family.

### *The Parents*

The reaction of parents to the birth of a child with OI is determined by their previous experiences, although their immediate reactions may be related to the degree of visible deformity and apparent disability of the child. In families with no previous exposure to OI, initial shock and psychological immobility may be followed by feelings of anger, confusion, fear of the unknown and the future, fear of others' perceptions, loneliness, and concern about physician competence and knowledge about OI. The feeling parents most often expressed is guilt, a feeling that has added meaning when the disability is a genetic condition.

Many parents must go through a bereavement process and mourn the loss of the "normal" child they expected. In addition to coming to terms with their feelings about the disability, parents have to face the usual concerns of having a new baby as well as the physical, medical, and financial concerns relating to disability.

When the diagnosis is not made at birth, it is likely that the child will suffer repeated fractures before the OI is confirmed. The unexplained fractures may bring accusations of child abuse from health care professionals. For these parents, a diagnosis brings relief as well as vindication, although then, still need to deal with their feelings about the OI.

Parents may go through a variety of phases as they come to accept their child and the child's disability. Having conflicting emotions about the baby at this time is normal, as many parents may feel the need to completely deny the disability or may need to see the disability as completely identifying the child. They also must face the problem of how to describe what is going on to their extended families. Some family members may deny the disorder, while others may overreact and show inappropriate or undue concern for the affected child. There will be variations in the length of time that it takes individual family members to come to terms with the disability. It is essential that parents realize they have limited amounts of energy and that the child is their first priority. They must set limits on how much interaction they have with the extended family if family members become too demanding of their time.

As they begin to experience full awareness of the disability and its implications, many parents feel lonely, resentful, angry, and/or sad. Eventually, however, most parents learn routines, see their children survive, and have their confidence begin to build. They also experience a sense of healing. They begin to see their child as a person "with" a disability as opposed to a disabled child. At this point, the parents begin to take control of their lives.

Parents who have difficulty moving through these normal stages of grieving should be encouraged to contact other parents of children with OI and/or seek professional assistance.

As the child begins to grow, most parents learn to cope with new fractures, although it takes an enormous amount of patience and courage. They must learn how to explain their child's limitations to others, even when they themselves are uncertain whether fractures will occur from the disorder or as part of everyday toddler activity. These parents learn to live in an atmosphere of unending crisis management.

### The Siblings

The arrival of a new baby can lead to sibling rivalry in any family. These problems are magnified when the new child has OI, because caring for such a child is complicated and time-consuming. Too often, other children are unintentionally neglected. Even very young children can sense their parents' distress and preoccupation with the new baby, although they may not understand why their parents are reacting this way. Usually, older children help in feeding, changing and bathing the baby; with OI, this is usually not possible because of the extreme care that must be taken when handling a baby with OI. If the child with OI is older, he or she may not be physically able to interact with the new baby. In either case, the siblings are unable to form a physical relationship and a gap may be created between them. Many families with OI have found that one way to promote the bonding between siblings is to allow the unaffected child to hold the new baby on a pillow and feed him or her while a parent remains close by for safety.

It is very important for parents to be sensitive to the emotional needs of their unaffected children. By observing them at play and by playing with them, they can try to learn if certain situations are causing unrest in the child. If the child seems angry and frustrated, different methods of relieving that frustration, such as punching bags and kicking a ball, might help relieve tension. The parents should also set aside special times to be with the unaffected children. Although this may be difficult, this quality time is very important. It is especially important for parents to consider the feelings of a sibling who may have been the cause of a fracture. For a sibling who is already having negative feelings toward the child with OI, causing a fracture may result in feelings of guilt and remorse. As the child gets older, frank discussions can be very beneficial.

In these situations, parents need to be encouraged to reserve energy to deal with the needs of all their children, although this may never be equal. They need to weigh the complaints of siblings the same way as they would for typical sibling interactions, trying to determine what is normal and what is due to the impact of the disability. Parents must take extra precautions to ensure that all their children feel loved and appreciated and that open lines of communication exist among all family members.

### *The Child with OI*

**Early childhood.** Parents generally strive throughout their childrens' formative years to teach them principles and skills that will enable them to lead self-sufficient, productive lives, as independent of parental influence as possible. For the parent of a child with OI, this can be somewhat of a challenge. While parents realize the value of teaching their children to be independent, they also tend to protect them by pulling the children closer to them. Finding the right balance is the key.

Since many children with OI experience much pain in their early years, they often become frightened of sudden movements, of being touched (especially by strangers), or by unfamiliar situations. If a parent can provide as many positive experiences in these situations as possible, the fear can be overridden with confidence. Teach your child that others can be trusted to lift or touch him.

It is important to allow others to care for your child while you leave for limited periods of time. Not only does this provide some much needed "alone" time for you as parents, but it teaches your child that he/she can function independently without you. You need to teach your child independence and you, in turn, need to let go.

**Going to school.** Starting school may be particularly difficult for children with OI and their parents, who must accept that the benefits of academic and social growth outweigh the physical risks. Children with OI will find it harder to realize these benefits if they are excluded from all activities and interactions with their peers.

Some parents may have difficulty working with school personnel, particularly when they have had previous negative experiences with human service providers. A particular concern of parents of mildly affected children who appear "normal," but who are at risk for fractures, is the fear that if people are aware of their child's disorder, they will treat the whole child as "different" and not just different in relation to risk of fracture. Teachers and other school personnel who lack accurate information about OI may place inappropriate and unnecessary restrictions on this child. It is best to start with a positive attitude and to provide information about OI so that these individuals can understand the child and learn the most effective methods of helping him or her in the school setting.

**Adolescence.** Older children who use a wheelchair are often concerned about immobility, the social problems associated with short stature, and the pain and specific immobility due to recurrent fractures, which may be more prevalent at the time of the adolescent growth spurt.

During adolescence, concerns about physical appearance and peer acceptance are heightened. Depression and feelings of inadequacy may be particularly problematic for teenagers with OI. Being shorter in stature, using an orthopedic appliance, often being encased in a cast, or having different features will be most pronounced and hurtful during the teen years.

There are many different social strategies that can be used to promote appropriate adaptation to disabling conditions like OI. Those that are self-limiting, such as withdrawal and concealment, tend to promote loss of self-esteem. One productive coping strategy is increased assertiveness, in which the individual becomes more socially active. One of the best mechanisms for promoting an adolescent's self-esteem is to foster participation in activities that interest him or her—find out what they like, such as politics, religion, sports, painting, etc., and encourage them to pursue this interest. Adolescents should also be encouraged to engage in regular teenage activities, such as dancing. Even in a wheelchair, people with OI can enjoy the thrill of moving to different rhythms! People with OI can also participate in sports such as bowling, sailing, cross country skiing, tennis, swimming, and more.

Following high school, the transition to college or the work world is an extremely challenging time, particularly when the person is not completely independent. Balancing parental concerns and the young adult's desires for autonomy creates tension within the family. It is especially difficult for parents to think of "letting" go of a child who has always needed their help and support. Some adolescents may have a particularly difficult time breaking away, because the family, has done so much for them. These adolescents will benefit from thoughtful and careful counseling—designed to help them through their difficult entry into adulthood and independence.

Other issues that should be addressed at this stage include dating, sexuality, marriage, and having, children. While some parents may, have difficulty discussing these topics with their children, it would be a mistake to treat your child's sexual development as a non-issue. Most people with OI can have satisfying sexual relationships, get married, and have children. They need to know about safe sex, sexually transmitted diseases, and AIDS. Everyone needs to learn how to take responsibility for themselves and for their partners.

**Adulthood.** For the individual who is severely affected by OI, problems of immobility and social and financial dependence often become most troublesome in young adulthood. Affected adults may be dependent on family, friends, and neighbors for mobility, although some of these people may be deterred from assisting those in greatest need, fearing that they will be responsible for new fractures. It is important to note, however, that with the technology that is available today, even individuals who are severely affected are able to live on their own with limited assistance from home care providers.

Less than ideal accessibility may contribute to physical and social isolation and restrict occupational and educational choices. Discrimination in the work place is sometimes prevalent, and fair financial compensation for work done is not always received. The real problems arising from the physically disabling aspects of OI, hindrances perceived by employers, acquaintances, and members of the opposite sex, place great barriers between the adult with OI and his/her life goals. Adults face the likelihood of new fractures and hospital stays. In a busy and aggressive society, they must compete on an equal basis with their physically healthy counterparts but may experience difficulty in obtaining health insurance or receiving dispensation for legitimate absences from work.

People with milder forms of OI have unique problems arising from the conflict between their outwardly normal appearance and their underlying fragility. "Who do I tell about my condition? Will it help me or hinder me to explain my absence from work related to OI by explaining the nature of the condition? When do I tell my date or my significant other?" These questions are increasingly faced by adults with OI in today's world.

**The Family**. For the family with OI, the ability to balance the reality of the disability and the rest of life is essential. Because of the on-going concern for and reality of recurrent bone breaks and other medical complications, families need added psychological resiliency to maintain equilibrium. Preparing a child with a disability to manage on his own requires greater thought and foresight than a non-disabled child. According to a model that was developed by Kay Harris Kriegsman, Ph.D., parents must address four factors that will help their child prepare for adulthood:

**Experience:** Children with disability often miss out on experiences such as riding a bike, weeding a garden, or hiking in the woods. It is important for children to feel the rain, wind, or snow.

**Risk taking:** Experiences such as going to a sleep away camp or a school dance are often denied to children with OI. But these types of experiences are important if the child is to learn limits and the cost of consequences.

139

**Responsibility:** When children are needed in a family they feel valued and competent. They should be assigned tasks, such as answering the telephone, wiping the dishes, or setting the table. Responsibility, to the larger community is learned through volunteering for a charitable or religious organization.

**Socialization:** Socialization involves the give and take of normal interaction. Some children with OI are always in the spotlight and do not learn to shift attention to others. Socialization also involves learning how to deal on the same level as one's peers; sometimes, children with OI deal primarily with adults and the medical community and they miss out on the important developmental peer interactions.

The family will remain balanced if all members work as a unit and each family member accepts his or her responsibility to the family system.

## Child Abuse

Osteogenesis imperfecta (OI) is characterized by bones that break easily. A minor accident may result in a fracture; some fractures may occur while a child is being diapered, lifted, or dressed. It is possible for a person with OI to break a bone without being aware of it. Children who are not diagnosed at birth often suffer a series of painful fractures before health care professionals are able to diagnose the condition.

Child abuse is also characterized by broken bones. In recent years, Americans have become increasingly aware of this problem and major efforts have been undertaken to protect children. Child abuse is a pattern of behavior that often is passed down from one generation to the next. Many abusive parents were themselves abused as children. Open, honest discussion of the issue not only can ensure the safety of countless children but can also encourage parents who wish to break the cycle of abusive behavior to seek the help they need.

### Diagnosis: OI or Child Abuse?

False accusations of child abuse may occur in families with children who have milder forms of OI and/or in whom OI has not previously been diagnosed. Types of fractures that are typically observed in both child abuse and OI include:

- fractures in multiple stages of healing

- rib fractures

- spinal fractures

- fractures for which there is no adequate explanation of trauma.

When the fracture seems incompatible with the reported cause of the injury, child abuse is often suspected. And, unfortunately, when false accusations of child abuse occur, families become victimized.

The following practical advice, together with competent legal advice from a family law attorney, is intended to help parents who have been accused of child abuse.

1.  Each state has its own policy for dealing with child abuse cases. We strongly suggest that you secure the advice and, if possible, the services of a family law attorney as soon as charges of child abuse are brought. Attorney referral services are generally offered by each state's Bar Association. If you are not satisfied with the services that your attorney is providing, don't be afraid to find another attorney to handle your case.

2.  Remember, physicians and social services case workers are doing their jobs; whoever reported the suspected child abuse to the social services authorities may be bound by law to do so. Everyone involved is concerned about what is best for the child.

3.  Seek the best medical diagnosis available. It is of utmost importance that the health care professional (including, but not limited to, an orthopedist familiar with OI) conducting the evaluation have considerable experience in both diagnosing and treating OI.

4.  A consultation with a geneticist familiar with OI may reveal a family history of mild OI if symptoms such as blue-tinted sclera (the white part of the eye), presenile hearing loss, rickets, dental problems, short stature, and/or a history of broken bones are identified.

5.  Most often, child abuse is suspected when the explanation given by the child or parent does not appear to match the injury found by the treating physicians and other medical

personnel. The decisions of the social services agency are based heavily on the medical information given to the agency by the physician.

6. Unless you advise the case worker, do not change the hospital or physicians who are providing medical services to your child. Changes made without the knowledge of the case worker may be interpreted as an attempt to hide the child abuse.

7. Keep the case worker up to date on what is happening. Attempt to confirm with the case worker that he/she understands what you have told them. Demonstrate that you truly want to work together for what is best for your child. Resistance toward the case worker may be interpreted as guilt.

8. If your child is being taken from your home, you may request that he or she be taken to the home of a grandparent or other relative.

9. When the problem is resolved, insist that the charges be taken off all records, including computerized records. If this is not done, you may be registered as an abusive parent until your youngest child is 18 years of age.

For other information about OI and child abuse, contact the Osteogenesis Imperfecta Foundation at (800) 981-2663. Please note: The OI Foundation is not able to provide legal referrals.

## *Education*

As the parent of a child with osteogenesis imperfecta (OI), you need to become familiar with the federal and state services that are available to provide your child with a free and appropriate education designed specifically to meet his or her needs. You should be aware of and take an active role in obtaining these services, which are available as soon as your child is born and continue through age 21.

### *Background*

The federal law that supports special education and related service programming for children and youth with disabilities is called the Individuals with Disabilities Education Act (IDEA). Under this law, which was originally enacted in 1975, all eligible school-aged children and youth with disabilities are entitled to receive a free appropriate public education (FAPE) in the least restrictive environment. The least restrictive environment would entitle most children with OI to be educated with non-disabled children, to the maximum extent possible, where they can benefit from the stimulation and social contact and where appropriate supportive supplementary assistance is provided when necessary. In addition to this law, amendments were passed in 1986 that include:

- provisions to help states develop early intervention programs for infants and toddlers with disabilities, and

- special funding incentives for states that make a free appropriate public education available for all eligible preschool children with disabilities ages three through five.

It is important for you to become familiar with your state special education law. The IDEA is a federal law and, as such, provides minimum requirements that states must meet to receive federal funds to assist in providing special education and related services. Your state law and regulations may go beyond the federal requirements, and it is important to know their specifics. You may want to contact your State Department of Education, Office of Special Education, and ask for a parent handbook on special education.

## *Early Intervention Services*

Early intervention services for infants and toddlers are designed to identify and treat a problem as early as possible. These services are offered through a public or private agency and are provided in different settings, such as the home, a clinic, a neighborhood daycare center, hospital, or the local health department. Often, they are provided at no cost to the family.

Each state decides which of its agencies will be the lead agency in charge of early intervention services for infants and toddlers with special needs. The first contact person in any state may be an early interventionist (an early childhood specialist working with infants and toddlers), someone with the lead agency, or someone in your state's Child Find office.

To find out who can help in your area, call the National Information Center for Children and Youth with Disabilities (NICHCY) at 1-800-695-0285 to obtain a State Resource Sheet. Explain that you want

143

to find out about early intervention services for your child and ask for a name in your area. (Be sure to keep a record of names and telephone numbers for everyone you contact.) The Resource Sheet will also list the names and contact information for support groups, parent groups, and groups concerned with specific disabilities. NICHCY also has the following brochures available: "Accessing Programs for Infants, Toddlers, and Preschoolers with Disabilities" and "Parents' Guide to Accessing Parent Programs."

You can also obtain information from your Superintendent of Schools or by getting the name of the Director of Special Education.

### *Obtaining Special Education Services for Your School-age Child*

The first step in obtaining special education services for your school-age child is to arrange for your child to receive an evaluation by the district's Committee on Special Education (CSE). This refers to the total process of gathering and using information to determine whether a child has a disability and the nature and extent of the special education and related services that the child needs. The public schools are required to conduct this evaluation of your child at no cost to you.

The evaluation process should look at the "whole child" and include information about your child's total environment. Performed by a multidisciplinary team (including two or more appropriately selected specialists, such as a school psychologist, speech/language pathologist, occupational therapist, physical therapist, medical specialist, educational diagnostician, classroom teacher, and others), the evaluation process includes observations by professionals who have worked with your child, your child's medical history, and information and observations from the family.

There are at least three ways for your child to receive an evaluation: You can request an evaluation; the school may ask permission to evaluate your child; or a teacher or doctor may suggest that your child be evaluated.

Following the evaluation, if your child is found to be eligible, the evaluation results will form the basis for developing your child's Individualized Education Program (IEP). This is a written statement of the educational program designed to meet a child's special needs. It is designed to (1) establish the learning goals for your child; and (2) state the services that the school district will provide for your child. It is developed by a multidisciplinary team that must include one teacher or other specialist who is knowledgeable about OI, along with the child's teacher(s), a representative of the school system, the parents, and the child (when appropriate).

A child's IEP should include statements of the child's strengths and weaknesses and should describe the instructional program developed specifically for him or her. This plan shows the child's current educational level, short-and long-term goals, and any special means or needs to achieve these goals. It also includes transportation and any related services your child will require. Accessible transportation, physical therapy, occupational therapy, adapted physical education, and the services of a "mobility facilitator" or "aide" are generally included for children with OI. The IEP may also call for adaptive equipment or assistive technology. As long as the equipment is used only at school, it should be provided at the district's expense, not yours. It is very important for parents to be entirely satisfied with the IEP prior to signing it as this document will direct the services your child will receive. Remember, however, that the IEP can be changed. You may request a review or revision of the IEP at any time.

If you are unable to reach agreement with the school on the placement of your child, a specific procedure is available called Due Process. This is a procedure that is guaranteed upon request if a disagreement arises concerning identification, assessment, or placement of a child. You should be notified of this process in writing when the school advises you of their recommended placement of your child.

### Tips for Parents

There are a number of things you can do to ease your child's transition into the classroom.

- Meet with your child's teachers to explain OI and provide pamphlets and brochures from the OI Foundation.

- Explain that fractures may occur and when they do, no one—including the teachers and other children—should feel that they are at fault. Emphasize that the benefits gained by the child's participation in a regular school program far outweigh the risk of a fracture, which could occur wherever the child may be. Provide a telephone number should an emergency arise, along with other instructions should a fracture occur.

- Ask the teacher to explain to the other children about your child's condition. If your child is comfortable talking about him/

herself and OI, the child could be present to hear the explanation and possibly participate in explaining or answering questions. However, if this would be embarrassing for the child, ask the teacher to talk about OI to the class when the child is not present.

- Explain to the teachers that it is best for your child to be treated the same as the other students, equally and without special favor or attention. It is most beneficial if the teachers understand the child's strengths and limitations and know that they have the full support of the parents.

- Arrange for an ambulatory child with OI to change classes a few minutes before the bell rings to prevent unnecessary physical contact in crowded halls.

- Keep a separate set of books at home for the student to use to avoid the need to carry heavy books for homework.

- Modifications can be made in the curriculum so that a child can participate in regular programs, including gym, to the fullest extent possible.

- Many schools hire a full-time aide to assist a child using a wheelchair to get around. However, once a child has reached second grade, other classmates can sometimes be enlisted to assist the student in getting around or with other activities, when appropriate.

- If your child uses special equipment to accomplish a necessary activity, you can offer to provide the same equipment for use in school.

After your child turns 16, the IEP must include mention of transition services. Transition services are defined by the IDEA as a coordinated set of activities for a student that promotes movement from school to postsecondary activities, including: education, vocational training, adult services, and independent living.

### College

In most cases, the only deterrent facing the student with OI in choosing a college is optimum accessibility of both the learning and living facilities. Many colleges and universities have support services to assist in the accommodation of students with disabilities. Personnel providing these services can often be helpful in providing information to help prospective students determine whether the college will meet their needs. A visit to any college being considered is imperative to judge the degree of accessibility.

### Additional Sources of Information

State Department of Education
Division of Special Education
State Capital

National Information Center for Children and Youth with Disabilities
P.O. Box 1492
Washington, D.C. 20013
(800) 695-0285 (Voice/TTY)
(202) 884-8200 (Voice/TTY)

ERIC Clearinghouse on Disabilities and Gifted Education Council for Exceptional Children
1920 Association Drive
Reston, VA 20191-1589 (800) 328-0272

HEATH Resource Center (National Clearinghouse on Postsecondary Education for Individuals with Disabilities)
One Dupont Circle, NW, Suite 800
Washington, D.C. 20036-1193
(800) 544-3284, (202) 939-9320

### Additional Readings

Anderson, W., Chitwood, S., & Hayden, D. (in press). *Negotiating the special education maze: A guide for parents and teachers* (3rd ed.). Bethesda, MD: Woodbine.

NICHCY (1997, Feb.). Parenting a child with special needs: A guide to reading and resources. 2nd ed., NICHCY News Digest.

# Chapter 18

# *Fibrous Dysplasia*

## Definition

Fibrous dysplasia is a chronic disorder of the skeleton that causes expansion of one or more bones due to abnormal development of fibrous tissue within the bone. The abnormality causes uneven growth, pain, brittleness, and deformity in affected bones.

Any bone can be affected by fibrous dysplasia. However, some patients have only one bone involved (monostotic), while others have numerous affected bones (polyostotic). The most common sites of disease are the femur (thigh bone), tibia (shin bone), ribs, skull, facial bones, humerus (upper arm), and pelvis. The vertebrae of the spine are less frequently involved. Although many bones can be affected at once, fibrous dysplasia is not a disease that spreads from one bone to another. Multiple affected bones are often found on one side of the body. Some individuals with fibrous dysplasia develop hormonal problems and a distinct type of skin pigmentation; this condition is referred to as McCune-Albright syndrome. Patients with fibrous dysplasia in only one bone usually do not develop this syndrome.

## Cause

The exact cause of fibrous dysplasia is not known, but recent studies indicate that it may be caused by a chemical abnormality in a protein

"Fast Facts on Fibrous Dysplasia," © 1999. Reprinted with permission of Osteoporosis And Related BoneDiseases-National Resource Center. Available at http://www.osteo.org/fibdys.htm.

in the bone which leads to an overgrowth of the cells that produce fibrous tissue. The chemical abnormality occurs because of a mutation (change) in the structure of the gene that produces the protein. Fibrous dysplasia is thought to be a congenital disorder, meaning that individuals who have it probably had it when they were born.

## Prevalence

Fibrous dysplasia is usually diagnosed in children and young adults. If the disease involves more than one bone, it is more likely to produce problems before the age of 10 years. The disease is found equally in males and females and does not appear to vary in incidence among the races. It is a very uncommon disorder; the exact incidence is not established.

## Symptoms

The most common symptoms are:

- **Bone pain**—Pain may be present as a consequence of the expanding fibrous tissue in the bone. Bone that has been sufficiently weakened by this gradual expansion may signal an impending fracture by the onset of pain. A fracture may cause a sudden increase in severe pain. Less commonly, abnormal bone could produce pain by pressing on an adjacent nerve. In patients with considerable deformity of the weight-bearing long bones (thighs and shins), arthritis can develop in the hips and knees.

- **Bone deformity**—Fibrous dysplasia bone is weaker than regular bone and is easily deformed. Because fibrous dysplasia can affect any bone, bone deformity can occur anywhere in the skeleton. However, bone deformity caused by fibrous dysplasia is most obvious when it occurs in the skull and facial bones. Fibrous dysplasia of the skull may cause loss of vision and hearing.

- **Fracture**—When a bone is affected by fibrous dysplasia, the fibrous tissue expands while the surrounding bone breaks down. As a result, although the fibrous tissue is thick, the bone becomes thin and fragile and fractures can occur, particularly in the long bones of the legs, which makes walking difficult.

## Diagnosis

The bones affected by fibrous dysplasia usually have a characteristic appearance on x-ray. When there is a doubt about the diagnosis, a doctor may obtain a small bone specimen for examination by a pathologist. In some patients, an elevation of the enzyme alkaline phosphatase is found in the blood; however, elevated alkaline phosphatase does not always mean a person has fibrous dysplasia.

## Prognosis

There is a great variability in the clinical course of the disorder. Young patients who have fibrous dysplasia in many bones may have more problems than patients with few lesions who may have mild symptoms or no symptoms at all.

Fibrous dysplasia is not usually a fatal disease. It has seldom been thought to have been the cause of death in a patient. A very small percentage of patients with fibrous dysplasia have died from a malignant bone tumor that developed in an affected bone.

## Treatment

**Surgical treatment:** Surgery is often used to treat fibrous dysplasia. In the past, radiation therapy was also used. Because of a theoretical risk of provoking malignancy, radiation should not be used. Some of the surgical procedures commonly used are:

- removal of affected bone followed by bone grafting in patients with persistent bone pain;

- removal of bone wedge with placement of nails or pins and bone grafts to correct a deformity;

- removal of bone wedge in tibia with fixation and/or bone grafts to correct a deformity.

- placement of a rod down the shaft of a bone to bridge the fibrous dysplasia lesion and thereby prevent the fracture of a weak bone.

Surgery is recommended for fibrous dysplasia to relieve intractable bone pain; to improve mobility that may be impaired due to skeletal deformity; to facilitate the healing of fractures; to relieve local pressure on the spinal cord, spinal nerves or brain; and to treat the unusual complication of bone sarcoma. The results of these surgical procedures may vary.

**Nonsurgical treatment:** Pamidronate (Aredia®) is a drug previously approved by the Food and Drug Administration for control of high blood calcium levels in patients with malignancies and for Paget's disease of bone, a disease that superficially resembles fibrous dysplasia. Preliminary studies with pamidronate suggest that some fibrous dysplasia patients may have considerable benefit from this therapy, even though it is not specifically approved for the treatment of this disease. Multiple intravenous infusions of pamidronate have been reported to relieve bone pain and improve x-rays in some patients with fibrous dysplasia. Physicians specializing in bone and mineral disorders who treat Paget's disease are likely to have the most relevant experience with pamidronate.

## Specialists in Fibrous Dysplasia

Patients with fibrous dysplasia are most often evaluated and treated by orthopedic surgeons. Craniofacial or plastic surgeons are needed to correct facial deformities, and neurosurgeons are needed for treatment of brain or spinal complications.

## Exercise

Exercise is very important in maintaining skeletal health and appropriate exercise is recommended for patients with fibrous dysplasia. It is helpful in avoiding weight gain and in maintaining mobility of the joints. Any exercise program should be carefully supervised by a physician.

## Additional Information

For more information, contact The Paget Foundation, 120 Wall Street, Suite 1602, New York, NY 10005, (voice) 212-509-5335 (fax) 212-509-8492.

ORBD–NRC is supported by the National Institute of Arthritis and Musculoskeletal and Skin Diseases, National Institutes of Health

Osteoporosis and Related Bone Diseases–National Resource Center
1150 17th St., NW, Suite 500
Washington, DC 20036
202-223-0344 or 800-624-BONE
TTY (202) 466-4315
E-Mail: orbdnrc@nof.org

# Chapter 19

# *Gaucher Disease*

### *What is Gaucher disease?*

Gaucher disease is an inherited metabolic disorder in which harmful quantities of a fatty substance called glucocerebroside accumulate in the spleen, liver, lungs, bone marrow, and, in rare cases, the brain. Three clinical forms (phenotypes) of Gaucher disease are commonly recognized. The first category, called type 1, is by far the most common. Patients in this group usually bruise easily and experience fatigue due to anemia, low blood platelets, enlargement of the liver and spleen, weakening of the skeleton, and in some instances, lung and kidney impairment. There are no signs of brain involvement. The onset of clinical manifestations may be early in life, or delayed until adulthood. The second group is classified as type 2. In this form, liver and spleen enlargement are apparent by 3 months of age. In addition, there is extensive and progressive brain damage. These patients usually die by 2 years of age. In the third category, called type 3, liver and spleen enlargement is variable, and signs of brain involvement such as seizures gradually become apparent. All of these patients exhibit a deficiency of an enzyme called glucocerebrosidase that catalyzes the first step in the biodegradation of glucocerebroside. Except for the brain, glucocerebroside arises mainly from the biodegradation of old red and white blood cells. In the brain, glucocerebroside arises

"Gaucher's Disease," National Institute of Neurological Disorders and Stroke (NINDS), reviewed June 27, 2000. Available at http://www.ninds.nih.gov.

from the turnover of complex lipids during brain development and the formation of the myelin sheath of nerves.

### Is there any treatment?

Highly effective enzyme replacement therapy is available for patients with type 1 Gaucher disease. This therapy decreases liver and spleen size, reduces skeletal abnormalities, and successfully reverses other manifestations of the disorder including abnormal blood counts. There is currently no effective treatment for severe brain damage that may occur in patients with types 2 and 3.

### What is the prognosis?

There is no permanent cure for Gaucher disease. The majority of individuals with this disorder need enzyme replacement therapy.

### What research is being done?

The NINDS is currently conducting a study to examine the skeletal response to enzyme replacement therapy in patients with type 1 whose spleens have been removed and its effect in patients with type 3 Gaucher disease. NINDS will conduct an enzyme therapy trial in patients with type 2 Gaucher disease.

## Selected References

Metabolism of Glucocerebrosides. II. Evidence of an Enzymatic Deficiency in Gaucher's Disease, *Biochemistry and Biophysical Research Communications*, 18; 221-225 (1965)

Replacement Therapy for Inherited Enzyme Deficiency—Macrophage-targeted Glucocerebrosidase for Gaucher's Disease, *The New England Journal of Medicine*, 324:21; 1464-1470 (1991)

Enzyme Replacement Therapy for Gaucher's Disease: Skeletal Responses to Macrophage-Targeted Glucocerebrosidase, *Pediatrics*, 96; 629-637 (1995)

Gaucher Disease Chapter 86 in *The Metabolic and Molecular Bases of Inherited Disease*, 7th edition, McGraw-Hill, Inc. New York, pp 2641-2670 (1995)

NIH Technology Assessment Panel on Gaucher Disease Gaucher Disease—Current Issues in Diagnosis and Treatment, *The*

*Journal of the American Medical Association*, 275:7; 548-553 (February 21, 1996)

Prospective study of neurological responses to treatment with macrophage-targeted glucocerebrosidase in patients with type 3 Gaucher disease *Annals of Neurology*, 42; 613-621 (1997)

## Organizations

### National Gaucher Foundation
11140 Rockville Pike, Suite 350
Rockville MD 20852-3106
E-mail: ngf@gaucherdisease.org
Tel: 301-816-1515
Toll Free: 800-GAUCHER (428-2437)
Fax: 301-816-1516

### National Organization for Rare Disorders (NORD)
P.O. Box 8923
(100 Route 37)
Fairfield CT 06812-8923
E-mail: orphan@rarediseases.org
Tel: 203-746-6518
Toll-Free: 800-999-NORD (-6673)
Fax: 203-746-6481

### National Tay-Sachs and Allied Diseases Association
2001 Beacon Street, Suite 204
Brookline MA 02146
E-mail: NTSAD-boston@worldnet.att.net
Tel: 617-277-4463
Toll Free: 800-90-NTSAD (906-8723)
Fax: 617-277-0134

# Chapter 20

# *Hypophosphatasia*

## *Definition*

Hypophosphatasia is an inherited metabolic (chemical) bone disease that results from low levels of an enzyme called alkaline phosphatase (ALP). Enzymes are proteins that act in the body's chemical reactions by breaking down other chemicals. ALP is normally present in large amounts in bone and liver. In hypophosphatasia, abnormalities in the gene that makes ALP lead to production of inactive ALP. Subsequently, several chemicals—including phosphoethanolamine, pyridoxal 5'-phosphate (a form of vitamin B6) and inorganic pyrophosphate—accumulate in the body and are found in large amounts in the blood and urine. It appears that the accumulation of inorganic pyrophosphate is the cause of the characteristic defective calcification of bones in infants and children (rickets) and in adults(osteomalacia).

Nevertheless, the severity of hypophosphatasia is remarkably variable from patient-to-patient. The most severely affected fail to form a skeleton in the womb and are stillborn. The most mildly affected patients may show only low levels of ALP in the blood, yet never suffer bony problems.

In general, patients are categorized as having "perinatal," "childhood" or "adult" hypophosphatasia depending on the severity of the disease which in turn is reflected by the age at which bony manifestations are first detected. Odontohypophosphatasia refers to children and adults who have only dental, but not skeletal, problems (premature loss of teeth).

The x-ray changes are quite distinct to the trained eye. Similarly, the diagnosis of hypophosphatasia is largely substantiated by measuring ALP in the blood (a routine test) that is low in hypophosphatasia. However, it is important that the doctors use appropriate age ranges for normals when interpreting an ALP level.

## Prevalence

It has been estimated that severe forms of hypophosphatasia occur in approximately one per 100,000 live births. The more mild childhood and adult forms are probably somewhat more common. About one out of every 200 individuals in the United States may be a carrier for hypophosphatasia

## Prognosis

The outcome following a diagnosis of hypophosphatasia is very variable. In general, the earlier the diagnosis is made the more severe the skeletal manifestations. Cases detected in the womb or with severe deformity at birth almost always have a lethal outcome within days or weeks. When the diagnosis is made before six months of age, some infants have a downhill and fatal course, others survive and may even do well. When diagnosed during childhood, there can by presence or absence of skeletal deformity from underlying rickets, but premature loss of teeth (less than five years of age) is the most common manifestation. Adults may be troubled by recurrent fractures in their feet and painful, partial fractures in their thigh bones.

## Symptoms

Depending on the severity of the skeletal disease, there may be deformity of the limbs and chest. Pneumonia can result if chest distortion is severe. Recurrent fractures can occur. Teeth may be lost prematurely, have wide pulp (inside) chambers, and thereby be predisposed to cavities.

## Inheritance Factors

The severe perinatal and infantile forms of hypophosphatasia are inherited as autosomal recessive conditions. The patient receives one defective gene from each parent. Some more mild (childhood or adult) hypophosphatasia cases are also inherited this way. Other mild adult and odontohypophosphatasia cases seem to be inherited in an autosomal dominant pattern (the patient gets just one defective gene, not two, transmitted from one of his/her parents). In this form, mild hypophosphatasia can occur from generation-to-generation. The perinatal form of hypophosphatasia can often be detected during pregnancy by ultrasound and by measuring ALP activity in chorionic villus samples from amniocentesis.

Individuals with hypophosphatasia and parents of children with hypophosphatasia are encouraged to seek genetic counseling to explain the likelihood and severity of hypophosphatasia recurring in their families.

## Treatments

As yet, there is no cure for hypophosphatasia and no proven medical therapy. Some medications are being evaluated. Treatment is generally directed towards preventing or correcting the symptoms or complications.

Expert dental care and physical therapy are recommended. An orthopaedic procedure called "rodding" may be especially helpful for adults with painful partial fractures in their thigh bones. Severely affected infants may manifest increased levels of calcium in their blood that may be treated with calcitonin and certain diuretics. Doctors should avoid the temptation to give calcium supplements or vitamin D unless there is clear-cut deficiency.

*−by Michael P. Whyte, M.D., Medical Director,*
*Metabolic Research Unit,*
*Shriners Hospital,*
*St. Louis, Missouri.*

### The Magic Foundation for Children's Growth

This article is for informational purposes only. Neither the MAGIC Foundation nor the contributing medical specialists assumes any liability for its content. Consult you physician for diagnosis and treatment.

The MAGIC Foundation is a national nonprofit organization created to provide support services for the families of children afflicted with a wide variety of chronic and/or critical disorders, syndromes and diseases that affect a child's growth. Some of the diagnoses are quite common while others are very rare.

**MAGIC Foundation**
1327 N. Harlem Avenue
Oak Park, IL 60303
Tel: 708-383-0808
Fax: 708-383-0899
Website: http://www.magicfoundation.org

# Chapter 21

# *Myeloma Bone Disease*

Myeloma means, literally, a "tumor composed of cells normally found in bone marrow." The majority of patients with myeloma develop destructive bone lesions, also known as osteolytic bone lesions. These lesions occur primarily in the vertebrae, the ribs, the pelvis, and the skull. They occur in the red bone marrow where nests of myeloma cells accumulate. Myeloma cells do not have a direct effect on the skeleton; rather, they cause bone destruction by producing signals that activate normal osteoclasts to resorb bone. Why this occurs is not clearly understood. There is currently, however, a large amount of research directed at understanding the mechanisms by which bone is destroyed by myeloma cells.

The skeletal lesions that occur in myeloma not only result in pain, pathological fractures, and hypercalcemia, but sometimes deformity and occasionally nerve compression syndromes. The lesions occur most commonly in the vertebrae. The appearance of the vertebral spine may resemble osteoporosis radiologically although the histologic abnormalities are quite different.

## Incidence

The incidence of myeloma is 3-4/100,000 in the U.S., which translates into approximately 13,500 new cases of myeloma in the U.S. each year. Myeloma is more common in blacks than whites, and the male/female ratio is 3:2. The incidence varies from country to country, with a higher incidence found in most Western industrialized countries. Over the past 30 years there has been a 400 percent increase in the incidence of the disease. This apparent increase is probably due to better diagnostic techniques and the higher average age of the general population. However, more frequent myeloma in patients under age 55 may indicate environmental causative factors over the past three decades.

## Clinical Symptoms

Approximately 70 percent of myeloma patients experience pain of varying intensity, often in the lower back. Sudden severe pain can be a sign of fracture or collapse of a vertebra. Patients also have general malaise and vague complaints. Hypercalcemia (too much calcium in the blood), which is present in 30 percent of patients, can cause tiredness, thirst, and nausea, and usually occurs when a patient has impaired kidney function.

## Treatment

It is not yet possible to cure myeloma, although it is possible to improve the clinical status and the survival in patients through the use of chemotherapy, alpha interferon and, possibly, bone marrow transplants.

For myeloma patients with hypercalcemia, the goal is to treat the hypercalcemia and its potentially dangerous complications. In these patients, hypercalcemia is always associated with increased bone resorption and frequently with impaired kidney function. The best approach is to treat the myeloma itself and to treat the hypercalcemia with drugs that inhibit bone resorption, such as bisphosphonates, and the careful use of intravenous fluids. Bisphosphonates have been very effective in the treatment of hypercalcemia of myeloma.

The more common situation is the patient with myeloma bone disease who does not have hypercalcemia. Until recently, these patients have been treated for the bone disease with symptomatic therapy, namely: analgesics for pain, orthopedic treatment for fractures, or local radiation therapy for localized bone pain. Recent studies have indicated that potent bisphosphonates, such as pamidronate and clodronate, may have beneficial effects in patients with myeloma. In some patients, pain is reduced, the need for analgesics is less, episodes of fracture and hypercalcemia are reduced, and the need for radiation therapy for bone pain is lessened. As a consequence, pamidronate has received FDA approval in the U.S. for treatment of not just hypercalcemia in myeloma, but also myeloma bone disease in the absence of hypercalcemia. Further studies are ongoing to determine the effects of bisphosphonates on survival of patients, the ideal dose and duration, and whether other new and more potent bisphosphonates have similar beneficial effects. One important and unanswered question is whether bisphosphonates should be used in patients who do not as yet have symptoms or evidence of bone disease.

Other points are important in the management of patients with myeloma bone disease. These include the management of severe bone pain and the avoidance of fractures. Patients with severe pain that is localized often do well with a course of local radiation therapy, particularly when the bone disease is localized in the vertebral spine. Analgesic use is warranted as needed for severe bone pain. Patients will do best when they have an understanding of their bone disease and what activities put them at risk for further complications. The same principles that apply to patients with osteoporosis also apply to those with myeloma bone disease. Patients should avoid those lifestyle situations that are potentially dangerous (e.g., climbing ladders or slipping on ice or loose bathroom rugs).

## Organizational Resources

The International Myeloma Foundation (IMF), founded in 1990, is dedicated to improving the quality of life for multiple myeloma patients and, ultimately, to preventing and curing myeloma. IMF focuses on patients with multiple myeloma and their family members as well as physicians and health professionals with specific clinical or research interests in myeloma. IMF holds educational conferences for both patients and physicians. The IMF can be contacted at 2120 Stanley Hills Drive, Los Angeles, CA 90046, (800) 452-CURE, <http://www.myeloma.org/imfis.html>.

The Osteoporosis and Related Bone Diseases—National Resource Center (NIH ORBD—NRC) also has fact sheets on coping with fractures and pain as well as general information on treatment with bisphosphonates. For patients in the United Kingdom, similar information is available from the National Osteoporosis Society, Radstock, Bath.

This information was obtained from:

Mundy, G.R. Myeloma bone disease. *Myeloma Today,* September-October 1995.

Durie, B.G.M. "Multiple myeloma: A concise review of the disease and treatment options." Dr. Durie is the director of Research and Myeloma Programs for the Intercenter Cancer Research Group, Cedars-Sinai Comprehensive Cancer Center, Los Angeles, CA.

National Institutes of Health
Osteoporosis and Related Bone Diseases–National Resource Center
1150 17th St., NW, Suite 500
Washington, D.C. 20036
202-223-0344 or 800-624-BONE
Fax: (202) 223-2237
TTY: (202) 466-4315
E-Mail: orbdnrc@nof.org

The Osteoporosis and Related Bone Diseases–National Resource Center is supported by the National Institute of Arthritis and Musculoskeletal and Skin Diseases, with contributions from the National Institute of Child Health and Human Development, National Institute of Dental and Craniofacial Research, National Institute of Environmental Health Sciences, NIH Office of Research on Women's Health, Office of Women's Health, PHS, and the National Institute on Aging.

# Chapter 22

# *Paget's Disease of Bone*

## Definition

Paget's disease of bone is a chronic disorder that typically results in enlarged and deformed bones in one or more regions of the skeleton. Excessive bone breakdown and formation cause the bone to be dense but fragile. As a result, bone pain, arthritis, noticeable deformities, and fractures can occur.

## Causes

The cause of Paget's disease is unknown. Recent studies, however, have suggested that the disease may be caused by a "slow viral" infection of bone, a condition that is present for many years before symptoms appear. In addition, there is also a hereditary factor, since the disease may appear in more than one member of a family. The hereditary factor may lead to susceptibility among family members to the suspected viral infection.

## Prevalence

Paget's disease is most common in Caucasian people of European descent, but it also occurs in African-Americans. It is rare in those of

"Paget's Disease of Bone," © March 1997. Reprinted with permission of Osteoporosis and Related Bone Diseases–National Resource Center. Available at http://www.osteo.org/paget.htm.

Asian descent. Paget's disease is rarely diagnosed in people under 40 but may occur in up to 3 percent of the American population over 60. Both men and women are affected.

## Symptoms

Bone pain is the most common symptom. The pain may occur in any bone affected by Paget's disease and often localizes to areas adjacent to the joints (e.g., hip pain may occur when the pelvis or thigh bone is involved). Headaches and hearing loss may occur when Paget's disease affects the skull. Pressure on nerves may also occur when the skull or spine is affected. Deformities of bone, such as an increase in head size, bowing of a limb, or curvature of the spine, may occur in advanced cases. These deformities are due to enlargement or softening of the affected bones.

Although Pagetic lesions may occur in multiple sites, it does not spread from bone to bone. When it is in the hip, however, damage to the cartilage of joints adjacent to the affected bone may lead to arthritis. Pagetic bone is susceptible to fractures with even moderate stress.

## Diagnosis

Bones affected with Paget's disease have a characteristic appearance on x-rays. Sometimes, the patient's doctor is alerted to the possibility of Paget's disease when a blood test reveals an elevated level of alkaline phosphatase. In this case, more specific tests, such as the bone-specific alkaline phosphatase test, x-rays, and bone scans, are done. After the age of 40, siblings and children of someone with Paget's disease may wish to have a standard alkaline phosphatase blood test every two or three years.

## Hearing Loss in Paget's Disease

When Paget's disease affects the skull and the temporal bone (the bone that surrounds the inner ear), severe and progressive loss of hearing may occur. This may involve both sides or one side predominantly. If the loss of hearing is progressive and due to Paget's disease, treating the underlying Paget's disease may slow or stop the progression of the hearing loss. Hearing aids may sometimes be helpful.

## Exercise

Exercise is very important in maintaining skeletal health and is recommended for some patients with Paget's disease. Before beginning any exercise program, it is wise to discuss the program with your physician, since undue stress on affected bones should be avoided. Exercise is also helpful in avoiding weight gain that may put additional stress on the bones and in maintaining the mobility of the joints.

## Medical Treatment

Two classes of drugs are approved by the FDA for the treatment of this disease. Both classes of drugs suppress the abnormal bone remodeling that is associated with Paget's disease:

**Bisphosphonates.** Bisphosphonates are drugs that inhibit abnormal bone resorption. Three bisphosphonates are approved in the U.S. for treatment of Paget's disease:

- **Alendronate sodium (Fosamax®)**, which is given in tablet form;

- **Etidronate disodium (Didronel®)**, which is also given in tablet form; and

- **Pamidronate disodium (Aredia®),** which is given intravenously.

**Calcitonin.** Calcitonin is a hormone secreted by the thyroid gland that also inhibits abnormal bone resorption. Synthetic salmon calcitonin is taken by injection; the brand names for this drug are **Calcimar®, Miacalcin®**, and **Osteocalcin®**. At this time, **Cibacalcin®** (synthetic human calcitonin), which is another drug approved by the FDA for treating Paget's disease, can only be obtained if a physician requests it directly from the manufacturer.

Talk to your physician about the treatment that is most appropriate for you.

## Surgical Treatment

There are generally three major complications of Paget's disease for which surgery may be recommended. The first complication occurs when Pagetic bone fractures. Surgical fixation of Pagetic fractures may allow the fracture to heal in better position. The second complication occurs when the patient develops severe degenerative arthritis. If medication and physical therapy are no longer helpful, and if disability is severe, surgery may be considered as an option. Total joint replacement of the hips and knees should be reserved for the most severe cases of arthritis, when other methods of treatment are no longer effective. The third situation involves bone deformity, especially of the tibia. The surgical cutting and realignment of a Pagetic bone may help painful weight-bearing joints, especially the knees. Medical therapy prior to surgery is recommended to decrease bleeding during surgery and to prevent other complications during and after surgery.

## Quality of Life

Some of the same issues that affect patients with osteoporosis and other chronic disorders affect patients with Paget's disease. There has, however, been little research on the impact of Paget's disease on quality of life. A study by Dr. Deborah Gold et al. that was published in the *Journal of Bone and Mineral Research* entitled "Paget's Disease of Bone and Quality of Life" (vol. 11, no. 12, pp. 1897-1903) addressed the psychological, social, and physical consequences of Paget's disease as well as the impact they had on quality of life. This study was based on previous studies of patients with another prevalent chronic skeletal disorder—osteoporosis—because many of the physical consequences of these two disorders are similar.

Results of the study suggest that a substantial portion of the individual's perception of quality of life depends on his or her physical condition and disease state. The greater the illness-related problems, the worse the quality of life. Income and education enhanced self-reported quality of life as did excellent self-rated health and health that had improved from five years previous. From this study, the researchers concluded that Paget's disease of bone affects the psychological functioning of its sufferers considerably, and this finding may have an impact on treatment of Paget patients. If physicians and other health care professionals are aware of the likelihood of psychological issues, they may tailor treatment plans to include psychological outcomes, which may ultimately improve quality of life for patients with Paget's disease of bone.

## Specialists in Paget's Disease

Endocrinologists (physicians that specialize in hormonal and metabolic disorders) and rheumatologists (physicians that specialize in joint and muscle disorders) are internists that are generally knowledgeable about treating Paget's disease. Also, orthopedic surgeons, otolaryngologists (physicians that specialize in ear, nose, and throat disorders) and neurologists may be called upon to evaluate specialized symptoms in Paget's disease.

## Addtitional Information

For more information, contact:

The Paget Foundation
120 Wall Street, Suite 1602
New York, NY 10005
(voice) 212-509-5335
(fax) 212-509-8492

ORBD–NRC is supported by the National Institute of Arthritis and Musculoskeletal and Skin Diseases, National Institutes of Health

Osteoporosis and Related Bone Diseases–National Resource Center
1150 17th St., NW, Suite 500
Washington, DC 20036
202-223-0344 or 800-624-BONE
TTY (202) 466-4315
E-Mail: orbdnrc@nof.org

# Chapter 23

# *Hearing Loss and Bone Disorders*

For people with metabolic bone disorders such as Paget's disease of bone or osteogenesis imperfecta, hearing loss is an often overlooked yet serious handicap. To understand the nature of hearing loss in individuals with metabolic bone disorders, it is important to first understand the basic mechanism of hearing.

## *Anatomy of the Ear*

The ear is divided into three sections: the external, middle, and inner ear (see Figure 23.1). The external ear includes the outer ear and the ear canal, at the end of which is the ear drum. Behind the ear drum is a small chamber called the middle ear. The middle ear contains three tiny bones (the incus, the malleus, and the stapes) that connect the ear drum and the inner ear; they act in series to transmit airborne sound through the middle ear to the cochlea in the inner ear. Once the sound (or vibration) reaches the cochlea, it is converted into nerve impulses and transmitted by the auditory nerve to the brain, where it is interpreted. A person with a hearing impairment might have a problem in the middle ear, inner ear, auditory nerve, brain, or in more than one of these areas.

© August 1996. Reprinted with permission of Osteoporosis and Related Bone Diseases–National Resource Center. Available at http://www.osteo.org/hear.htm.

## Types of Hearing Loss

The three primary types of hearing impairment are: conductive, sensorineural, or mixed. When hearing loss is caused by a physical problem in the external ear or in the middle ear, it is referred to as a conductive hearing loss. Sensorineural hearing loss occurs when a sound is conducted normally from the exterior ear through the eardrum to the middle ear, but the inner ear does not transmit the sound normally to the brain. When the middle ear and the inner ear are involved, the hearing loss is referred to as a mixed hearing loss. Hearing loss is also classified according to degree of severity—mild, moderate, severe, or profound—and according to whether the hearing loss affects low, high, or all frequencies of sound.

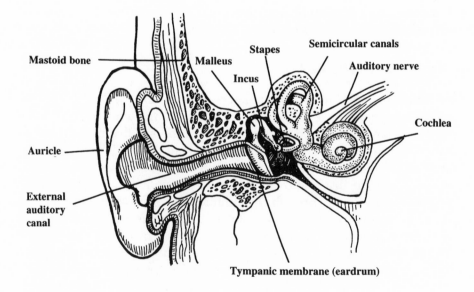

**Figure 23.1.** *Anatomy of the Ear*

*(From Edwin M. Monsell, M.D., Ph.D., Head, Division of Otology and Neurotology, Department of Otolaryngology–Head and Neck Surgery, Henry Ford Hospital, Detroit, MI. Reproduced by permission)*

## Hearing Loss in Osteogenesis Imperfecta

As many as 50 percent of people with osteogenesis imperfecta (OI) experience hearing loss beginning early in adulthood. It generally appears as a conductive loss in the late teens or twenties due to problems with the small bones in the middle ear. They may be fragile or malformed, or the footplate of the stapes may become fixed and rigid and no longer capable of transmitting sound effectively to the inner ear. Changes can also be also observed in other areas of the middle and inner ear. A sensorineural (nerve) loss may also develop. There is much variation in the severity of the hearing loss; some people may be deaf in old age, while others may be hard of hearing. Some people with OI never develop significant hearing problems.

## Management

It is recommended that any child with OI, and especially those who demonstrate speech problems, speech delay, or recurrent ear infections, should undergo a formal audiologic assessment. Young adults should have baseline assessment for later comparison, and adults experiencing tinnitus (ringing), often an early symptom of a fixed stapes, should undergo audiologic assessment. For either conductive, sensorineural, or mixed hearing loss, hearing aids that provide adequate amplification can help individuals of all ages.

Individuals with conductive loss that is severe and progressive may be helped with a surgical procedure known as a stapedectomy. In this procedure, the fixed foot process of the stapes is replaced by a prosthesis that allows for the normal propagation of sound waves to the inner ear. It should be noted, however, that this surgery should not be considered routine in OI because of tissue fragility. There are also many other pre- and post-operative issues that need to be assessed, discussed, and clarified before any individual with OI may be considered a "good candidate" for surgery. As a general rule, patients should seek treatment centers where the otologists (doctors with a subspecialty in ear disorders) have considerable experience with stapes surgery.

## Hearing Loss in Paget's Disease of Bone

Although many people lose some degree of hearing as part of the aging process, individuals with Paget's disease are more likely than other people the same age to have a hearing loss. Research studies have shown that Paget's disease causes hearing loss when the temporal bone is involved (i.e., the bone surrounding the inner ear), and this hearing loss is usually not due to compression or other effects on the auditory nerve. Paget's disease affects the cochlea, the coiled structure of the inner ear that converts sound vibration into nerve impulses. A change in the bone density of the cochlear capsule has also been observed in patients with Paget's disease who have a hearing loss, and this change may be associated with hearing loss in Paget's. When the temporal bone is involved, a more severe and progressive hearing loss may occur that may involve both sides or one side predominantly.

The type of hearing loss in Paget's disease may be conductive, sensorineural, or both. Some causes of the conductive component of the hearing loss may be correctable through surgery; however, this type of surgery has been found overall to be less effective than it is when the cause is other than Paget's disease.

## Management

If a hearing loss is progressive and is due to Paget's disease, treating the underlying Paget's disease may slow the progression of the hearing loss. Any loss of hearing should be investigated as a medical condition because it may be due to serious or correctable problems such as perforation of the eardrum, infection, or even tumor in rare cases. It is especially important to investigate the cause of hearing loss when it involves one side more than the other because the presence of a tumor is more likely.

It is recommended that persons with Paget's disease and hearing loss, or with Paget's disease involving the skull, undergo a baseline hearing test and evaluation by an ear, nose, and throat specialist or an otologist. The doctor may also want to study the temporal bone with special tests to determine whether Paget's disease is present in the ear.

Hearing loss can cause individuals to miss important communications and to withdraw from full participation in life. Even if hearing loss cannot be corrected with medication or surgery, most hearing loss can be overcome with a hearing aid. Other devices may be used along with hearing aids and are available through hearing aid specialists and ear, nose, and throat doctors.

## Additional Resources

There are many organizations that can be contacted for information about hearing devices and available services. Some of these are:

### American Academy of Otolaryngology–Head and Neck Surgery (AAO–HNS)
1 Prince Street
Alexandria, VA 22314
703-836-4444

The AAO-HNS is the not-for-profit professional, educational, and research association for ear, nose, and throat specialists. They have fact sheets on hearing loss and can also provide patients with a list of specialists.

### American Speech-Language-Hearing Association (ASHA)
10801 Rockville Pike
Rockville, MD 20852
888-321-ASHA

ASHA is the national professional, scientific, and credentialing association for speech-language pathologists and audiologists. Part of its mission is to ensure that individuals with hearing disorders have access to high quality services to help them communicate more effectively. A toll-free HELPLINE is available for those seeking information. ASHA can also provide a list of certified audiologists.

### National Institute on Deafness and Other Communication Disorders (NIDCD) Clearinghouse
31 Center Drive, MSC 2320
Bethesda, MD 20892-2320
301-496-7343

The NIDCD Clearinghouse is a national resource center for information about the normal and disordered mechanisms of hearing, balance, smell, taste, voice, speech, and language. It provides an information service to respond to professional and public inquiries; develops and distributes publications such as fact sheets, bibliographies, information packets, and organization directories; and maintains a database of references to journal articles, books, audiovisual materials, brochures, facts sheets, and other educational materials.

### Self-Help for Hard of Hearing People, Inc. (SHHH)
7910 Woodmont Avenue, Suite 1200
Bethesda, MD 20814
(301) 657-2248

SHHH is a national self-help organization for those who are hard of hearing. SHHH can help with information on coping with hearing loss. ORBD—NRC is supported by the National Institute of Arthritis and Musculoskeletal and Skin Diseases, National Institutes of Health

### *ORBD Osteoporosis and Related Bone Diseases–National Resource Center*
1232 22nd St., NW,
Washington, D.C. 20037-1292
202-223-0344 or 800-624-BONE
TTY (202) 466-4315
E-Mail: orbdnrc@nof.org

# Chapter 24

# *Osteopetrosis*

One of the less common metabolic bone disorders is osteopetrosis. Osteopetrosis is an inherited disease caused by a defect in bone resorption—the process in which old bone is broken down and removed so that new bone can be added to the skeleton. Osteoclasts are the cells responsible for bone resorption. In osteopetrosis the osteoclasts do not perform normally, either because there are too few of them or because they are ineffective in removing bone. This flaw in bone resorption results in bones that are abnormally dense, yet are easily broken. Men and women are equally affected by the disease.

The increased bone mass in individuals with osteopetrosis can limit the amount of available bone marrow space. Since the bone marrow is responsible for the production of blood cells, impaired bone marrow function can produce several clinical problems. For example, interference with red blood cell production can lead to anemia. Impairment of white blood cell production can limit the body's ability to fight infection. When platelet production is suppressed, individuals are prone to bleeding since platelets are essential for clotting blood. Anemia, infection, and bleeding are just some of the symptoms that individuals with osteopetrosis can experience—blindness, deafness and even stroke can occur when the skeleton is so dense that blood vessels and nerves cannot pass through the bones.

Three major types of osteopetrosis have been identified in humans:

From *ORBD—NRC News* Vol. III, No. 7; May 12, 1997. © 1997. Reprinted with permission of Osteoporosis and Related Bone Diseases–National Resource Center. Available at http://www.osteo.org/understand.htm.

**Malignant infantile form.** This type of osteopetrosis is usually discovered in the first months of life. In addition to having many of the above symptoms of the disease, children with this condition often have significant delays in psychomotor and tooth development. The malignant infantile form of the disease can be severe and frequently results in death from infection or bleeding. In fact, 30 percent of children with this form of the disease will die during the first ten years of life. This form of the disease is inherited as an autosomal recessive trait—thereby affecting some brothers and sisters.

**Adult form.** The adult form of osteopetrosis is milder than the infantile form. This type of the disease is benign and generally does not alter life expectancy. Many of the individuals with the adult form of osteopetrosis have few or no symptoms. It is inherited from generation to generation as an autosomal dominant trait.

**Intermediate form.** This type of the disease is found in children younger than ten years of age. It tends to be less severe than the malignant infantile form, but more severe than the adult form. Individuals with this type of osteopetrosis generally do not have a reduced life expectancy.

The diagnosis of osteopetrosis is usually made when dense bones are discovered on x-rays. A bone biopsy can confirm the presence of the disease, while supplemental tests are usually performed to evaluate any potential complications. Confirming the specific subtype of the disease is important so that individuals can receive the most appropriate treatment.

Various therapies have been used in the treatment of osteopetrosis. Bone marrow transplantation (BMT) allows the abnormal osteoclasts to be replaced with normal cells. BMT is the only approach that has resulted in a cure of the malignant infantile form of the disease. Because of its high failure rate and because of its side-effects, BMT tends to be reserved for only the most severe cases of osteopetrosis. According to The Paget Foundation, survival rates after BMT in children with osteopetrosis range from 40-70 percent.

High doses of calcitrol (the active form of vitamin D) have been used to stimulate osteoclast function in individuals with osteopetrosis. Calcitrol has been shown to significantly reduce symptoms in people who have mild or severe forms of the disease, though it is not approved by the Food and Drug Administration for this purpose. Similarly, experimental use of interferon gamma 1-b treatment has been reported to decrease infection rate and improve blood abnormalities in severely affected patients. Another type of medication that may be used to treat patients with osteopetrosis are glucocorticoids. Large doses of glucocorticoid drugs (such as prednisone) may be given for short periods of time to patients with impaired red blood cell or platelet production.

Research efforts are underway in an attempt to identify the gene defects that cause osteopetrosis.

Two documents on osteopetrosis have recently been developed by the Resource Center and the Paget Foundation: a patient information brochure and an annotated bibliography for professionals. For further information on these educational resources, please contact the NIH ORBD–NRC at 202-223-0344.

National Institutes of Health
Osteoporosis and Related Bone Diseases–National Resource Center
1150 17th St., NW, Suite 500
Washington, DC 20036
202-223-0344 or 800-624-BONE
Fax (202) 223-2237
TTY (202) 466-4315
E-Mail: orbdnrc@nof.org

The Osteoporosis and Related Bone Diseases–National Resource Center is supported by the National Institute of Arthritis and Musculoskeletal and Skin Diseases, with contributions from the National Institute of Child Health and Human Development, National Institute of Dental and Craniofacial Research, National Institute of Environmental Health Sciences, NIH Office of Research on Women's Health, Office of Women's Health, PHS, and the National Institute on Aging.
The Resource Center is operated by the National Osteoporosis Foundation, in collaboration with The Paget Foundation and the Osteogenesis Imperfecta Foundation.

Chapter 25

# *Hypercalcemia*

**Important:** *This information is intended for use by doctors and other health care professionals. If you are a cancer patient, your doctor can explain how it applies to you, or you can call the Cancer Information Service at **1-800-422-6237**.*

## *Overview*

Hypercalcemia is the most common life-threatening metabolic disorder associated with neoplastic diseases, occurring in an estimated 10 percent-20 percent of all persons with cancer. Carcinomas of the breast, lung, head and neck, kidney, and certain hematologic malignancies, particularly multiple myeloma, are most frequently associated with hypercalcemia.[1] Although early diagnosis followed by hydration and treatment with agents that decrease serum calcium concentrations (hypocalcemic drugs) can produce symptomatic improvements within a few days, diagnosis may be complicated because symptoms may be insidious at onset and can be confused with those of many malignant and nonmalignant diseases. It should be emphasized, however, that diagnosis and timely interventions are not only lifesaving in the short term but may enhance patients' compliance with primary and supportive treatments and may improve quality of life.[2]

---

National Cancer Institute (NCI) PDQ Statement, May 1998. Available at http://cancernet.nci.nih.gov/clinpdq/supportive/Hypercalcemia_Physician.html.

## Laboratory Assessment

Normal serum calcium levels are maintained within narrow and constant limits, approximately 9.0-10.3 mg/dL (= 4.5-5.2 mEq/L or 2.25-2.57 mmol/L) for men and 8.9-10.2 mg/dL (= 4.4-5.1 mEq/L or 2.22-2.54 mmol/L) for women. Hypercalcemia exists when the serum calcium level exceeds 11.0 mg/dL (>5.5 mEq/L or 2.74 mmol/L).

Specific numerical criteria for normal serum calcium concentrations vary between institutions; however, therapeutic intervention is considered urgent for symptomatic patients and for those with serum calcium concentrations greater than 12.0 mg/dL (>6.0 mEq/L or 2.99 mmol/L).[3] To optimally assess serum calcium, it is crucial to correct patients' measured total calcium values for coexisting hypoalbuminemia (i.e., serum albumin <4 g/dL).

### Correction of Serum Calcium Level in Patients with Concurrently Low Albumin[3]

For each gram per deciliter decrease in serum albumin (<4.0 g/dL) serum calcium concentrations are corrected by adding 0.8 mg/dL (or 0.4 mEq/dL or 0.2 mmol/L, depending on the units in which calcium is reported) to the measured serum calcium value.

Correct serum calcium concentrations in hypoalbuminemia by adding the following values to patients' measured serum calcium (select the equation appropriate for units reported by your laboratory):

- (Calcium in mg/dL) = (base albumin concentration [4.0 mg/dL]— measured serum albumin concentration [g/dL]) x 0.8 mg/dL

- (Calcium in mEq/L) = (base albumin concentration [4.0 mg/dL]— measured serum albumin concentration [g/dL]) x 0.4 mEq/L

- (Calcium in mmol/L) = (base albumin concentration [4.0 mg/dL]—measured serum albumin concentration [g/dL]) x 0.2 mmol/L

## Normal Calcium Homeostasis

### Hormonal Influences

Although calcium homeostasis is maintained by two hormones, parathormone (parathyroid hormone or PTH) and calcitriol (1,25-dihydroxy vitamin D), minute- to-minute regulation of serum ionized calcium is regulated by PTH. PTH secretion is stimulated when ambient serum ionized calcium is decreased. PTH acts on peripheral target cell receptors, increasing the efficiency of renal tubular calcium reabsorption. In addition, PTH enhances calcium resorption from mineralized bone and stimulates conversion of vitamin D to its active form, calcitriol, which subsequently increases dietary calcium absorption.

In healthy persons, vitamin D-mediated daily dietary calcium intake approximates the amount of calcium excreted in urine, feces, and sweat. In hypercalcemia of malignancy, calcitriol concentrations and intestinal calcium absorption are generally suppressed, therefore, "humoral hypercalcemia" is most frequently due to aberrant mediators such as parathyroid hormone-related protein (PTHrP; see "Mechanisms of cancer-associated hypercalcemia," below).[4,5] In contrast, circulating vitamin D metabolite concentrations may be increased in some hematologic tumors (e.g., lymphomas), thereby, enhancing intestinal calcium absorption and causing or exacerbating hypercalcemia.[6]

*Renal Function*

Normal healthy kidneys are capable of filtering large amounts of calcium that are subsequently reclaimed by tubular reabsorption. The kidneys are capable of increasing calcium excretion by nearly fivefold to maintain homeostatic serum calcium concentrations. However, hypercalcemia may occur when the concentration of calcium present in the extracellular fluid overwhelms the kidneys' compensatory mechanisms.

Although calcium reabsorption is linked to sodium and fluid reabsorption in the proximal renal tubules, fine regulation occurs in the distal renal tubules primarily under the influence of PTH. Tumors that are capable of producing a substance similar to normal PTH such as PTH-related peptide (see "Mechanisms of cancer-associated hypercalcemia," below) drive the renal tubules to increase calcium reabsorption. Under these circumstances, hypercalcemia and high calcium concentrations in urine (hypercalciuria) impair sodium and water reabsorption, causing polyuria (a "calcium diuresis") with subsequent loss of circulating fluid volume (dehydration). As a consequence of dehydration, renal blood flow and the glomerular filtration rate decrease and proximal tubular calcium and sodium reabsorption increase leading to further increases in serum calcium concentrations. Anorexia, nausea, and vomiting associated with circulating volume contraction exacerbates dehydration.[7] Immobilization caused by weakness and lethargy may exacerbate calcium resorption from bone. The kidneys may be irreversibly compromised if the concentration of calcium in the glomerular filtrate exceeds its solubility, resulting in calcium precipitation in the renal tubules (nephrocalcinosis).

*Bone Resorption*

In healthy adults before midlife, bone formation and resorption are in dynamic balance. Even though 99 percent of total body calcium is contained in bone, bone seems to have a minor function in the daily maintenance of plasma calcium levels. The normal daily exchange between bone and extracellular fluid is quite small.[8]

## Mechanisms of Cancer-associated Hypercalcemia

The fundamental cause of cancer-induced hypercalcemia is increased bone resorption with calcium mobilization into the extracellular fluid and secondarily, inadequate renal calcium clearance. Two types of cancer-induced hypercalcemia have been described: osteolysis by primary or metastatic tumor infiltrating bone and humoral hypercalcemia of malignancy mediated by circulating factors secreted by malignant cells without evidence of bony disease.[9,10] Humoral hypercalcemia and local osteolysis are not exclusive; both mechanisms may be operative.[11]

A PTH-like protein known as parathyroid hormone-related protein or peptide (PTHrP) has been isolated and characterized. PTHrP is a primitive protein that appears to have important roles in calcium transport and developmental biology. It shares partial amino acid sequence and conformational homology with normal PTH, binds with the same receptors on skeletal and renal target tissues, and affects calcium and phosphate homeostasis as does PTH.[10,12,13]

Circulating growth factors produced by solid tumors (especially squamous cell carcinoma of the lung, head, neck, and kidney, and breast cancers) may also mediate hypercalcemia. Potential mediators include transforming growth factor alpha, transforming growth factor beta, interleukin-1, tumor necrosis factors (TNF) alpha and beta, and interleukin-6.[14]

It is also possible that osteolytic lesions may secrete factors that are the same as or different from those that are implicated in humoral hypercalcemia of malignancy. Some tumors produce prostaglandin E2, a potent stimulator of osteoclastic bone resorption. Hematologic malignancies may stimulate osteoclastic bone resorption through the production of cytokines such as TNF (alpha and beta) and interleukins 1 and 6, formerly referred to as osteoclast-activating factor(s). [7,8,10,15]

## *References:*

1. Muggia FM: Overview of cancer-related hypercalcemia: epidemiology and etiology. *Seminars in Oncology* 17(2, Suppl 5): 3-9, 1990.

2. Theriault RL: Hypercalcemia of malignancy: pathophysiology and implications for treatment. *Oncology* (Huntington NY) 7(1): 47-50, 1993.

3. Bajorunas DR: Clinical manifestations of cancer-related hypercalcemia. *Seminars in Oncology* 17(2, Suppl 5): 16-25, 1990.

4. Schilling T, Pecherstorfer M, Blind E, et al.: Parathyroid hormone-related protein (PTHrP) does not regulate 1,25-dihydroxy vitamin D serum levels in hypercalcemia of malignancy. *Journal of Clinical Endocrinology and Metabolism* 76(3): 801-803, 1993.

5. Stewart AF, Horst R, Deftos LJ, et al.: Biochemical evaluation of patients with cancer-associated hypercalcemia: evidence for humoral and nonhumoral groups. *New England Journal of Medicine* 303(24): 1377-1383, 1980.

6. Breslau NA, McGuire JL, Zerwekh JE, et al.: Hypercalcemia associated with increased serum calcitriol levels in three patients with lymphoma. *Annals of Internal Medicine* 100(1): 1-7, 1984.

7. Mundy GR, Ibbotson KJ, D'Souza SM, et al.: The hypercalcemia of cancer: clinical implications and pathogenic mechanisms. *New England Journal of Medicine* 310(26): 1718-1727, 1984.

8. Mundy GR: Pathophysiology of cancer-associated hypercalcemia. Seminars in Oncology 17(2, Suppl 5): 10-15, 1990.

9. Mundy GR, Martin TJ: Hypercalcemia of malignancy: pathogenesis and management. *Metabolism* 31(12): 1247-1277, 1992.

10. Broadus AE, Mangin M, Ikeda KL, et al.: Humoral hypercalcemia of cancer: identification of a novel parathyroid hormone-like peptide. *New England Journal of Medicine* 319(9): 556-563, 1988.

11. Bertolini DR, Nedwin GE, Bringman TS, et al.: Stimulation of bone resorption and inhibition of bone formation in vitro by human tumour necrosis factors. *Nature* 319(6053): 516-518, 1986.

12. Horiuchi N, Caufield MP, Fisher JE, et al.: Similarity of synthetic peptide from human tumor to parathyroid hormone in vivo and in vitro. *Science* 248(4833): 1566-1568, 1987.

13. Suva LJ, Winslow GA, Wettenhall RE, et al.: A parathyroid hormone-related protein implicated in malignant hypercalcemia: cloning and expression. *Science* 237(4817): 893-896, 1987.

14. Dodwell DJ: Malignant bone resorption: cellular and biochemical mechanisms. *Annals of Oncology* 3(4): 257-267, 1992.

15. Warrell RP: Etiology and current management of cancer-related hypercalcemia. *Oncology* (Huntington NY) 6(10): 37-43, 1992.

### Incidence of Hypercalcemia by Cancer Type

Calcemia occurs more frequently in some malignancies (e.g., squamous cell cancers of the lung, head and neck, and esophagus) than in others. Within each disease type, the incidence of hypercalcemia varies greatly in reported series.

### Lung

Persons with lung cancer make up 25 percent-35 percent of reported cases of cancer-induced hypercalcemia. Hypercalcemia is rarely reported in small cell carcinoma and adenocarcinoma but occurs more frequently among patients with epidermoid and large cell bronchogenic carcinoma histologies. Dainer suggested that hypercalcemia in persons with small cell histology malignancies is very often related to altered parathyroid function and/or ectopic parathyroid hormone (PTH) production.[1] Hypercalcemia in lung cancer is usually not an early or presenting symptom but occurs more often during advanced disease stages.

## Breast

Twenty percent to forty percent of reported cases of cancer-induced hypercalcemia occur among women with breast cancer. Hypercalcemia during breast cancer is more likely to occur after hormonal therapy using estrogens, androgens, progestins, or antiestrogens. Although its occurrence is not predictable, approximately 75 percent of women with stage III breast cancer and significant bone destruction will develop hypercalcemia.[2]

Some breast cancer cells secrete prostaglandins. Prostaglandins have been associated with increased bone resorption following hormonal therapy. An increased risk of developing hypercalcemia has also been observed among patients with breast cancer following treatments with estrogens or antiestrogens. The fact that bone-resorbing activity is inhibited by indomethacin implicates prostaglandins as mediators of bone destruction and hypercalcemia.[3]

## Head and Neck

The incidence of hypercalcemia with cancers affecting regions of the head and neck varies with the site of primary involvement but ranges from 2.9 percent to 25 percent. Cancers of the oropharynx, hypopharynx, tongue, larynx, the floor of the mouth, and tonsillar fossa are associated with a 37 percent, 24.3 percent, 21.5 percent, 18.7 percent, 17.6 percent, and 15.7 percent incidence of hypercalcemia, respectively.[2]

## Multiple Myeloma

More than one third of all persons with multiple myeloma develop hypercalcemia. Generally, hypercalcemia in patients with multiple myeloma strongly correlates with bone destruction. Immobility and renal failure also contribute to developing hypercalcemia in this population. Among patients with multiple myeloma, approximately 50 percent have some degree of renal insufficiency and are, therefore, predisposed to developing hypercalcemia.[3]

As in other hematologic malignancies, the release of a cytokine, such as the lymphotoxin associated with myeloma, correlates with the appearance of hypercalcemia. In vitro, lymphotoxin causes hypercalcemia when infused or injected. Not all bone resorption in myeloma, however, can be blocked by antisera to lymphotoxin. This suggests that lymphotoxin does not act alone in mediating hypercalcemia in myeloma. Other suspect mediators include IL-1 and IL-6, PTHrP, and vitamin D metabolites.

### T-cell Lymphoma

Overall, hypercalcemia is a rare complication of lymphoma. Hypercalcemia is especially prevalent, however, among persons with T-cell lineage lymphomas.[2] Almost all persons with human T-cell lymphotropic virus type I (HTLV-1)-associated leukemia/lymphoma develop hypercalcemia.

### Parathyroid

Hypercalcemia is the major cause of morbidity and mortality in individuals with parathyroid cancer. Most persons with recurrent parathyroid cancer die of complications of hypercalcemia compared with those whose death is directly related to local tumor invasion or metastatic disease.[4]

### Potentiating Factors

Immobility is associated with an increase in resorption of calcium from bone. Dehydration and anorexia, nausea, and vomiting that exacerbate dehydration reduce renal calcium excretion (see the Overview section above).

Hormonal therapy (estrogens, antiestrogens, androgens, and progestins) may precipitate hypercalcemia. Thiazide diuretics increase renal calcium reabsorption and may precipitate or exacerbate hypercalcemia.[5]

**Table 25.1.** Incidence of Hypercalcemia by Cancer Type

| Tumor Type | Percentage of Patients Who Develop Hypercalcemia |
|---|---|
| Lung | 27.0 percent |
| Breast | 25.0 percent |
| Multiple Myeloma | 7.3 percent |
| Head and Neck | 6.9 percent |
| Unknown Primary | 4.7 percent |
| Lymphoma/Leukemia | 4.3 percent |
| Renal | 4.3 percent |
| Gastrointestinal | 4.1 percent |

## References:

1. Dainer PM: Octreotide acetate therapy for hypercalcemia complicating small cell carcinoma of the lung. *Southern Medical Journal* 84(10): 1250-1254, 1991.

2  Muggia FM: Overview of cancer-related hypercalcemia: epidemiology and etiology. *Seminars in Oncology* 17(2, Suppl 5): 3-9, 1990.

3. Mundy GR: Pathophysiology of cancer-associated hypercalcemia. *Seminars in Oncology* 17(2, Suppl 5): 10-15, 1990.

4. Warrell RP, Israel R, Frisone M, et al.: Gallium nitrate for acute treatment of cancer-related hypercalcemia: a randomized, double-blind comparison to calcitonin. *Annals of Internal Medicine* 108(5): 669-674, 1988.

5. Coleman RE: Bisphosphonate treatment of bone metastases and hypercalcemia of malignancy. *Oncology* (Huntington NY) 5(8): 55-60, 1991.

## *Manifestations of Hypercalcemia*

There is little correlation between the presenting symptoms of hypercalcemia and serum calcium concentrations. Symptoms associated with hypercalcemia, however, are characteristically nonspecific, easily attributed to chronic or terminal illness, and may therefore complicate rapid diagnosis.[1,2] Symptom severity may be, at least in part, due to confounding factors such as previous cancer treatment, drug-disease state interactions, or comorbid pathologies.

Few patients experience all the symptoms that have been associated with hypercalcemia (see Table 25.2), and some may have none at all; however, patients with corrected total serum calcium concentrations greater than 14 mg/dL (>7.0 mEq/L or 3.49 mmol/L) are generally symptomatic.[1] It must be emphasized that clinical manifestations are closely related to the rapidity of hypercalcemia onset. Some patients develop signs and symptoms when calcium is only slightly elevated, while others with long-standing hypercalcemia may tolerate serum calcium levels greater than 13 mg/dL (>6.5 mEq/L or 3.24 mmol/L) with few symptoms. Neuromuscular manifestations are generally more marked in elderly than in young individuals.

Ralston, et al. observed that malaise and fatigue were the most common complaints at patient presentation, followed (in order of decreasing prevalence rate) by varying degrees of obtundation, anorexia, pain, polyuria-polydipsia, constipation, and nausea or vomiting.[3]

Reasons for seeking hospitalization when hypercalcemia was diagnosed included constipation, declining performance status, altered mental status, anorexia, vomiting, weight loss, and weakness.[2,4]

Clinical manifestations can be categorized according to body systems and functions.

## *Neurologic Symptoms*

Calcium ions have a major rôle in neurotransmission. Increased calcium levels decrease neuromuscular excitability, which leads to hypotonicity in smooth and striated muscle. Symptom severity correlates directly with the magnitude and inversely with the rate of change in serum ionized calcium concentrations. Neuromuscular symptoms include weakness and diminished deep tendon reflexes. Muscle strength is impaired, and respiratory muscular capacity may be decreased. Central nervous system impairment may manifest as altered personality, cognitive difficulty, apathy, impaired concentration, confusion, fatigue, lethargy, or psychotic behavior. Obtundation is progressive as serum calcium concentrations increase and may

**Table 25.2.** Symptoms prevalence among patients treated for hypercalcemia of malignancy stratified by corrected serum total calcium concentrations at presentation[3]

| Symptoms | Serum Calcium Concentration | |
| --- | --- | --- |
| | <3.5 mmol/L | >/= 3.5 mmol/L |
| CNS symptoms | 41 percent | 80 percent |
| constipation | 21 percent | 25 percent |
| malaise-fatigue | 65 percent | 50 percent |
| anorexia | 47 percent | 59 percent |
| nausea and/or vomiting | 22 percent | 30 percent |
| polyuria and/or polydipsia | 34 percent | 35 percent |
| pain | 51 percent | 35 percent |

progress to stupor or coma.[1,2] Local neurologic signs are not common, but hypercalcemia has been documented to increase cerebrospinal fluid protein, which may be associated with headache. Headache can be exacerbated by vomiting and dehydration.[2] Abnormal electroencephalograms are seen in patients with marked hypercalcemia.[1]

## Cardiovascular Symptoms

Hypercalcemia is associated with increased myocardial contractility and irritability. Electrocardiographic changes are characterized by slowed conduction, including prolonged P-R interval, widened QRS complex, shortened Q-T interval, S-T segments may be shortened or absent, and the proximal limb of T waves may slope abruptly and peak early. Hypercalcemia enhances patients'sensitivity to the pharmacologic effects of digitalis glycosides (e.g., digoxin). When serum calcium concentrations exceed 16 mg/dL (>8.0 mEq/L or 3.99 mmol/L), T waves widen, secondarily increasing the Q-T interval. As calcium concentrations increase, bradyarrhythmias and bundle branch block may develop. Incomplete or complete AV block may develop at serum concentrations around 18 mg/dL (9.0 mEq/L or 4.49 mmol/L) and may progress to complete heart block, asystole, and cardiac arrest.[1,2]

## Gastrointestinal Symptoms

Gastrointestinal symptoms are probably related to the depressive action of hypercalcemia on the autonomic nervous system and resulting smooth muscle hypotonicity. Increased gastric acid secretion often accompanies hypercalcemia and may intensify gastrointestinal manifestations. Anorexia, nausea, and vomiting are intensified by increased gastric residual volume. Constipation is aggravated by dehydration that accompanies hypercalcemia. Abdominal pain may progress to obstipation and can be confused with acute abdominal obstruction.

## Renal Symptoms

Hypercalcemia causes a reversible tubular defect in the kidney resulting in the loss of urinary concentrating ability and polyuria. Decreased fluid intake and polyuria lead to symptoms associated with dehydration, including thirst, dry mucosa, diminished or absent sweating, poor skin turgor, and concentrated urine. Decreased proximal reabsorption of sodium, magnesium, and potassium occur as a result of salt and water depletion that is caused by cellular dehydration and hypotension. Renal insufficiency may occur as a result of diminished glomerular filtration, a complication observed most often in patients with myeloma.

Although nephrolithiasis and nephrocalcinosis are usually not associated with hypercalcemia of malignancy, calcium phosphate crystals can precipitate within renal tubules to form renal calculi as a consequence of long-standing hypercalciuria. When they occur, coexisting primary hyperparathyroidism should be considered.

### Bone Symptoms

Hypercalcemia of malignancy can result from osteolytic metastases or humorally-mediated bone resorption, with secondary fractures, skeletal deformities, and pain.

### Pain

Increased serum calcium concentrations do not produce painful sensations. However, it has been suggested that hypercalcemia may lower the pain threshold.[5]

### References:

1.  Bajorunas DR: Clinical manifestations of cancer-related hypercalcemia. *Seminars in Oncology* 17(2, Suppl 5): 16-25, 1990.

2.  Mahon SM: Signs and symptoms associated with malignancy-induced hypercalcemia. *Cancer Nursing* 12(3): 153-160, 1989.

3.  Ralston SH, Gallacher SJ, Patel U., et al.: Cancer-associated hypercalcemia: morbidity and mortality. Clinical experience in 126 treated patients. *Annals of Internal Medicine* 112(7): 499-504, 1990.

4.  Mahon SM: Symptoms as clues to calcium levels. *American Journal of Nursing* 87(3): 354-356, 1987.

5.  Mundy GR, Martin TJ.: The hypercalcemia of malignancy: pathogenesis and management. *Metabolism* 31(12): 1247-1277, 1982.

## Assessment of Hypercalcemia

Only the ionized or free fraction of calcium is physiologically significant. A change in the protein-bound fraction with or without a change in serum total calcium will cause an inverse change in the ionized serum calcium concentration. A number of clinical conditions alter calcium protein binding and must be considered during patient assessment. Clinicians should beware of falsely accepting a normal or slightly elevated serum total calcium level as being of no clinical significance in patients who have decreased serum albumin concentrations. For this reason, serum total calcium values must be corrected for decreased serum albumin concentrations (refer to the Correction of Serum Calcium Level in Patients with Concurrently Low Albumin subsection in the Overview section above).

Calcium also binds to globulins in blood. Although in contrast with hypoalbuminemia, hypogammaglobulinemia has a relatively small effect on calcium protein binding. Serum total calcium concentration can be corrected for changes in globulins as follows: total serum calcium concentration varies directly by 0.16 mg/dL, 0.08 mEq/L, or 0.04 mmol/L with each 1 g/dL change in globulin concentration. In clinical practice, changes in serum globulin concentrations rarely effect clinically significant changes in the ionized calcium fraction.

Acid-base status also affects the interpretation of serum calcium values. While acidosis decreases the protein-bound fraction, consequently increasing the ionized calcium fraction, protein binding is increased in alkalosis. Serum total calcium concentration can be corrected for changes in pH as follows: total serum calcium concentration varies inversely by 0.12 mg/dL, 0.06 mEq/L, or 0.03 mmol/L with each 0.1 unit change in pH. Unlike changes in serum albumin concentration, alterations in blood pH rarely effect clinically significant changes in the ionized calcium fraction.[1]

Primary assessment should include the following:[2,3]

Clinical status (refer to the Manifestations of Hypercalcemia section above):

- Neuromuscular (evaluate muscular strength, muscle tone, decreased deep tendon reflexes)

- Neurologic (fatigue, apathy, depression, confusion, restlessness)

- Cardiovascular (hypertension, EKG changes, arrhythmias, digitalis toxicity)

- Renal (urine output polyuria, nocturia, glucosuria, polydipsia)
- Gastrointestinal (anorexia, nausea, abdominal pain, constipation, decreased bowel sounds, abdominal distention)
- Miscellaneous (musculoskeletal pain, pruritus)

History:

- How rapidly have symptoms developed?
- Symptoms of malignancy are usually present when hypercalcemia is due to cancer
- Rapid symptom onset is more typical of hypercalcemia of malignancy than hypercalcemia associated with hyperparathyroidism and other diseases
- Is there radiographic evidence of primary or metastatic bony disease?
- Is the patient currently treated with or have they recently received treatment with tamoxifen or estrogenic or androgenic steroids?
- Is the patient taking digoxin?
- Is there an exogenous calcium source such as intravenous fluids or parenteral nutrition?
- Is the patient receiving thiazide diuretics, vitamins A or D, or lithium?
- Is there concurrent disease predisposing to dehydration or patient immobility?
- Are there potentially effective treatments for the patient's underlying malignancy?

Laboratory studies:

- Serum calcium concentration
- Serum albumin concentration
- Immunoreactive parathormone (iPTH)
- iPTH concentration is increased or rarely normal in hyperparathyroid disease; iPTH is typically decreased or undetectable in hypercalcemia of malignancy

- Parathormone-related peptide (PTHrP; if available)

- Serum 1,25-dihydroxy vitamin D concentration in patients with hematologic malignancies

- Blood urea nitrogen and creatinine concentrations (renal function)

- Other serum electrolytes concentrations (phosphate, magnesium)

### References:

1. Bajorunas DR: Clinical manifestations of cancer-related hypercalcemia. *Seminars in Oncology* 17(2, Suppl 5): 16-25, 1990.

2. Calafato A, Jessup AL.: Body fluid composition, alteration in: hypercalcemia. In: McNally JC, Somerville ET, Miaskowski C, et al., Eds.: *Guidelines for Oncology Nursing Practice*. Philadelphia: WB Saunders Company, 2nd Edition, 1991, pp 397-401.

3. Coward DD: Hypercalcemia knowledge assessment in patients at risk of developing cancer-induced hypercalcemia. *Oncology Nursing Forum* 15(4): 471-476, 1988.

## Management of Hypercalcemia

### Prevention

Individuals at risk of developing hypercalcemia may be the first to recognize symptoms. They should be advised about the ways in which it most frequently manifests (refer to the Manifestations of Hypercalcemia section above) and given guidelines advising them when to seek professional intervention.[1] Preventive measures include insuring adequate fluid (3-4 liters [100-140 fluid ounces] per day if not contraindicated) and salt intake, nausea and vomiting control, encouraging patients to walk and to generally be mobile, attention to febrile episodes, and cautiously using or eliminating drugs that may complicate management.[1-3]

Even though the gut has a role in normal calcium homeostasis, absorption is usually diminished in individuals with hypercalcemia, making dietary calcium restriction unnecessary.[4]

### Managing Hypercalcemia

Symptomatic treatment of hypercalcemia focuses first on correcting dehydration and enhancing renal calcium excretion, followed by specific hypocalcemic treatment with agents that inhibit bone resorption (e.g., calcitonin, bisphosphonates, gallium nitrate, and plicamycin).[5,6] Definitive treatment is that which effectively treats the malignant disease underlying hypercalcemia.[7]

The magnitude of hypercalcemia is typically the basis for determining whether treatment is indicated. Immediate aggressive hypocalcemic treatment is warranted in patients with a corrected total serum calcium greater than 14 mg/dL (>7 mEq/L or 3.5 mmol/L) (refer to the Laboratory Assessment subsection in the Overview section above). In patients with total corrected serum calcium concentration between 12-14 mg/dL (6-7 mEq/L or 3.0-3.5 mmol/L), clinical manifestations should guide the type of therapy and the urgency with which it is implemented.[5] Treatment response is indicated by resolution of symptoms attributable to hypercalcemia and by diminishing serum calcium concentrations and urinary calcium and hydroxyproline excretion.

Aggressive treatment is not generally indicated in patients with mild hypercalcemia (corrected total serum calcium <12 mg/dL [<6 mEq/L or 3.0 mmol/L]). Clear treatment decisions are problematic, however, for patients with mild hypercalcemia and coexistent central nervous system symptoms, especially for younger patients in whom hypercalcemia is generally better tolerated. It is very important to evaluate other causes for altered central nervous system function before attributing them solely to hypercalcemia.[5]

Hypocalcemic treatment can provide marked improvement of distressing symptoms. Polyuria, polydipsia, central nervous system symptoms, nausea and vomiting, and constipation are more likely to be managed successfully than are anorexia, malaise, and fatigue. Pain control may be improved for some patients who achieve normocalcemia.[8] Effective calcium-lowering therapy usually improves symptoms, enhances the quality of life, and may allow patients to be managed in a subacute, ambulatory, or home care setting.

After normocalcemia is achieved, urinary and serum calcium should be monitored serially with the frequency determined by anticipated response duration for any particular hypocalcemic regimen.

### *Mild Hypercalcemia*

(corrected total serum calcium <12 mg/dL [<6 mEq/L or 3.0 mmol/L]) Hydration followed by observation is an option for asymptomatic patients with tumors that are likely to respond to antineoplastic treatment (e.g., lymphoma, breast cancer, ovarian cancer, head and neck carcinoma, and multiple myeloma) if treatment is about to be implemented.[9]

In symptomatic patients or when tumor response is expected to occur slowly, hypocalcemic therapy should be implemented to manage symptoms and stabilize patients' metabolic states. Additional ancillary interventions should be directed toward nausea and vomiting control, encouraging mobility, attention to febrile episodes, and minimal use of sedating medications.[9]

## Moderate to Severe Hypercalcemia

(corrected total serum calcium equal to 12-14 mg/dL [6-7 mEq/L or 3.0-3.5 mmol/L])

### Rehydration

Rehydration is the essential first step in treating moderate or severe hypercalcemia. Although fewer than 30 percent of patients achieve normocalcemia with hydration alone, replenishing extracellular fluid, restoring intravascular volume, and saline diuresis are fundamental to initial therapy. Adequate rehydration may require 3,000-6,000 mL 0.9 percent sodium chloride for injection (normal saline) within the first 24 hours to restore fluid volume. Restoring normal extracellular fluid volume will increase daily urinary calcium excretion by 100-300 mg. Clinical improvement in mental status and nausea and vomiting is usually apparent within 24 hours for most patients; however, rehydration is a temporizing intervention. If definitive cytoreductive therapies (surgery, radiation, or chemotherapy) are not forthcoming, hypocalcemic agents must be used to achieve long-term control.

### Diuretics

Thiazide diuretics are contraindicated because they increase renal tubular calcium absorption and may exacerbate hypercalcemia. Loop diuretics (e.g., furosemide, bumetanide, and ethacrynic acid) induce hypercalciuria by inhibiting calcium reabsorption in the ascending limb of the loop of Henle but should not be administered until volume expansion is achieved. Otherwise, loop diuretics can exacerbate fluid loss, further reducing calcium clearance. Because sodium and calcium clearance are closely linked during osmotic diuresis, loop diuretics will depress the proximal tubular resorptive mechanisms for calcium, increasing calcium excretion to 400-800 mg/day.

Moderate doses of furosemide, 20-40 mg every 12 hours, increase saline-induced urinary calcium excretion and are useful in preventing or managing fluid overload in adequately rehydrated patients. Aggressive treatment with furosemide (80-100 mg every 2-4 hours) is problematic because it requires concurrent administration of large volumes of saline to prevent intravascular dehydration.[10] This in turn requires intensive hemodynamic monitoring to avoid volume overload and cardiac decompensation as well as frequent serial urinary volume and electrolytes measurements to prevent life-threatening hypophosphatemia, hypokalemia, and hypomagnesemia.[9,11]

### Algorithms for initial management of hypercalcemia of malignancy

Asymptomatic patients with corrected serum total calcium <12 mg/dL (<6 mEq/L or <3 mmol/L):

- hydration with 3-4 L of 0.9 percent saline solution over 24 hours

- antineoplastic therapy

Symptomatic patients with corrected serum total calcium <12 mg/dL (<6 mEq/L or <3 mmol/L):

- hydration with 3-4 L of 0.9 percent of saline solution over 24 hours with or without furosemide

- salmon calcitonin at 4 IU/kg subcutaneously every 12 hours

### OR

- plicamycin at 25 micrograms/kg intravaneously over 15-30 minutes

- antineoplastic therapy

All patients (with intact renal function) with corrected serum total calcium >/= 12 mg/dL (>/= 6 mEq/L or >/= 3 mmol/L):

- hydration with 4-6 L of 0.9 percent saline over 24 hours with 40-160 mg/24 hours of furosemide given in divided doses (only after correcting dehydration)

- salmon calcitonin at 4 IU/kg subcutaneously every 12 hours plus 90 mg pamidronate intravenously over 4-24 hours

- plicamycin at 25 micrograms/kg intravaneously over 15-30 minutes plus 90 mg pamidronate intraveneously over 4-24 hours

- antineoplastic therapy

## *Pharmacologic Inhibition of Osteoclastic Bone Resorption*

### *Calcitonin*

Calcitonin is a peptide hormone secreted by specialized cells in the thyroid and parathyroid. Its synthesis and secretion normally increase in response to high serum ionized calcium concentrations and it opposes physiologic effects of PTH on bone and renal tubular calcium resorption; however, it is not known whether calcitonin has a significant role in calcium homeostasis. Nevertheless, calcitonin rapidly inhibits calcium and phosphorous resorption from bone and decreases renal calcium reabsorption. Calcitonin derived from salmon is much more potent and has a longer duration of activity than the human hormone. It is initially given subcutaneously at 4 IU/kg body weight per dose, administered subcutaneously or intramuscularly every 12 hours. Dose and schedule may be escalated after 1 or 2 days to 8 IU/kg every 12 hours and finally to 8 IU/kg every 6 hours if the response to lower doses is unsatisfactory. Unfortunately, tachyphylaxis commonly occurs. With repeated use, calcitonin's beneficial hypocalcemic effect wanes, even at the upper recommended limits of dose and schedule, so that its calcium-lowering effect persists for only a few days. There is evidence to suggest that the effect of calcitonin on bone resorption may be prolonged by concomitant glucocorticoid administration [12] and that when combined with bisphosphonates may hasten the onset and duration of hypocalcemic response.[13,14]

Calcitonin is usually well-tolerated; adverse effects include mild nausea, transient cramping abdominal pain, and cutaneous flushing. Calcitonin is most useful within the first 24-36 hours of treatment of severe hypercalcemia and should be used in conjunction with more potent but slower-acting agents.

### *Plicamycin*

Plicamycin (also referred to as mithramycin) is an inhibitor of osteoclast RNA synthesis. It has been shown to inhibit bone resorption in vitro and is clinically effective in the presence or absence of bone metastases. Onset of response occurs within 12 hours after a single intravenous dose of 25-30 micrograms/kg of body weight given either as a short infusion for 30 minutes or longer. Maximum response, however, does not occur until approximately 48 hours after administration and may persist for from 3-7 or more days after administration. Repeated doses may be given to maintain plicamycin's hypocalcemic effect but should not be given more frequently than every 48 hours to determine the maximum calcium-lowering effect produced by previous doses.[15] Multiple doses may control hypercalcemia for several weeks, but rebound hypercalcemia usually occurs without definitive treatment against the underlying malignancy.[16] Although single-dose treatment of hypercalcemia is generally well-tolerated with few adverse effects,[17] dysfibrinogenemia,[18] and nephrotoxicity [19] have been reported after single doses (20-25 micrograms/kg). Rapid intravenous administration is associated with nausea and vomiting.[16] High doses and repeated doses predispose to thrombocytopenia, a qualitative platelet dysfunction that may be associated with a bleeding diathesis, transient increases in hepatic transaminases, nephrotoxicity (decreased creatinine clearance, increased serum creatinine and BUN, potassium wasting, and proteinuria), hypophosphatemia, a flu-like syndrome, dermatologic reactions, and stomatitis.[16,19-24]

*Bisphosphonates*

Bisphosphonates are one of the most effective pharmacologic alternatives for controlling hypercalcemia. They bind to hydroxyapatite in calcified bone, rendering it resistant to hydrolytic dissolution by phosphatases, thereby inhibiting both normal and abnormal bone resorption.[25] Bisphosphonate treatment reduces the number of osteoclasts in sites undergoing active bone resorption and may prevent osteoclast expansion by inhibiting differentiation from their monocyte-macrophage precursors.[26-28] Bisphosphonates have variable effects on other aspects of bone remodeling such as new bone formation and mineralization. For example, etidronate at clinically relevant dosages (300-1,600 mg/day) inhibits new bone formation and mineralization.[29-31] With prolonged etidronate use, osteomalacia and pathologic fractures may occur.[30,32] In contrast, clodronate, pamidronate, and alendronate are 10, 100, and 1000 times, respectively, more potent inhibitors of bone resorption than etidronate and are clinically useful at dosages that are less likely to adversely affect new bone formation and mineralization.[33-36] Clinicians should note that many bisphosphonates may be useful in treating hypercalcemia of malignancy; however, only etidronate and pamidronate are approved in the United States for that indication.[37-39]

In comparison with etidronate, which requires daily administration for 3 or more days,[40-42] pamidronate is administered once over 4-24 hours (60 mg dose) or over 24 hours (90 mg dose).[43] With respect to serum calcium reduction and duration of hypocalcemic response, pamidronate (60 mg given intravenously as a single dose over 24 hours) has been demonstrated to be more effective than etidronate at 7.5 mg/kg body weight per day administered over 2 hours as a daily intravenous infusion for 3 consecutive days.[44,45]

Optimal pamidronate dosage and administration schedules have not been established; however, dosage selection may be indicated by the severity of hypercalcemia. In treating moderate hypercalcemia (corrected serum calcium <13.5 mg/dL, <6.75 mEq/L, or <3.37 mmol/L) 60 mg pamidronate administered intravenously over 24 hours has been demonstrated to be as effective as 90 mg.[46] For serum calcium levels >/= 13.5 mg/dL, 90 mg administered over 24 hours has been shown to be safe and somewhat more effective than 60 mg given by the same schedule.[46]

Onset of pamidronate's effects is apparent within 3-4 days, with maximal effects within 7-10 days after commencing treatment. Duration of effect may persist for 7-30 days.[47] Adverse effects include transient low-grade temperature elevations (1-2 degrees C) that typically occur within 24-36 hours after administration and persist for up to 2 days in up to 20 percent of patients. Other bisphosphonates (except clodronate) may also produce transient temperature elevations; the incidence of temperature elevation, nausea, anorexia, dyspepsia, and vomiting may be increased by rapid administration.[46,48] New onset hypophosphatemia and hypomagnesemia may occur; pre-existing abnormalities in the same electrolytes may be exacerbated by treatment. Serum calcium may overshoot below the normal range, and hypocalcemia (typically asymptomatic) may result. Renal failure has only been reported after rapid etidronate and clodronate injection, but rapid administration should be avoided with all bisphosphonates.[49] Intravenous pamidronate administration has been associated with acute-phase responses, including transiently decreased peripheral lymphocyte counts. Local reactions (thrombophlebitis, erythema, and pain) at the infusion site have been reported.[46]

Calcitonin and plicamycin have a more rapid hypocalcemic effect than bisphosphonates; however, pamidronate has several advantages over nonbisphosphonate therapies. In comparison with plicamycin, response rates are greater among patients treated with pamidronate.[50] Pamidronate more frequently reduces serum calcium concentrations to normocalcemic ranges than either calcitonin or plicamycin.[50,51] In addition, pamidronate's hypocalcemic effect is dose-related and sustained after repeated administration and generally persists for durations longer than are produced by either calcitonin or plicamycin therapies.[47] With respect to safety, pamidronate lacks the renal, hepatic, and platelet toxic effects associated with plicamycin.

*Gallium Nitrate*

Gallium nitrate was developed as an antineoplastic agent that was coincidentally found to produce a hypocalcemic effect. It has been shown to be superior to etidronate in the percentage of patients who achieve normocalcemia and in the duration of normocalcemia.[52] Drawbacks to its use include a continuous 5-day intravenous infusion schedule (200 mg/square meter body surface area/day)[9] and the potential for nephrotoxicity, particularly when used concurrently with other potentially nephrotoxic drugs (e.g., aminoglycosides and amphotericin B) (Fujisawa-Ganite package insert, 1991).

Gallium nitrate has also been given by daily subcutaneous injection to prevent bone resorption and maintain bone mass in patients with multiple myeloma.[53]

*Gallocorticoids*

Glucocorticoids have efficacy as hypocalcemic agents primarily in steroid-responsive tumors (e.g., lymphomas and myeloma) and in patients whose hypercalcemia is associated with increased vitamin D synthesis or intake (sarcoidosis and hypervitaminosis D).[54-56] Glucocorticoids increase urinary calcium excretion and inhibit vitamin D-mediated gastrointestinal calcium absorption. However, response is typically slow; 1-2 weeks may elapse before serum calcium concentrations decrease. Oral hydrocortisone (100-300 mg) or its glucocorticoid equivalent may be given daily; however, complications of long-term steroid use limit its usefulness even in responsive patients.

*Phosphate*

Phosphate offers a minimally effective chronic oral treatment for mild to moderate hypercalcemia. It is most useful after successful initial reduction of serum calcium with other agents and should probably be reserved for patients who are concurrently hypercalcemic and hypophosphatemic. The usual treatment is 250-375 mg per dose given four times daily (1-1.5 g elemental phosphorus/day) to minimize the potential for developing hyperphosphatemia.[57] Supranormal phosphate administration results in decreased renal calcium clearance and presumably decreases serum calcium concentrations by precipitating calcium into bone and soft tissues.[58,59] Extraskeletal precipitation of calcium in vital organs may have adverse consequences and is especially significant after intravenous administration.[9,60,61] Intravenous administration produces a rapid decline in serum calcium concentrations but is rarely used because there are safer and more effective antiresorptive agents for life-threatening hypercalcemia (calcitonin and plicamycin). Hypotension, oliguria, left ventricular failure, and sudden death can occur as a result of rapid intravenous administration. Contraindications for phosphate include normophosphatemia, hyperphosphatemia, and renal insufficiency. Oral phosphate should be given at the lowest dose possible to maintain serum phosphorous concentrations less than 4 mg/dL 1-2 hours after administration.

The use of phosphates is limited by individual patient tolerance and toxicity; 25 percent-50 percent of patients cannot tolerate oral phosphates.[11] Oral phosphate-induced diarrhea may be initially advantageous in patients who have experienced constipation secondary to hypercalcemia; it is the predominant and dose-limiting adverse effect for oral therapy and frequently prevents dosage escalation greater than 2 g neutral phosphate per day.[9]

## Dialysis

Dialysis is an option for hypercalcemia that is complicated by renal failure. Peritoneal dialysis with calcium-free dialysate fluid can remove 200-2,000 mg of calcium in 24-48 hours and decrease the serum calcium concentration by 3-12 mg/dL (1.5-6 mEq/L or 0.7-3 mmol/L). Ultrafilterable calcium clearance may exceed that of urea with calcium-free dialysate exchanges of 2 L each every 30 minutes.[62] Hemodialysis is equally effective.[63,64] Because large quantities of phosphate are lost during dialysis and phosphate loss aggravates hypercalcemia, serum inorganic phosphate should be measured after each dialysis session and phosphate should be added to the dialysate during the next fluid exchange or to the patient's diet.[65] It is recommended, however, that phosphate replacement should be limited to restoring serum inorganic phosphate concentrations to normal rather than supranormal.[57]

*Others*

Other less well-proven interventions include prostaglandin synthesis inhibitors, cisplatin, octreotide acetate, and amifostine.

Prostaglandin synthesis inhibitors such as the nonsteroidal antiinflammatory drugs may have some efficacy in the management of cancer-induced hypercalcemia. The E-series prostaglandins mediate bone resorption. Despite experimental evidence, however, aspirin and other nonsteroidal drugs have demonstrated only modest clinical response rates in controlling hypercalcemia. For patients who are unresponsive to or unable to tolerate other agents, aspirin may be given to produce a serum salicylate concentration equal to 20-30 mg/dL or 25 mg indomethacin may be given orally every 6 hours.[66-69]

Serum calcium was normalized for a median of 34 (range: 4-115) days in nine of 13 patients with various solid tumors given cisplatin at 100 mg/square meter body surface area intravenously over 24 hours. Patients were re-treated as frequently as every 7 days if necessary to maintain serum calcium concentrations less than 11.5 mg/dL (<5.75 mEq/L or 2.87 mmol/L). Four of seven patients responded to repeated treatment. Responders achieved a statistically significant difference in serum calcium levels from baseline on the 10th day after treatment, which continued thereafter. Serial tumor measurements revealed that the hypocalcemic response did not correlate with tumor shrinkage; there was no detectable antitumor response in any measurable or evaluable disease.[70]

Amifostine (formerly known as ethiofos and WR-2721) is currently being evaluated as a myeloprotective agent against ionizing irradiation and alkylating chemotherapy. Amifostine suppresses PTH secretion, inhibits bone resorption, and interferes with renal tubular reabsorption of calcium. Hypocalcemia was reported as an adverse reaction in early clinical studies, but amifostine may have some effectiveness in managing cancer-related hypercalcemia.

Octreotide acetate has shown some activity in cancer-related hypercalcemia in two anecdotal reports. It is thought that octreotide interferes with the ectopic secretion of PTH or parathyroid-like hormones. Octreotide may be useful when other interventions fail or are inappropriate. In one report, octreotide was administered at 150 micrograms subcutaneously three times per day for 6 days. Normocalcemia occurred within 24 hours after the first dose and persisted until 1 day after octreotide was discontinued.[1]

Future pharmacologic management is likely to combine osteoclastic inhibitors with cytotoxic or endocrine therapy.[71] Studies using oral bisphosphonates in combination with systemic chemotherapy in patients with advanced breast cancer demonstrated reduced radiotherapy and analgesic requirements, fewer complications, and less disease progression in the study group.[2,4]

### *Patient and Family Education*

Because hypercalcemia compromises the quality of life and can be life-threatening if not promptly recognized and treated, individuals at risk and their caregivers should be made aware that it is a possible complication of their disease. Patients and their significant others should be advised about the type of symptoms that may occur, preventive measures, exacerbating factors, and when to seek medical assistance.[72]

## *Supportive Care*

Despite encouraging developments in pharmacologic management, the prognostic implications related to hypercalcemia remain relatively grim. Only patients for whom effective anticancer therapy is possible can be expected to experience a longer survival.

Recurrence of hypercalcemia is likely when control of the underlying disease is not possible. Self-care measures to diminish the occurrence of symptoms of hypercalcemia should be taught and implemented. Such measures include maintenance of mobility and ensuring adequate hydration.

- Care givers need to prevent or recognize and manage adverse effects of therapy. Fluid overload and electrolyte imbalance can occur during initial therapy. Serum sodium, potassium, calcium, phosphate, and magnesium concentrations may be markedly decreased. Electrolyte levels should be monitored at least daily, and clinical signs and symptoms should be assessed at least every 4 hours when implementing hydration or specific hypocalcemic drug treatments.

- Symptom management is crucial. Preventing accidental or self-inflicted injury as a consequence of the patient's altered mental status is a priority during acute management. Until serum calcium decreases, additional pharmacologic interventions may be necessary to control nausea, vomiting, and constipation

.• Supportive management of delirium, agitation, or mental-status changes occurs in patients with hypercalcemia. Primary treatment of hypercalcemia and/or its underlying etiology will eventually lead to the resolution of mental-status changes in most of these patients. Some patients will present with clinically significant and distressing mental-status changes, agitation, or delirium that warrant management or control (refer to the PDQ Delirium summary). Neuroleptic medications such as haloperidol (0.5-5.0 mg given intravenously or orally twice a day to four times a day) alone or in combination with benzodiazepines (i.e., 0.5-2.0 mg lorazepam given intravenously or orally twice a day to four times a day) are effective in controlling agitation; this enhances patient and family comfort and allows for easier institution of primary therapies. The use of benzodiazepines in these situations should be reserved for those instances where sedation and not improvement in mental status is the primary goal of the intervention. Whether these interventions will improve mental status is highly variable and depends on a number of factors, including the degree to which the delirium is multifactorial in nature and how many other possible and controllable etiologies are present (sepsis, multiple medications, other metabolic abnormalities, and the presence of central nervous system disease). Often, while control of agitation is a readily attainable goal, the resolution of mental-status changes may not be possible until the hypercalcemia resolves. Moreover, the relationship between mental status and serum calcium levels is variable. Some patients will not manifest improvement in mental status until days to a week or more after serum calcium levels are in the normal range; others will display improvement, for example, when hydrated, before laboratory values catch up.

• Many times, lethargy is a presenting symptom of hypercalcemia. At the time, such patients are mistakenly viewed as depressed by family members (and by staff on occasion) before the actual etiology of the mental-status changes becomes known. The differential diagnosis is generally straightforward in that many of these patients will lack the cognitive or ideational symptoms of a mood disorder (hopelessness, helplessness, anhedonia, guilt, worthlessness, or thoughts of suicide) and instead will appear mainly lethargic and apathetic, while formal mental-status testing is likely to reveal cognitive deficits.

- The possibility of pathologic fractures must be considered. Many health care facilities institute fracture precautions that include gentle handling when moving or transferring patients and fall-prevention strategies. Maximum mobility and weight-bearing exercises are desirable.

- Supportive care in terminal stages will likely consist of comfort measures for patients and their significant others. Changes in mentation and behavior may be especially distressing to family members.

### *Prognosis*

Hypercalcemia generally develops as a late complication of malignancy; its appearance has grave prognostic significance. It remains unclear, however, whether death is associated with hypercalcemic crisis (uncontrolled or recurrent progressive hypercalcemia) or with advanced disease. Currently available hypocalcemic agents have little effect in decreasing the mortality rate among patients with hypercalcemia of malignancy. Although there is some disagreement among investigators who have evaluated survival among patients with cancer-related hypercalcemia,[73-76] it has been observed that 50 percent of patients with hypercalcemia die within 1 month and 75 percent within 3 months after starting hypocalcemic treatment. In the same study, patients with hypercalcemia who responded to specific antineoplastic treatment were found to have a slightly greater survival advantage over nonresponders. Other prognostic variables shown to correlate with improved survival duration included serum albumin concentration (direct correlation), serum calcium concentrations after treatment (inverse correlation), and age (inverse correlation).[8] In contrast with their modest effect on survival, Ralston, et al. observed marked but differential response rates after hypocalcemic treatments as a factor of symptom type. The most substantial improvements occurred in renal- and central nervous system-related symptoms, nausea and vomiting, and constipation. Symptoms of anorexia, malaise, and fatigue improved, but less completely.[8]

### *References:*

1. Coward DD: Hypercalcemia knowledge assessment in patients at risk of developing cancer-induced hypercalcemia. *Oncology Nursing Forum* 15(4): 471-476, 1988.

2.  Calafato A, Jessup AL.: Body fluid composition, alteration in: hypercalcemia. In: McNally JC, Somerville ET, Miaskowski C, et al., Eds.: *Guidelines for Oncology Nursing Practice*. Philadelphia: WB Saunders Company, 2nd Edition, 1991, pp 397-401.

3.  Twycross RG, Lack SA: *Therapeutics in Terminal Cancer*. London: Pitman Publishing Ltd., 1984.

4.  Coombes RC, Ward MK, Greenberg PB, et al.: Calcium metabolism in cancer: studies using calcium isotopes and immunoassays for parathyroid hormone and calcitonin. *Cancer* 38(5): 2111-2120, 1976.

5.  Bilezikian JP: Management of acute hypercalcemia. *New England Journal of Medicine* 326(18): 1196-1203, 1992.

6.  Theriault RL: Hypercalcemia of malignancy: pathophysiology and implications for treatment. *Oncology* (Huntington NY) 7(1): 47-50, 1993.

7.  Mundy GR: Pathophysiology of cancer-associated hypercalcemia. *Seminars in Oncology* 17(2, Suppl 5): 10-15, 1990.

8.  Ralston SH, Gallacher SJ, Patel U., et al.: Cancer-associated hypercalcemia: morbidity and mortality. Clinical experience in 126 treated patients. *Annals of Internal Medicine* 112(7): 499-504, 1990.

9.  Ritch PS: Treatment of cancer-related hypercalcemia. *Seminars in Oncology* 17(2, Suppl 5): 26-33, 1990.

10. Suki WN, Yium JJ, Von Minden M, et al.: Acute treatment of hypercalcemia with furosemide. *New England Journal of Medicine* 283(16): 836-840, 1970.

11. Ignoffo RJ, Tseng A: Focus on pamidronate: a biphosphonate compound for the treatment of hypercalcemia of malignancy. *Hospital Formulary* 26(10): 774-786, 1991.

12. Binstock ML, Mundy GR: Effect of calcitonin and glucocorticoids in combination on the hypercalcemia of malignancy. *Annals of Internal Medicine* 93(2): 269-272, 1980.

13. Thiebaud D, Jacquet AF, Burckhardt P: Fast and effective treatment of malignant hypercalcemia: combination of suppositories of calcitonin and a single infusion of 3-amino

1-hydroxypropylidene-1-bisphosphonate. *Annals of Internal Medicine* 150(10): 2125-2128, 1990.

14. Ralston SH, Gallacher SJ, Dryburgh FJ, et al.: Treatment of severe hypercalcaemia with mithramycin and aminohydroxypropylidene bisphosphonate. *Lancet* 2(8604): 277, 1988.

15. Parsons V, Baum M, Self M: Effect of mithramycin on calcium and hydroxyproline metabolism in patients with malignant disease. *British Medical Journal* 1(538): 474-477, 1967.

16. Kennedy BJ: Metabolic and toxic effects of mithramycin during tumor therapy. *American Journal of Medicine* 49(4): 494-503, 1970.

17. Perlia CP, Gubisch NJ, Wolter J, et al.: Mithramycin treatment of hypercalcemia. *Cancer* 25(2): 389-394, 1970.

18. Ashby MA, Lazarchick J: Acquired dysfibrinogenemia secondary to mithramycin toxicity. *American Journal of the Medical Sciences* 292(1): 53-55, 1986.

19. Benedetti RG, Heilman KJ, Gabow PA: Nephrotoxicity following single dose mithramycin therapy. *American Journal of Nephrology* 3(5): 277-278, 1983.

20. Fillastre JP, Maitrot J, Canonne MA, et al.: Renal function and alterations in plasma electrolyte levels in normocalcaemic and hypercalaemic patients with malignant diseases, given an intravenous infusion of mithramycin. *Chemotherapy* 20(5): 280-295, 1974.

21. Purpora D, Ahern MJ, Silverman N: Toxic epidermal necrolysis after mithramycin. *New England Journal of Medicine* 299(25): 1412, 1978.

22. Bashir Y, Tomson CR: Cardiac arrest associated with hypokalaemia in a patient receiving mithramycin. *Postgraduate Medical Journal* 64(749): 228-229, 1988.

23. Ahr DJ, Scialla SJ, Kimball DB: Acquired platelet dysfunction following mithramycin therapy. *Cancer* 41(2): 448-454, 1978.

24. Margileth DA, Smith FE, Lane M: Sudden arterial occlusion associated with mithramycin therapy. *Cancer* 31(3): 708-712, 1973.

24. Bisaz S, Jung A, Fleisch H: Uptake by bone of pyrophosphate, diphosphonates and their technetium derivatives. *Clinical Science and Molecular Medicine* 54(3): 265-272, 1978.

26. Chambers TJ: Diphosphonates inhibit bone resorption by macrophages in vitro. *Journal of Pathology* 132(3): 255-262, 1980.

27. Cecchini MG, Fleisch H: Bisphosphonates in vitro specifically inhibit, among the hematopoietic series, the development of the mouse mononuclear phagocyte lineage. *Journal of Bone and Mineral Research* 5(10): 1019-1027, 1990.

28. Cecchini MG, Felix R, Fleisch H, et al.: Effect of bisphosphonates on proliferation and viability of mouse bone marrow-derived macrophages. *Journal of Bone and Mineral Research* 2(2): 135-142, 1987.

29. McCloskey EV, Yates AJ, Beneton MN, et al.: Comparative effects of intravenous diphosphonates on calcium and skeletal metabolism in man. *Bone* 8(Suppl 1): S35-S41, 1987.

30. Flora L, Hassing GS, Cloyd GG, et al.: The long-term skeletal effects of EHDP in dogs. *Metabolic Bone Disease and Related Research* 3(4-5): 289-300, 1981.

31. King WR, Francis MD, Michael WR: Effect of disodium ethane-1-hydroxy-1, 1-diphosphonate on bone formation. *Clinical Orthopaedics and Related Research* 78: 251-270, 1971.

32. Mautalen C, Gonzalez D, Blumenfeld EL, et al.: Spontaneous fractures of uninvolved bones in patients with Paget's disease during unduly prolonged treatment with disodium etidronate (EHDP). *Clinical Orthopaedics and Related Research* 207: 150-155, 1986.

33. Fleisch H: Bisphosphonates: pharmacology and use in the treatment of tumour-induced hypercalcaemic and metastatic bone disease. *Drugs* 42(6): 919-944, 1991.

34. Fenton AJ, Gutteridge DH, Kent GN, et al.: Intravenous aminobisphosphonate in Paget's disease: clinical, biochemical, histomorphometric and radiological responses. *Clinical Endocrinology* (Oxford) 34(3): 197-204, 1991.

35. Adamson BB, Gallacher SJ, Byars J, et al.: Mineralisation defects with pamidronate therapy for Paget's disease. *Lancet* 342(8885): 1459-1460, 1993.

36. Boyce BF, Adamson BB, Gallacher SJ, et al.: Mineralisation defects after pamidronate for Paget's disease. *Lancet* 343(8907): 1231-1232, 1994.

37. Nussbaum SR, Warrell RP, Rude R, et al.: Dose-response study of alendronate sodium for the treatment of cancer-associated hypercalcemia. *Journal of Clinical Oncology* 11(8): 1618-1623, 1993.

38. Zysset E, Ammann P, Jenzer A, et al.: Comparison of a rapid (2-h) versus a slow (24-h) infusion of alendronate in the treatment of hypercalcemia of malignancy. *Bone and Mineral* 18(3): 237-249, 1992.

39. Rizzoli R, Buchs B, Bonjour JP: Effect of a single infusion of alendronate in malignant hypercalcaemia: dose dependency and comparison with clodronate. *International Journal of Cancer* 50(5): 706-712, 1992.

40. Singer FR, Ritch PS, Lad TE, et al.: Treatment of hypercalcemia of malignancy with intravenous etidronate: a controlled, multicenter study: the Hypercalcemia Study Group. *Archives of Internal Medicine* 151(3): 471-476, 1991.

41. Jacobs TP, Gordon AC, Silverberg SJ, et al.: Neoplastic hypercalcemia: physiologic response to intravenous etidronate disodium. *American Journal of Medicine* 82(2A): 42-50, 1987.

42. Ryzen E, Martodam RR, Troxell M, et al.: Intravenous etidronate in the management of malignant hypercalcemia. *Archives of Internal Medicine* 145(3): 449-452, 1985.

43. Sawyer N, Newstead C, Drummond A, et al.: Fast (4-h) or slow (24-h) infusions of pamidronate disodium (aminohydroxypropylidene disphosphonate (APD)) as single shot treatment of hypercalcaemia. *Bone and Mineral* 9(2): 121-128, 1990.

44. Ralston SH, Gallacher SJ, Patel U, et al.: Comparison of three intravenous bisphosphonates in cancer-associated hypercalcemia. *Lancet* 2(8673): 1180-1182, 1989.

45. Gulcalp R, Ritch P, Wiernik PH, et al.: Comparative study of pamidronate disodium and etidronate disodium in the treatment of cancer-related hypercalcemia. *Journal of Clinical Oncology* 10(1): 134-142, 1992.

46. Nussbaum SR, Younger J, Vandepol CJ, et al.: Single-dose intravenous therapy with pamidronate for the treatment of hypercalcemia of malignancy: comparison of 30-, 60-, and 90-mg dosages. *American Journal of Medicine* 95(3): 297-304, 1993.

47. Elomaa I, Blomqvist C, Porkka L, et al.: Diphosphonates for osteolytic metastases. *Lancet* I(8438): 1155-1156, 1985.

48. Burckhardt P, Thiebaud D, Perey L, et al.: Treatment of tumor-induced osteolysis by APD. *Recent Results in Cancer Research* 116: 54-66, 1989.

49. Bounameaux HM, Schifferli J, Montani JP, et al.: Renal failure associated with intravenous diphosphonates. *Lancet* 1(8322): 471, 1983.

50. Ostenstad B, Andersen OK: Disodium pamidronate versus mithramycin in the management of tumour-associated hypercalcemia. *Acta Oncologica* 31(8): 861-864, 1992.

51. Ralston SH, Gardner MD, Dryburgh FJ, et al.: Comparison of aminohydroxypropylidene diphosphonate, mithramycin, and corticosteroids/calcitonin in the treatment of cancer-associated hypercalcaemia. *Lancet* 2(8461): 907-910, 1985.

52. van Holten-Verzantvoort AT, Bijvoet OL, Cleton FJ, et al.: Reduced morbidity from skeletal metastases in breast cancer patients during long-term bisphosphonate (APD) treatment. *Lancet* 2(8566): 983-985, 1987.

53. Warrell RP, Lovett D, Dilmanian FA, et al.: Low-dose gallium nitrate for prevention of osteolysis in myeloma: results of a pilot randomized study. *Journal of Clinical Oncology* 11(12): 2443-2450, 1993.

54. Tashjian AH, Voelkel EF, Levine L: Effects of hydrocortisone on the hypercalcemia and plasma levels of 13,14-dihydro-15-keto-prostaglandin E2 in mice bearing the HSDM1 fibrosarcoma. *Biochemical and Biophysical Research Communications* 74(1): 199-207, 1977.

55. Mundy GR, Rick ME, Turcotte R, et al.: Pathogenesis of hypercalcemia in lymphosarcoma cell leukemia: role of an osteoclast activating factor-like substance and a mechanism of action for glucocorticoid therapy. *American Journal of Medicine* 65(4): 600-606, 1978.

56. Ralston SH, Fogelman I, Gardiner MD, et al.: Relative contribution of humoral and metastatic factors to the pathogenesis of hypercalcemia in malignancy. *British Medical Journal Clinical Research* Edition 288(6428): 1405-1408, 1984.

57. Potts JT: Diseases of the parathyroid gland and other hyper- and hypocalcemic disorders. In: Isselbacher KJ, Braunwald E, Wilson JD, et al. Eds.: *Principles of Internal Medicine*. New York: McGraw-Hill, 1994, pp 2151-2171.

58. Massry SG, Mueller E, Silverman AG, et al.: Inorganic phosphate treatment of hypercalcemia. *Archives of Internal Medicine* 121(4): 307-312, 1968.

59. Hebert LA, Lemann J, Petersen JR, et al.: Studies of the mechanism by which phosphate infusion lowers serum calcium concentration. *Journal of Clinical Investigation* 45(12): 1886-1894, 1966.

60. Shackney S, Hasson J: Precipitous fall in serum calcium, hypotension, and acute renal failure after intravenous phosphate therapy for hypercalcemia: report of two cases. *Annals of Internal Medicine* 66(5): 906-916, 1967.

61. Goldsmith RS, Ingbar SH: Inorganic phosphate treatment of hypercalcemia of diverse etiologies. *New England Journal of Medicine* 274(1): 1-7, 1966.

62. Nolph KD, Stoltz M, Maher JF: Calcium free peritoneal dialysis: treatment of vitamin D intoxication. *Archives of Internal Medicine* 128(5): 809-814, 1971.

63. Cardella CJ, Birkin BL, Rapoport A: Role of dialysis in the treatment of severe hypercalcemia: report of two cases successfully treated with hemodialysis and review of the literature. *Clinical Nephrology* 12(6): 285-290, 1979.

64. Schreiner GE, Teehan BP: Dialysis of poisons and drugs—annual review. *Transactions—American Society for Artificial Internal Organs* 18(0): 563-599, 1972.

65. Stoltz ML, Nolph KD, Maher JF: Factors affecting calcium removal with calcium-free peritoneal dialysis 78(3): 389-398, 1971.

66. Seyberth HW, Segre GV, Morgan JL, et al.: Prostaglandins as mediators of hypercalcemia associated with certain types of cancer. *New England Journal of Medicine* 293(25): 1278-1283, 1975.

67. Seyberth HW, Segre GV, Hamet P, et al.: Characterization of the group of patients with the hypercalcemia of cancer who respond to treatment with prostaglandin synthesis inhibitors. *Transactions—American Society for Artificial Internal Organs* 89: 92-104, 1976.

68. Coombes RC, Neville AM, Bondy PK, et al.: Failure of indomethacin to reduce hydroxyproline excretion or hypercalcemia in patients with breast cancer. *Prostaglandins* 12(6): 1027-1035, 1976.

69. Brenner DE, Harvey HA, Lipton A, et al.: A study of prostaglandin E2, parathormone, and response to indomethacin in patients with hypercalcemia of malignancy. *Cancer* 49(3): 556-561, 1982.

70. Lad TE, Mishoulam HM, Shevrin DH, et al.: Treatment of cancer-associated hypercalcemia with cisplatin. *Archives of Internal Medicine* 147(2): 329-332, 1987.

71. Warrell RP: Etiology and current management of cancer-related hypercalcemia. *Oncology* (Huntington NY) 6(10): 37-43, 1992.

72. List A.: Malignant hypercalcemia: the choice of therapy. *Archives of Internal Medicine* 151(3): 437-438, 1991.

73. Warrell RP, Israel R, Frisone M, et al.: Gallium nitrate for acute treatment of cancer-related hypercalcemia: a randomized, double-blind comparison to calcitonin. *Annals of Internal Medicine* 108(5): 669-674, 1988.

74. Blomqvist CP: Malignant hypercalcemia—a hospital survey. *Acta Medica Scandinavica* 220(5): 455-463, 1986.

75. Mundy GR, Martin TJ.: The hypercalcemia of malignancy: pathogenesis and management. *Metabolism* 31(12): 1247-1277, 1982.

76. Fisken RA, Heath DA, Bold AM: Hypercalcaemia—a hospital survey 49(196): 405-418, 1980.

# Chapter 26

# *Bone Density, Osteoporosis, and Inflammatory Bowel Disease*

Make no bones about it. Osteoporosis is a serious medical problem. This disease, which is characterized by loss of bone mass and density affects over 75 million persons in the U.S., Europe, and Japan; a figure expected to double by the year 2020. By the time it is clinically apparent up to 30 percent of bone mass may be lost. As the bones lose the material of which they are composed, they become weaker and more brittle; the result is pain, deformity, and eventually fractures.

An estimated 1.3 million osteoporosis-related fractures occur each year in the United States. The annual cost of these osteoporosis-related fractures is over $10 billion/year. The most common osteoporosis-related fractures are those involving the hip (proximal femur), back (vertebral body), and wrist (distal forearm). Of these sites, hip fracture has the greatest effect on morbidity and mortality; there is a 15-20 percent reduction in expected survival in the first year following this fracture.

IBD patients are especially at risk to develop osteoporosis, and studies have found evidence of this in between 30 percent-60 percent of cases; this may occur even without steroid use, especially in Crohn's Disease. The exact reason why these bone abnormalities happen so frequently in IBD is not clear, but here are some possibilities:

- The chemicals mediators involved in chronic inflammation called "cytokines" may effect the daily normal process of bone remodeling;

- Decreased Calcium absorption is another possibility as is;

- Decreased Calcium & Vitamin D intake along with Malnutrition;

- Lastly the effects of Steroids on bone formation as well as decreased Vitamin D absorption is of great importance.

Steroids cause bone loss by influencing the normal balance between bone formation and destruction; they also inhibit calcium absorption by the intestinal tract. Steroid induced bone loss is greatest during the first 6-12 months of therapy. Studies suggest that the chance of developing steroid-induced bone fractures is increased if the daily dose is higher than 15 mg/day *or* if total life time dose is over 30 grams.

Postmenopausal women make up the largest of the groups at risk; in fact, women are four times more likely than men to develop osteoporosis. Additional risk factors for osteoporosis can be divided into *genetic*, *hormone-related* and *lifestyle-related*. They include:

- Caucasian or Asian race;

- Family history of the disease;

- Age (greatly increased risk over the age of 70);

- Early onset of menopause (before age of 45);

- Failure/surgical removal of ovaries, resulting in lower level of estrogen production;

- Estrogen deficiency due to certain conditions like anorexia nervosa, malnutrition, or over-exercise;

- Certain types of diseases like chronic liver disease, IBD, hyperparathyroidism, hyperthyroidism;

- Lack of exercise;

- Cigarette smoking;

- Excessive alcohol consumption;

- Inadequate calcium intake;

- Transplant surgery;

- Small body build.

Fortunately, progress is being made in the prevention, diagnosis, and treatment of this debilitating disease. Within the last several years it has become possible to measure bone density by x-ray techniques. These new x-ray techniques are easy, safe, and quick to perform; more importantly, they are precise, accurate, and predict the risk of fractures. They require no patient preparation, expose the patient to less radiation than a chest x-ray, and take only 10-15 minutes to perform.

The onset of osteoporosis and an increased risk for subsequent fractures in postmenopausal women correlates with a low bone density. In both men and women without any risk factors, bone density decreases by about 1 percent per year after age 30; this loss reaches 2-5 percent per year in women during the first five years after menopause. A Bone Mineral Density(BMD) scan is thus indicated in most patients who have significant risk factors for osteoporosis; repeat studies can be used to follow the success of therapy.

Prevention is the best treatment, and there are a variety of means to do this. You should check with your physician as to which is best for you. Here are some general guidelines

1.  Do not be sedentary—get some form of exercise.

2.  Decrease or eliminate risk factors such as tobacco and alcohol.

3.  Adjust calcium and Vitamin D intake according to your age, sex and medical condition(calcium intake in doses of up to 1500 mg/day may be needed for postmenopausal women). Calcium levels may need to be monitored by your physician.

4.  Estrogen is protective in postmenopausal women; the benefit of this needs to be weighed against the potential downsides such as increased risk of Uterine and Breast Cancer. This hormone can decrease the rate of subsequent osteoporosis related fractures by 50 percent.

Other therapies are available, ranging from the recently FDA approved medication Fosomax (Alendronate), to the hormone *Calcitonin*. Fosomax may be the first medication capable of reversing the bone changes that lead to osteoporosis. The pros and cons of the various treatment regimens should be considered carefully, aiming to insure adequate bone mass before it's too late.

# Part Five

# Osteoporosis Risk Factors and Prevention

# Chapter 27

# *Genes and Osteoporosis*

## *Gene Predicts Bone Density, Those at Risk for Osteoporosis*

Researchers have found a gene that may help to identify, early in life, individuals at high risk for osteoporosis. This gene strongly influences bone density, an important determinant of the risk of osteoporosis. Osteoporosis (porous, weak bone) affects more than 25 million people in the U.S.; it is the major underlying cause of bone fractures in postmenopausal women and the elderly. Osteoporosis usually results from two factors: the peak bone strength (density) attained in early life, and how rapidly a person loses bone in later life. "The prospect of having a genetic marker of bone density that would permit early intervention to prevent osteoporosis is extremely exciting," says Dr. Lawrence E. Shulman, Director of the National Institute of Arthritis and Musculoskeletal and Skin Diseases at the National Institutes of Health, which funded the study.

Although heredity has long been suspected of playing a role in bone density, until now genes responsible for this trait have not been identified. As reported in the January 20th issue of the scientific journal *Nature*, Dr. John A. Eisman and colleagues at the Garvan Institute of Medical Research in Sydney, Australia, have now found that a single

"Gene Predicts Bone Density, Those at Risk for Osteoporosis," *NIAMS Research News*, January 19, 1994, National Institute of Arthritis and Musculoskeletal and Skin Diseases (NIAMS). Available at http://www.nih.gov/niams/news/bmdgene.htm.

gene can account for up to 75 percent of the total genetic effect on bone density. This gene codes for the vitamin D receptor (VDR), a protein that enables vitamin D to exert its actions on bone and on calcium metabolism. Non-genetic factors such as hormones, calcium intake, and exercise also influence the density of bone.

Eisman and his colleagues measured bone densities in 70 pairs of identical twins and 55 nonidentical twins. The researchers found that identical twins, who share 100 percent of their genes, had more similar bone densities than did nonidentical twins, who do not share all genes. The researchers also found that there are two forms (alleles) of the VDR gene, one called "B" and the other called "b." Normal people have one copy of the VDR gene from each parent, and thus may have either the BB, Bb, or bb combination. The researchers then looked at the effect of the two forms of the VDR gene on bone density. They found a strong link between the "B" version of the VDR gene and low bone density in the spine and femur (thigh bone at the hip). Bone density was lowest in those with the BB combination, intermediate in those with Bb, and highest in those with bb. Nonidentical twins that had the same alleles of the VDR gene were similar to identical twins in this regard, thus strengthening the importance of these receptor genes to bone density. It is not yet clear how the difference between the two forms of the VDR gene could affect bone density.

The researchers also examined 311 unrelated healthy women from the Sydney area. In this second population, the vitamin D receptor gene was also found to be a strong predictor of bone density, and again the "B" allele was associated with lower bone density. Eisman and colleagues predict that women with BB, having low bone density in early life, will, when they start to lose bone as they age, reach the "fracture threshold" of low bone density in the spine 11 years earlier, and in the hip 8 years earlier, than those with bb. The latter translates to a four-fold increase in the risk of hip fracture for BB individuals as compared to those with bb.

These findings need to be extended to other and larger populations in the United States and elsewhere. They may provide an important explanation for the wide variation in bone density, not only among individuals, but also among various ethnic groups. African-American women in the United States, for example, develop approximately 10 percent greater peak bone mass by age 35 than do Caucasian women.

Research is also needed to uncover the precise role of the vitamin D receptor in regulating bone density. These investigations open new frontiers in research on the underlying causes of osteoporosis, and in particular the critical role of vitamin D in bone formation and metabolism. They could also pave the way for developing new targeted approaches to the prevention and treatment of this common and debilitating disease, a major public health problem in the United States.

The National Institute of Arthritis and Musculoskeletal and Skin Diseases, a component of the National Institutes of Health, leads and coordinates the Federal research effort in osteoporosis and related bone disorders by supporting research projects, research training, clinical trials, and epidemiological studies, and by disseminating information on research results.

**Reference:** Nigel A. Morrison et al. *Nature* 367: 284-287. January 20, 1994.

# Chapter 28

# Menopause and the Long-Term Effects of Estrogen Deficiency

## What to Expect

Menopause is an individualized experience. Some women notice little difference in their bodies or moods, while others find the change extremely bothersome and disruptive. Estrogen and progesterone affect virtually all tissues in the body, but everyone is influenced by them differently.

### Hot Flashes

Hot flashes, or flushes, are the most common symptoms of menopause, affecting more than 60 percent of menopausal women in the U.S. A hot flash is a sudden sensation of intense heat in the upper part or all of the body. The face and neck may become flushed, with red blotches appearing on the chest, back, and arms. This is often followed by profuse sweating and then cold shivering as body temperature readjusts. A hot flash can last a few moments or 30 minutes or longer.

Hot flashes occur sporadically and often start several years before other signs of menopause. They gradually decline in frequency and intensity as you age. Eighty percent of all women with hot flashes have them for two years or less, while a small percentage have them for more than five years. Hot flashes can happen at any time. They

National Institutes of Health, NIH Web Publication available at http://www.nih.gov/health/chip/nia/menop/men3.htm.

can be as mild as a light blush, or severe enough to wake you from a deep sleep. Some women even develop insomnia. Others have experienced that caffeine, alcohol, hot drinks, spicy foods, and stressful or frightening events can sometimes trigger a hot flash. However, avoiding these triggers will not necessarily prevent all episodes.

Hot flashes appear to be a direct result of decreasing estrogen levels. In response to falling estrogen levels, your glands release higher amounts of other hormones that affect the brain's thermostat, causing body temperatures to fluctuate. Hormone therapy relieves the discomfort of hot flashes in most cases.

Some women claim that vitamin E offers minor relief, although there has never been a study to confirm it. Aside from hormone therapy, which is not for everyone, here are some suggestions for coping with hot flashes:

- Dress in layers so you can remove them at the first sign of a flash.

- Drink a glass of cold water or juice at the onset of a flash.

- At night keep a thermos of ice water or an ice pack by your bed.

- Use cotton sheets, lingerie and clothing to let your skin "breathe."

### *Vaginal/Urinary Tract Changes*

With advancing age, the walls of the vagina become thinner, dryer, less elastic and more vulnerable to infection. These changes can make sexual intercourse uncomfortable or painful. Most women find it helpful to lubricate the vagina. Water-soluble lubricants are preferable, as they help reduce the chance of infection. Try to avoid petroleum jelly; many women are allergic, and it damages condoms. Be sure to see your gynecologist if problems persist.

Tissues in the urinary tract also change with age, sometimes leaving women more susceptible to involuntary loss of urine (incontinence), particularly if certain chronic illnesses or urinary infections are also present. Exercise, coughing, laughing, lifting heavy objects or similar movements that put pressure on the bladder may cause small amounts of urine to leak. Lack of regular physical exercise may contribute to this condition. It's important to know, however, that incontinence is not a normal part of aging, to be masked by using adult diapers. Rather, it is usually a treatable condition that warrants medical evaluation. Recent research has shown that bladder training is a simple and effective treatment for most cases of incontinence and is less expensive and safer than medication or surgery.

Within four or five years after the final menstrual period, there is an increased chance of vaginal and urinary tract infections. If symptoms such as painful or overly frequent urination occur, consult your doctor. Infections are easily treated with antibiotics, but often tend to recur. To help prevent these infections, urinate before and after intercourse, be sure your bladder is not full for long periods, drink plenty of fluids, and keep your genital area clean. Douching is not thought to be effective in preventing infection.

## Menopause and Mental Health

A popular myth pictures the menopausal woman shifting from raging, angry moods into depressive, doleful slumps with no apparent reason or warning. However, a study by psychologists at the University of Pittsburgh suggests that menopause does not cause unpredictable mood swings, depression, or even stress in most women.

In fact, it may even improve mental health for some. This gives further support to the idea that menopause is not necessarily a negative experience. The Pittsburgh study looked at three different groups of women: menstruating, menopausal with no treatment, and menopausal on hormone therapy. The study showed that the menopausal women suffered no more anxiety, depression, anger, nervousness or feelings of stress than the group of menstruating women in the same age range. In addition, although more hot flashes were reported by the menopausal women not taking hormones, surprisingly they had better overall mental health than the other two groups. The women taking hormones worried more about their bodies and were somewhat more depressed.

However, this could be caused by the hormones themselves. It's also possible that women who voluntarily take hormones tend to be more conscious of their bodies in the first place. The researchers caution that their study includes only healthy women, so results may apply only to them. Other studies show that women already taking hormones who are experiencing mood or behavioral problems sometimes respond well to a change in dosage or type of estrogen.

Studies indicate that women of childbearing age, particularly those with young children at home, tend to report more emotional problems than women of other ages.

The Pittsburgh findings are supported by a New England Research Institute study which found that menopausal women were no more depressed than the general population: about 10 percent are occasionally depressed and 5 percent are persistently depressed. The exception is women who undergo surgical menopause. Their depression rate is reportedly double that of women who have a natural menopause.

Studies also have indicated that many cases of depression relate more to life stresses or "mid-life crises" than to menopause. Such stresses include: an alteration in family roles, as when your children are grown and move out of the house, no longer "needing" mom; a changing social support network, which may happen after a divorce if you no longer socialize with friends you met through your husband; interpersonal losses, as when a parent, spouse or other close relative dies; and your own aging and the beginning of physical illness. People have very different responses to stress and crisis. Your best friend's response may be negative, leaving her open to emotional distress and depression, while yours is positive, resulting in achievement of your goals. For many women, this stage of life can actually be a period of enormous freedom.

## What about Sex?

For some women, but by no means all, menopause brings a decrease in sexual activity. Reduced hormone levels cause subtle changes in the genital tissues and are thought to be linked also to a decline in sexual interest. Lower estrogen levels decrease the blood supply to the vagina and the nerves and glands surrounding it. This makes delicate tissues thinner, drier, and less able to produce secretions to comfortably lubricate before and during intercourse. Avoiding sex is not necessary, however. Estrogen creams and oral estrogen can restore secretions and tissue elasticity. Water-soluble lubricants can also help.

While changes in hormone production are cited as the major reason for changes in sexual behavior, many other interpersonal, psychological, and cultural factors can come into play. For instance, a Swedish study found that many women use menopause as an excuse to stop sex completely after years of disinterest. Many physicians, however, question if declining interest is the cause or the result of less frequent intercourse.

Some women actually feel liberated after menopause and report an increased interest in sex. They say they feel relieved that pregnancy is no longer a worry.

For women in perimenopause, birth control is a confusing issue. Doctors advise all women who have menstruated, even if irregularly, within the past year to continue using birth control. Unfortunately, contraceptive options are limited. Hormone-based oral and implantable contraceptives are risky in older women who smoke. Only a few brands of IUD are on the market. The other options are barrier methods—diaphragms, condoms, and sponges—or methods requiring surgery such as tubal ligation.

### *Is My Partner Still Interested?*

Some men go through their own set of doubts in middle age. They, too, often report a decline in sexual activity after age 50. It may take more time to reach ejaculation, or they may not be able to reach it at all. Many fear they will fail sexually as they get older. Remember, at any age sexual problems can arise if there are doubts about performance. If both partners are well informed about normal genital changes, each can be more understanding and make allowances rather than unmeetable demands. Open, candid communication between partners is important to ensure a successful sex life well into your seventies and eighties.

For most women, natural menopause is not a major crisis and does not influence their opinion of their general health.

In a society that places so much value on youth and beauty, it's not much fun to think about menopause. But when you get there, you find it doesn't really make that much difference; you concentrate on how you feel about yourself, not on how you think others see you. I continue trying to improve myself, to keep learning and keep active. It's not your age that counts, it's how you handle it.

## *Long-Term Effects of Estrogen Deficiency*

### *Osteoporosis*

One of the most important health issues for middle-aged women is the threat of osteoporosis. It is a condition in which bones become thin, fragile, and highly prone to fracture. Numerous studies over the past 10 years have linked estrogen insufficiency to this gradual, yet debilitating disease. In fact, osteoporosis is more closely related to menopause than to a woman's chronological age.

Bones are not inert. They are made up of healthy, living tissue which continuously performs two processes: breakdown and formation of new bone tissue. The two are closely linked. If breakdown exceeds formation, bone tissue is lost and bones become thin and brittle. Gradually and without discomfort, bone loss leads to a weakened skeleton incapable of supporting normal daily activities.

Each year about 500,000 American women will fracture a vertebrae, the bones that make up the spine, and about 300,000 will fracture a hip. Nationwide, treatment for osteoporotic fractures costs up to $10 billion per year, with hip fractures the most expensive. Vertebral fractures lead to curvature of the spine, loss of height, and pain. A severe hip fracture is painful and recovery may involve a long period of bed rest. Between 12 and 20 percent of those who suffer a hip fracture do not survive the six months after the fracture. At least half of those who do survive require help in performing daily living activities, and 15 to 25 percent will need to enter a long-term care facility. Older patients are rarely given the chance for full rehabilitation after a fall. However, with adequate time and care provided in rehabilitation, many people can regain their independence and return to their previous activities.

For osteoporosis, researchers believe that an ounce of prevention is worth a pound of cure. The condition of an older woman's skeleton depends on two things: the peak amount of bone attained before menopause and the rate of the bone loss thereafter. Hereditary factors are important in determining peak bone mass. For instance, studies show that black women attain a greater spinal mass and therefore have fewer osteoporotic fractures than white women. Other factors that help increase bone mass include adequate intake of dietary calcium and vitamin D, particularly in young children prior to puberty; exposure to sunlight; and physical exercise. These elements also help slow the rate of bone loss. Certain other physiological stresses can quicken bone loss, such as pregnancy, nursing, and immobility. The biggest culprit in the process of bone loss is estrogen deficiency. Bone loss quickens during perimenopause, the transitional phase when estrogen levels drop significantly.

**Table 28.1.** Influences on Bone Development

| Increases bone formation | Speeds bone loss |
|---|---|
| Dietary calcium | Estrogen deficiency |
| Vitamin D | Pregnancy |
| Exposure to sunlight | Nursing |
| Exercise | Lack of exercise |

Doctors believe the best strategy for osteoporosis is prevention because currently available treatments only halt bone loss—they don't rebuild the bone. However, researchers are hopeful that in the future, bone loss will be reversible. Building up your reserves of bone before you start to lose it during perimenopause helps bank against future losses. The most effective therapy against osteoporosis available today for postmenopausal women is estrogen (see Managing Menopause). Remarkably, estrogen saves more bone tissue than even very large daily doses of calcium. Estrogen is not a panacea, however. While it is a boon for the bones, it also affects all other tissues and organs in the body, and not always positively. Its impact on the other areas of the body must be considered.

## Cardiovascular Disease

Most people picture an older, overweight man when they think of a likely candidate for cardiovascular disease (CVD). But men are only half the story. Heart disease is the number one killer of American women and is responsible for half of all the deaths of women over age 50. Ironically, in past years women were rarely included in clinical heart studies, but finally physicians have realized that it is as much a woman's disease as a man's.

CVDs are disorders of the heart and circulatory system. They include thickening of the arteries (atherosclerosis) that serve the heart and limbs, high blood pressure, angina, and stroke. For reasons unknown, estrogen helps protect women against CVD during the childbearing years. This is true even when they have the same risk factors as men, including smoking, high blood cholesterol levels, and a family history of heart disease. But the protection is temporary. After menopause, the incidence of CVD increases, with each passing year posing a greater risk. The good news, though, is that CVD can be prevented or at least reduced by early recognition, lifestyle changes and, many physicians believe, hormone replacement therapy.

Menopause brings changes in the level of fats in a woman's blood. These fats, called lipids, are used as a source of fuel for all cells. The amount of lipids per unit of blood determines a person's cholesterol count. There are two components of cholesterol: high density lipoprotein (HDL) cholesterol, which is associated with a beneficial, cleansing effect in the bloodstream, and low density lipoprotein (LDL) cholesterol, which encourages fat to accumulate on the walls of arteries and eventually clog them. To remember the difference, think of the H in HDL as the healthy cholesterol, and the L in LDL as lethal. LDL cholesterol appears to increase while HDL decreases in postmenopausal women as a direct result of estrogen deficiency. Elevated LDL and total cholesterol can lead to stroke, heart attack, and death.

# Chapter 29

# *Pregnancy, Lactation and Osteoporosis*

## *Pregnancy-Associated Osteoporosis*

Pregnancy-associated osteoporosis was first reported more than forty years ago. At that time researchers had identified four post-pregnancy patients with varying degrees of spinal osteoporosis. In 1955, researchers reported five women who experienced vertebral fractures following delivery. While other cases of pregnancy-associated osteoporosis have since been identified, studies surrounding pregnancy and bone have offered conflicting results, including no changes in bone density, and even increases at specific sites. It appears that if pregnancy-associated osteoporosis does exist, it is probably quite rare. (By 1996, eighty cases had been reported in the literature.) It is also a condition that is difficult to adequately investigate, given the inability to perform maternal radiologic exams.

Pregnancy-associated osteoporosis tends to be identified in the postpartum period (56 percent) or the third trimester (41 percent). Affected women usually present with back pain, loss of height, and vertebral fractures. Hip pain and fracture of the femur are less common but have been reported. The condition usually appears during the first pregnancy, tends to be temporary and usually does not recur. It is not entirely clear whether this disorder is a consequence of pregnancy or whether it occurs because of pre-existing conditions in the pregnant woman. Studies have shown that only a minority of these patients have risk factors, such as heparin or glucocorticoid exposure. On the other hand, it is possible that genetic factors play a role in the development of pregnancy-associated osteoporosis. In a study by Dunne and associates, mothers of patients with the condition had significantly more fractures than controls.

Theoretically, pregnancy-associated osteoporosis is believed to occur because of the stress on maternal calcium stores and an increase in urinary calcium excretion. Yet, the intestinal absorption of calcium is increased during pregnancy—especially in the second and third trimesters. The body also responds to fetal calcium demands by increasing total 1,25-dihydroxyvitamin D levels. These two mechanisms help to satisfy the increased demand for calcium during pregnancy. Other physiologic changes during pregnancy that may actually be protective of bone include the third trimester estrogen surge and increased bone-loading due to weight gain. Clearly, there is much to be learned about bone remodeling during pregnancy and why some women become prone to bone loss and even fracture.

## Lactation and Bone Loss

Studies have shown that the majority of women with pregnancy-associated osteoporosis are breastfeeding at the time of diagnosis. Duration of lactation has ranged from one week to seven months. Bone loss tends to be greatest in skeletal sites with the highest concentration of trabecular bone. Reductions in bone density by three to five percent at the lumbar spine are common.

Two physiologic occurrences may be responsible for bone loss during lactation. First, there is an increased calcium demand from maternal bone. This demand varies from woman to woman based on the amount of breast milk produced and upon the duration of lactation. Secondly, because of elevated prolactin levels, women who breastfeed tend to be in a hypoestrogenic state.

Though significant amounts of bone mineral can be lost during breastfeeding, the loss of bone tends to be transient. Studies have consistently shown significant trends in bone loss during lactation, with full recovery of bone density by six months after weaning. Kalkwarf and Specker reported women who experience an earlier resumption of menses lose less bone during lactation and recover more bone after weaning. Other studies have identified similar trends in bone loss, with full recovery of bone density by six months following the cessation of breastfeeding.

## *Parity and Osteoporosis Risk*

Much of the research reports an increase in bone density with increasing parity (the number of pregnancies a woman delivers past 28 weeks gestation.) The positive effect on bone density has been seen in both pre and postmenopausal women. Parity appears to have a protective effect against fracture, as well. In an arm of the Leisure World study, Paganini-Hill and others concluded that women with three or more children had a 30-40 percent reduction in hip fracture risk when compared to nulliparous women (those who have never given birth). The validity of studies that use nulliparous women as controls has been criticized, however. Many have suggested that nulliparous women may not be appropriate studies of parity since they have not demonstrated the ability to conceive and to support fetal growth and development. Such women may have a hormonal environment that impedes conception and negatively impacts bone density.

The National Resource Center is supported by the National Institute of Arthritis and Musculoskeletal and Skin Diseases with contributions from the National Institute of Child Health and Human Development, National Institute of Dental and Craniofacial Research, National Institute of Environmental Health Sciences, NIH Office of Research on Women's Health, Office of Women's Health, PHS, and the National Institute on Aging.

The Resource Center is operated by the National Osteoporosis Foundation, in collaboration with The Paget Foundation and the Osteogenesis Imperfecta Foundation.

# Chapter 30

# *Depression and Fractures*

Clinicians may need to pay careful attention to depression among postmenopausal women at risk for osteoporotic fractures. According to a new study by M. A. Whooley, MD, et al., depression increases the risk of osteoporotic fractures by 40 percent among women over the age of 65. (See Whooley et al., 1997.)

"Depression is a significant risk factor for fracture among older women," according to Whooley et al. Whooley et al. evaluated 7518 women who were taking part in the Study of Osteoporotic Fractures. The subjects all completed the Geriatric Depression Scale at their second annual visit. They were classified as depressed if they scored at least six out of a possible 15 points on the scale.

Bone mineral density was assessed in the spine and hip via dual energy x-ray absorptiometry. The researchers ascertained fractures for five years, confirming all fracture reports radiographically.

A little over 6 percent of the women were depressed, according to the Geriatric Depression Scale. This group of women had 40 percent more fractures than the non-depressed women in the study.

"This association was not affected by adjusting for hip bone mineral density, benzodiazepine use, self-reported overall health, exercise, smoking, alcohol, steroid use, estrogen use, and prevalent vertebral fracture," according to the researchers. Controlling for falls explained part, but not all, of the association between depression and fractures.

From *The Back Letter*, November 1997, Vol. 12 No. 11 p.121(1), © 1997 Lippincott Williams and Wilkins. Reprinted with permission.

The researchers also found an association between depression and bone mineral density but only among women in the highest fertile [i.e., top third] of body mass index. "Among these women, each standard deviation decrease in hip bone mineral density was associated with a 25 percent increase in [the incidence] of depression." This association persisted after controlling for numerous confounding variables.

The reasons why depressed women suffer more fractures remain obscure and should be the focus of further studies. "Whether a common risk factor causes depression, low bone mineral density. and fracture, or whether depressive symptoms are associated with low bone mineral density and fracture through other mechanisms remains to be determined," according to Whooley et al.

## *Reference:*

Whooley MA et al., Depression is associated with low bone density and fracture in older women, presented at the annual meeting of the American Society for Bone and Mineral Research, Cincinnati, 1997; as yet unpublished.

# Chapter 31

# *Secondary Amenorrhea Leading to Osteoporosis*

## *Rapid Read*

- Female athletes are at an especially high risk for the development of eating disorders, amenorrhea, and osteoporosis. Nutritional counseling may be the key to adequate treatment.
  Nutritional counseling begins with such simple concepts as
  meeting recommended daily allowances, matching calorie in
  take with output, and obtaining important vitamins and minerals through common food sources.

- The treatment of anorexia is complex and often prolonged. A
  multidisciplinary approach is the hallmark of treatment and includes the nutritionist, psychiatrist, and primary care practitioner.
  Family members should be involved in the process whenever possible. Women receiving Depo-Provera, especially those with other
  risk factors such as family history, excessive alcohol intake, cigarette smoking, and/or low calcium intake, should be advised of the
  possible risk of osteoporosis as a result of amenorrhea.

## *Abstract*

Health care providers should educate themselves about the risk
factors and preventive measures concerning secondary amenorrhea,

Used with permission from McGee, C.: "Secondary Amenorrhea Leading to
Osteoporosis: Incidence and Prevention," in *The Nurse Practitioner*, 22(5:38-
64), © 1997 Springhouse Corporation/www.springnet.com.

or menstrual dysfunction, and related osteoporosis. Amenorrhea in adolescent and young adult women can lead to a reduction in bone density and eventual osteoporosis. Anorexia nervosa, oral contraceptives, and long-term, strenuous exercise can lead to amenorrhea. A physical assessment of patients with amenorrhea and possibly a prescribed change in diet and exercise routine can help prevent loss of bone density mass.

Osteoporosis is widely accepted as a "female disease" occurring primarily in postmenopausal women. The fact that this disease can affect premenopausal women experiencing menstrual dysfunction is less commonly known. Amenorrhea decreases bone density at an age when bone formation should still be occurring. The implications of this failure to attain sufficient bone density during the formative years are frightening. The adverse effects on skeletal strength may lead to devastating outcomes in this subgroup of women, either now or in the future. This article reviews causes, risk factors, and treatments associated with both osteoporosis and amenorrhea.

Three causes of secondary amenorrhea are discussed in detail: rigorous physical training, anorexia nervosa, and use of the contraceptive agent medroxyprogesterone acetate injection. A review of the literature is presented in order to establish the link between amenorrhea and osteoporosis. A great many young women may be unknowingly placing themselves at risk for developing osteoporosis. This article includes interventions that may decrease this risk and improve quality of life.

A 25-year-old marathon runner breaks her foot while playing basketball with her coworkers . . . A 21-year-old female with a 7-year history of anorexia nervosa suffers from chronic low back pain after a vertebral fracture . . . A 34-year-old woman receiving medroxyprogesterone acetate [Depo-Provera contraceptive injection] fractures two ribs when she falls while hiking . . . These cases all have one important commonality: They involve young women who are suffering from osteoporosis as a result of amenorrhea.

Bone formation and menstruation both depend on complex interactions of genetics, hormones, nutrition, and exercise. Osteoporosis is widely accepted as a "female disease" that occurs primarily in postmenopausal women. However, the link between osteoporosis and menstrual irregularities in premenopausal women is not as well established. Amenorrhea does decrease bone density [1]; furthermore, failure to attain sufficient bone density during the formative years can result in insufficient skeletal mass after menopause when the rate of bone loss exceeds that of bone formation [2]. Health care providers for adolescents and young adults should be aware of the fact that amenorrhea has potentially dangerous short- and long-term effects on bone density.

The process of developing a healthy skeleton actually begins before conception, with genetics playing the determinant role in the amount of bone density an individual will attain. During growth and development, nutrition and exercise are necessary for the formation of healthy bone [3]. Peak bone density is achieved by the third decade. A decrease in skeletal mass then begins and is accelerated in females after menopause [4]. Table 31.1 illustrates some of the factors that contribute to peak bone mass [5]; the other important risk factors are listed in the following section.

Remodeling is the continuous breakdown and buildup of the skeleton. The two bone cells that are active in this process are the osteoclasts and osteoblasts. Osteoclasts are responsible for the destruction and resorption of osseous tissue, while osteoblasts form new bone to fill in the excavated areas. Remodeling takes place throughout the life span and is also responsible for fracture repair [3,6].

## *Osteoporosis*

Osteoporosis is "a disease characterized [sic] by low bone mass, microarchitectural deterioration of bone tissue leading to enhanced bone fragility, and a consequent increase in fracture risk" [3]. Both intrinsic and extrinsic risk factors have been identified. Intrinsic risk factors include ethnicity (Caucasian or Asian), a positive family history, female gender, and certain medical disorders: thyrotoxicosis, Type I diabetes, rheumatoid arthritis, and Cushing's syndrome. A history of menstrual disturbances has also been implicated and includes late menarche, amenorrhea, and early menopause. Examples of extrinsic risk factors are smoking, excessive alcohol intake, lack of regular exercise, and insufficient intake of dietary calcium [3]. Osteopenia refers to a bone density of more than two standard deviations below the expected norm for individuals of the same sex and age [7]. This condition is also a risk factor for osteoporosis [8].

The statistics associated with postmenopausal osteoporosis are staggering. The disease affects more than 25 million people in the United States. It is the most common cause of fractures in postmenopausal women and the elderly, accounting for more than 1.5 million fractures each year [9]. Financial costs, including hospital stays, surgery, rehabilitation, and lost productivity, are estimated at $10 billion per 250 million people every year. This figure is expected to rise dramatically with the rising cost of health care and the increasing size of the elderly population. Personal costs include pain, loss of function, loss of independence, and fear of recurrent falls [10].

Osteoporosis is often diagnosed at the time of the first fracture [3]. Clinical indicators such as the presence of risk factors and loss of height have been suggested as a means of population screening [11]. Commonly used methods of determining bone mass are single- or dual-photon absorptiometry, dual energy X-ray absorptiometry, and computed tomography. Conventional X-rays will not detect osteoporosis until 30 percent to 50 percent of bone mass has been lost [12,13].

New technologies that allow for the measurement of biochemical indicators of bone remodeling are being developed. "Bone markers" are found in the blood and urine and promise exciting opportunities for diagnosing and monitoring osteoporosis. Bone resorption markers are released into the bloodstream as a result of osteoclast activity and are excreted in the urine. The Federal Drug Administration (FDA) has approved three immunoassays for biochemical markers of bone resorption that are performed as simple urine tests using the first or second void of the day. Values above normal indicate rapid bone loss. Markers for bone formation also exist and are measured in the serum. Examples are bone-specific alkaline phosphatase, osteocalcin, and procollagen I extension peptides. These tests are not yet available for clinical use in the detection or treatment of osteoporosis, although research is ongoing in this area [13].

Extensive research and clinical trials are also occurring in the treatment of postmenopausal osteoporosis. Current therapies include

**Table 31.1.** Determinants of Peak Bone Mass

**ENVIRONMENTAL FACTORS**
alcohol intake
cigarette smoking

**NUTRITIONAL FACTORS**
calcium
vitamin D

**MECHANICAL FACTORS**
regular weight-bearing exercises

**HORMONAL FACTORS**
ovaries
thyroid
parathyroid
adrenal glands

**GENETIC FACTORS**
both parents contribute

calcium supplementation and regular weight-bearing exercises. Hormone replacement therapy is often prescribed and is effective in preventing, but not replacing, loss of bone density. Often, some combination of these three is used [14].

Other pharmacological interventions are being studied and/or have been approved for use. Drugs used to treat osteoporosis fall into two categories: those that slow or inhibit bone resorption and those that accelerate bone formation. Estrogen and calcium fall into the first category. Another drug in this category is calcitonin, which has recently been approved for use in the United States in the form of a nasal spray (Miacalcin). This medication is indicated for women who are unable or unwilling to take estrogen, are more than five years postmenopausal, and have low bone density. Finally, the biphosphonates are powerful inhibitors of bone resorption. Alendronate sodium (Fosamax) is the first medication in this class to be approved by the FDA for the treatment of osteoporosis and is taken orally. At present, there are no drugs available for use that stimulate bone formation. Fluoride is the only medication in this class that has been widely tested. Trials to date have shown conflicting results; therefore further research must be done to establish the safety and efficacy of this drug [6,13]. These therapies all provide hope for the future in the treatment of this disabling disease; however, the best treatment for osteoporosis continues to be prevention.

## Amenorrhea

Amenorrhea is defined as a lack of menstruation during the reproductive years. It is said to be primary when a female has not experienced menarche by either 16 1/2 years of age or within two years after the development of secondary sexual characteristics. Secondary amenorrhea is the absence of menstruation for greater than six months in a woman with previously normal cycles [15]. Eumenorrhea is a menstrual cycle of 38 days or less; oligomenorrhea is the term for a menstrual cycle of greater than 38 but less than 90 days [16].

Amenorrhea may have many causes. The most common is physiologic amenorrhea due to pregnancy or nursing. Pathologic causes of primary amenorrhea include anatomic abnormalities, gonadal failure, and disorders of the hypothalamic-pituitary-ovarian axis. Disorders of this axis may also result in secondary amenorrhea; other factors that predispose women to this condition include age less than 25 years, a history of previous menstrual irregularities, certain medications, and extreme physical and/or emotional stress. Secondary amenorrhea may also occur in conjunction with such diseases as Cushing's syndrome, Addison's disease, and hyper- or hypothyroidism [15,17]. In certain young women, the most often seen pathologic amenorrhea is hypothalamic in nature [1].

Hypothalamic amenorrhea may occur in women who undergo rigorous physical training. This type of secondary amenorrhea is believed to be due to a combination of factors; no single factor has been definitely implicated. The physiologic cause is an interruption in the release of gonadotropin-releasing hormone (GNRH), resulting in decreased levels of circulating gonadotropins and consequent decreased levels of estrogen and progesterone [1]. Factors known to play a role include body composition (height, weight, and percent body fat); type, intensity, and frequency of exercise; nutritional status; and the presence of emotional or physical stressors [18].

Females with anorexia nervosa may also experience hypothalamic amenorrhea. Malnutrition complicates the picture; deficiencies in both calcium and vitamin D are especially critical in contributing to the

**Table 31.2.** Laboratory Studies in the initial Workup of Amenorrhea [12, 24]

| Laboratory Test | Normal Values | Comments |
|---|---|---|
| human chorionic gonadotropin | <3 mIU per ml | 3mIU per ml at 10 days post - conception |
| prolactin | 1.0 to 17.0 ng per ml | |
| thyroid stimulating hormone | 0.7-5.3 mIU per ml | |
| follicle stimulating hormone | 5 to 20 mIU per ml | midcylce peak increase twofold |
| luteinizing hormone | 5 to 20 mIU per ml | midcylce peak increases to threefold |

possibility of osteoporosis [12]. It is worth noting that many athletes are extremely weight-conscious and therefore prone to eating disturbances; the term "Female Athlete Triad" has been coined to describe the combination of amenorrhea, osteoporosis, and the presence of an eating disorder in a woman athlete. As many as 15 percent to 62 percent of female athletes may suffer from eating disorders as a result of self-imposed standards, as well as pressures from competitors, coaches, and parents [19].

Depo-Provera is a medication that often causes secondary amenorrhea. This contraceptive agent has been used for more than two decades in more than 90 countries around the world. It was approved by the FDA for use in the United States in 1993. Depo-Provera is reported to be more than 99 percent effective in preventing pregnancy when given intramuscularly (I.M.) every three months at a dose of 150 mg [20]. The medication inhibits the release of gonadotropins by the anterior pituitary, thereby suppressing ovarian production of estrogen. This hormonal imbalance results in atrophy of the uterine lining. The most common side effects are menstrual irregularities, ranging from amenorrhea to continuous menstrual bleeding. The majority of women on this medication do become amenorrheic [21].

## *Evaluation of Secondary Amenorrhea*

A thorough history and physical assessment must be done on any individual who presents with secondary amenorrhea. The interview should include menstrual and sexual histories, nutritional intake, type and amount of exercise, history of previous fractures, cigarette use, and alcohol intake. When conducting the physical examination, certain areas should be emphasized. Of particular importance is an accurate determination of body composition through measurements of height, weight, percent body fat, and body mass index. The subtle signs of hypothermia, abnormally low blood pressure, lanugo hair, and a history of fainting may indicate an eating disorder and should be noted [19]. Of course, a pelvic examination must be included. Dry vaginal mucosa, scant cervical mucus, and parabasal cells on vaginal cytology are signs of low estrogen. Conversely, high estrogen levels may be evidenced by abundant superficial cells on vaginal cytology [22].

In conjunction with the history and physical examination, a number of laboratory tests are indicated. A serum beta-hCG must be assessed to rule out pregnancy [17,22]. Sexually active females should be counseled that pregnancy may occur even in the presence of amenorrhea. Appropriate birth control measures are therefore indicated and should be practiced throughout the course of the workup [23]. Random estradiol levels may be misleading and are not usually included in the laboratory workup [22].

Table 31.2 lists the normal values of the included laboratory studies [22,24]. After pregnancy has been ruled out, the next step is to measure thyroid-stimulating hormone and prolactin levels. Hyerprolactinemia indicates a need for imaging studies of the anterior pituitary, while hypothyroidism should be treated as indicated. If these levels are normal, the practitioner should then evaluate relative estrogen status. This may be accomplished through administration of a progesterone challenge. The standard protocol for this procedure calls for 10 mg of medroxyprogesterone acetate by mouth every day for 10 days. Lack of withdrawal bleeding (a negative test) indicates inadequate estrogen stimulation, an incompetent outflow tract, or a nonreactive endometrium. Further workup may then include administration of an estrogen/progesterone challenge, an endometrial biopsy, or surgery. The procedure for an estrogen/progesterone challenge calls for 1.25 mg of conjugated equine estrogen to be taken orally for 21 consecutive days, with the addition of 5 to 10 mg of medroxyprogesterone acetate on the last five days of the cycle. Follicle-stimulating hormone (FSH) and luteinizing hormone (LH) levels are indicated in the presence of hypoestrogenic amenorrhea and a competent outflow tract. Elevated levels of FSH and LH suggest ovarian failure. Normal or decreased levels call for magnetic imaging of the sella turcica to rule out pituitary tumor. If no tumor is present, the amenorrhea is most likely hypothalamic in nature [22].

The workup of both primary and secondary amenorrhea may be simple and straight forward or complex and prolonged. The foregoing discussion is meant as an overview of the process that may be followed by the primary practitioner. In addition to performing tests, procedures, and examinations, the practitioner who is treating any client with amenorrhea should devote some time to health promotion and disease prevention.

## *Osteoporosis and Amenorrhea*

Statistics associated with osteoporosis in young people are not as extensively documented as those relating to postmenopausal women. However, the facts that have been reported are disturbing. Young amenorrheic women may lose as much as 2 percent to 6 percent of bone mass each year. Over time, an athlete in her twenties could lose as much as 25 percent of her bone density, resulting in a bone mass equal to that of a 60-year-old woman [19]. Weight-bearing exercise may provide some protection from bone loss [25,26]. However, losses in bone density may not be fully recovered, even in women who become eumenorrheic [25,27]. Experts generally agree that loss of bone density in premenopausal women is particularly dangerous.

## *Occurrence and Incidence*

A number of studies have been conducted that link physical activity, amenorrhea, and osteoporosis. Two studies involving ballet dancers produced interesting results. The first evaluated the frequency of stress fractures in ballet dancers. A total of 54 dancers were surveyed. Those who had experienced fractures were compared with those in the non-fracture group. The groups were significantly different in two areas. Those in the fracture group reported longer times spent dancing each day and were far more likely to be amenorrheic: 56 percent versus 17 percent in the non-fracture group [16]. The second study compared ballet dancers with sedentary subjects. Amenorrheic subjects in both groups had lower measurements of density in the bones of the spine, wrist, and metatarsal. Amenorrheic dancers did show an increase in spine mineral density in the first year of the study, suggesting that weight-bearing exercise may provide some protection from loss of bone mass. A disturbing finding was the fact that amenorrheic subjects who began regular menstrual cycles during the 2-year study continued to show bone densities lower than those of controls [25].

Another study compared gymnasts, runners, and nonathletic females. Amenorrhea was far more prevalent in the athletes: 15 percent for runners, 28 percent for gymnasts, and 0 percent for non-athletes. Among the runners and gymnasts, those with menstrual dysfunction had slightly lower measures of bone mineral density than those with normal menstrual patterns. Regardless of menstrual status, gymnasts exhibited higher femoral neck bone mineral density than all other subjects. This finding further supports the theory that weight-bearing exercise increases bone density [26].

## *Premenopausal Bone Loss and Depot Medroxyprogesterone Acetate Administration*

A 39-year-old woman who had been receiving Depo-Provera for 17 years was seen for evaluation of recurrent fractures. The patient had been diagnosed with endometriosis at age 16 and was initially treated with oral contraceptives with only minimal relief of symptoms. At age 22, she was switched to Depo-Provera at a dose of 150 mg I.M. every 10 weeks. She was diagnosed with osteoporosis in 1991 after fracturing her left wrist. Her bone density at that time was two standard deviations below that expected for a Caucasian woman of her age. She was in good general health at the time and denied a history of cigarette or alcohol abuse. Her daily calcium intake was estimated at 800 mg. Her family history was negative for osteoporosis. The patient elected to continue on Depo-Provera and experienced a pelvic fracture in 1992 and right wrist fracture in 1993. Repeated measures of bone density showed a continuing decline. She was placed back on oral contraceptives in 1993.

- Osteoporosis is often diagnosed at the time of the first fracture. Conventional X-rays will not detect osteoporosis until 30 percent to 50 percent of bone mass has been lost. New technologies that allow for the measurement of biochemical indicators of bone remodeling are being developed. The Federal Drug Administration (FDA) has approved three immunoassays for biochemical markers of bone resorption that are performed as simple urine tests using the first or second void of the day.

- Current therapies include calcium supplementation and regular weight-bearing exercises. Hormone replacement therapy is often prescribed and is effective in preventing, but not replacing, loss of bone density. Often, some combination of these three is used. Other pharmacological interventions are being studies and/or have been approved for use. Drugs used to treat osteoporosis fall into two categories: those that slow or inhibit bone resorption and those that accelerate bone formation. However, the best treatment for osteoporosis continues to be prevention.

- Amenorrhea is defined as a lack of menstruation during the reproductive years. It is said to be primary when a female has not experienced menarche by either 16 1/2 years of age or within two years after the development of secondary sexual characteristics. Secondary amenorrhea is the absence of menstruation for greater than six months in a woman with previously normal cycles. Amenorrhea may have many causes.

- A thorough history and physical assessment must be done on any individual who presents with secondary amenorrhea. The interview should include menstrual and sexual histories, nutritional intake, type and amount of exercise, history of previous fractures, cigarette use, and alcohol intake. When conducting the physical examination, certain areas should be emphasized. Of particular importance is an accurate determination of body composition through measurements of height, weight percent body fat, and body mass index.

- In conjunction with the history and physical examination, a number of laboratory tests are indicated.

- Statistics associated with osteoporosis in young people are not a extensively documented as those relating to menopausal women. However, the facts that have been reported are disturbing. Young amenorrheic women may lose as much as 2 percent to 6 percent of bone mass each year. A number of studies have been conducted that link physical activity, amenorrhea, and osteoporosis.

Other research focuses on the combination of anorexia nervosa, menstrual irregularities, and osteoporosis. Researchers in one study examined measurements of bone density in adolescent girls with anorexia nervosa. Eighteen subjects were compared with 25 controls. Anorectic subjects demonstrated significantly lower lumbar spine and whole body bone mineral densities than controls. Twelve of the 18 subjects were amenorrheic and had bone density readings that were two standard deviations below normal for their ages [28]. A follow-up study evaluated the bone mineral deficits of 15 anorectic patients from the previous study. Nine subjects who gained weight during this time demonstrated increases in whole body bone mineral density. Four of the remaining six subjects actually had decreases in spinal bone density [29].

Other researchers examined the incidence of fractures in 27 women with anorexia nervosa. All subjects were amenorrheic. Four of the participants suffered fractures during the 2-year study period and two had experienced prior fractures. This was a higher incidence of bone breaks than is expected for women in this age group. A return of regular menstrual cycles did occur in six women who reached 80 percent of ideal weight. However, this was not significantly related to increases in bone density [27].

Research reports linking Depo-Provera with osteoporosis are rare. Two studies that have been published were carried out in New

Zealand, where the dose is the same as that used in the United States. In the first, Depo-Provera users who had been on the medication for at least five years were found to have significantly lower bone densities of the lumbar spine and femoral neck than premenopausal controls. The subjects did demonstrate significantly greater bone density of the lumbar spine than postmenopausal controls [21]. Results of another study showed a gain in bone mineral density over two years after cessation of Depo-Provera. This finding was more dramatic in the spine than in the femoral neck [30]. These studies have been criticized on a number of points, including small sample size, failure to measure bone density prior to Depo-Provera use, and high incidence of smoking among Depo-Provera users [31,32].

The lack of a definite link between Depo-Provera usage and osteoporosis development is evident from these few studies. An interesting case study of a young woman who developed osteoporosis after 17 years of Depo-Provera treatment raises further questions (Case Study) [33]. Was there a causal relationship between the Depo-Provera use and the disease? If so, what are the long-term implications for women in the United States who began using this medication within recent years?

### Prevention and Health Education

Any practitioner who provides health care to women of childbearing age plays a critical role in identifying and educating those at risk of developing premenopausal osteoporosis related to secondary amenorrhea. Health teaching and nutritional counseling are low-cost interventions with the potential for preventing devastating outcomes, especially in certain individuals.

### The Female Athlete

Female athletes are at an especially high risk for the development of eating disorders, amenorrhea, and osteoporosis [19]. Recommendations for decreasing the intensity, duration, or frequency of exercise should be made. However, these individuals may not comply due to their desire to stay with their training programs [18]. Consequently, nutritional counseling may be the key to adequate treatment.

The nutritional histories of women who undergo rigorous physical training often reveal inadequate intake. Additionally, these individuals may lack an understanding of the importance of balancing calorie intake with energy expenditure. Nutritional counseling begins with such simple concepts as meeting recommended daily allowances, matching calorie intake with output, and obtaining important vitamins and minerals through common food sources.

The American Dietetic Association has published recommendations for adult athletes. Carbohydrates should comprise 60 percent to 65 percent of total calories. Daily intake of protein is calculated according to body weight: 1 to 1.5 grams per kilogram. Fats should make up no more than 30 percent of daily intake. These values should be adjusted according to type of exercise and intensity and frequency of training [34].

Beginning with the understanding that adequate calcium intake is crucial to the development of peak bone density, teaching would follow with identifying that 800 to 1,000 milligrams per day is the recommended daily allowance for adults. This number increases to 1,200 milligrams per day between the ages of 11 and 24 and in pregnant or lactating women [35]. Some amenorrheic athletes may require as much as 1,500 mg per day [36]. Dairy products are a major source of calcium; unfortunately, dairy products are often not consumed in adequate amounts by young women due to the cholesterol and fat contents of these foods. Skim milk, skim milk cheeses, and low-fat dairy products should be suggested along with other calcium-rich foods such as those listed in Table 31.3 [12]. Individuals should be counseled that calcium from vegetables is not readily absorbed from the intestine; therefore, vegetables should not be the sole source of calcium [35]. Lactose-intolerant individuals should be encouraged to try lactose-free products. Calcium supplements may be necessary for those who cannot or will not increase their dietary intake. Vitamin D is necessary for intestinal absorption of calcium. An adequate amount of this nutrient is obtained in most individuals through sun exposure

**Table 31.3.** Calcium Rich Nondairy Foods [12]

| Vegetables | Fish and Shellfish | Nuts and Seeds | Others |
|---|---|---|---|
| collards | canned sardines | almonds | soybeans |
| beets | canned salmon | peanuts | dry beans |
| turnips | oyster | sunflower seeds | tofu |
| kale | shrimp | | molasses |
| mustard greens | | | |
| spinach | | | |
| broccoli | | | |

[12]. The fact sheet "Suggestions for Increasing Your Calcium Intake" (Table 31.4) [9,35,37] summarizes these and other recommendations.

**Table 31.4.** Fact Sheet: Suggestions for Increasing Your Calcium Intake

| Food | Serving Size | Calcium: Content in mg |
|------|------|------|
| skim milk | 1 cup | 296 |
| skim milk powder | 1/3 cup (dry) | 293 |
| skim milk yogurt | 1 cup | 272 |
| skim milk hard cheeses | 100 grams | 400 to 1,200 |
| canned sardines (with bones) | 100 grams | 400 |
| canned salmon (with bones) | 6 ounces | 334 |
| collards | 1 cup | 290 |
| spinach | 1 cup | 212 |
| broccoli | 1 cup | 98 |
| calcium enriched orange juice | 8 ounces | 350 |
| orange | 1 whole | 54 |
| dried apricots | 1 cup | 87 |
| dried peaches | 1 cup | 77 |
| raisins | 1 cup | 90 |
| stewed rhubarb | 1 cup | 211 |
| canned baked beans | 1 cup | 138 |
| sunflower seeds | 1/2 cup | 87 |
| tofu | 3 ounces | 114 |

## Suggestions for Increasing Your Calcium Intake

Calcium is a very important mineral that your body needs to build strong bones and teeth. You get calcium through your diet, and the amount of calcium you need changes according to your age and gender. All women who are pregnant or breast-feeding and those between the ages of 11 and 24 should get at least 1,200 mg of calcium each day. Women between the ages of 25 and 50 need 1,000 mg; those who are over 50 need 1,000 to 1,500 mg each day.

This sounds like a lot of calcium, but don't let the numbers scare you. It is possible to get all the calcium you need through your diet if you know which foods to eat. Calcium supplements are also available, and your health care provider may instruct you to take a supplement along with trying the suggestions listed here. The foods that are listed have all been selected because they are high in calcium but low in fat. If you give your body the calcium it needs, your bones and teeth will thank you by staying strong and healthy.

*Tips for Adding Calcium to Your Diet Without Adding Fat*

1. Add nonfat powdered milk to almost everything. Every teaspoon of dried milk supplies 33 mg of calcium. Try adding it to homemade bread recipes, instant pudding, hot and cold cereals, pasta dishes, and anything else you can think of.

2. Try tofu. There are many interesting tofu recipes that are inexpensive, tasty, and healthy. Check your local bookstore for a recipe book.

3. Eat the bones in canned fish. This sounds strange, but remember that the bones are soft from having been cooked. Once the bones are chopped or mashed, you won't even know they are there.

4. Avoid canned fish that has been packed in oil, as this increases fat content.

5. Try the fat-free and reduced-fat dairy products that are now available. This includes ice cream, yogurt, sour cream, and many different types of cheeses. Fat-free cheeses may be better for cooking than for snacking, but try different brands and types to find the ones that you like for snacking.

6. Combine the dried fruits that are listed above for a low-fat snack that is high in fiber as well as calcium. Dried fruits are excellent to carry to work or school and on hikes or long runs.

7. Do not get all your calcium from one source. Choose from dairy products, fruits, vegetables, and so on. This helps your body to be able to absorb the maximum amount of calcium from the foods you eat.

8. If you have problems digesting milk products, try the lactose-free products that are available.

9. Sunflower seeds do contain fat, but not as much as many of the nuts that contain calcium.

This tool may be photocopied by health care professionals for use in their clinical practice. Institutions wishing to photocopy this material must first contact the Copyright Clearinghouse Center at (508) 750-8400. © 1997 Springhouse Corporation, Springhouse, PA 19477.

There are many other important factors in the nutritional counseling of the female athlete. The processes of growth and development as well as the physical demands of training place strenuous demands on the body. Specifics such as total calorie requirements, minimal ideal body fat, adequate fluid intake, and planning for pre-game meals may require the input of a sports nutritionist.

## The Anorectic Patient

The treatment of anorexia nervosa is complex and often prolonged. A multidisciplinary approach is the hallmark of treatment and includes the nutritionist, psychiatrist, and primary care practitioner. Family members should be involved in the process whenever possible. Outpatient treatment is the ideal. However, hospitalization is necessary in cases such as suicidal ideation, weight loss greater than 30 percent below normal, or failure to gain weight [38].

A thorough nutritional assessment should be obtained and nutritional counseling provided. A structured format for the interview with frequent encouragement may be helpful in obtaining information. Major goals of treatment include gradually increasing food intake, maintaining a balanced intake, and establishing regular eating patterns. Contracts outlining specific dietary guidelines may increase feelings of control in these patients [38].

Anorexia nervosa is a recognized psychiatric disorder and must be treated as such by a specialist in this area. In addition to psychotherapy and nutritional counseling, pharmacologic treatment may be indicated with such medications as tricyclic antidepressants, gastrointestinal stimulators, and appetite stimulants [38].

## The Depo-Provera User

Women receiving Depo-Provera, especially those with other risk factors such as family history, excessive alcohol intake, cigarette smoking, and/or low calcium intake, should be advised of the possible risk of osteoporosis as a result of amenorrhea. Despite a lack of concrete information regarding the long-term use of this medication, risk factor modification should be strongly encouraged. Regular follow-up should include monitoring for loss of height as an early indicator of decreasing bone density [11]. Nutritional counseling may also be indicated for these women.

It is important to note that Depo-Provera has been approved as a safe and effective contraceptive agent. Research linking this medication with decreased bone density is scarce. In fact, oral medroxyprogesterone acetate is sometimes prescribed in addition to estrogen replacement therapy for the treatment of osteoporosis [6]. However, the possibility of bone density losses resulting from Depo-Provera use is mentioned in the literature. Obtaining informed consent in this area is recommended. Another recommendation is that prospective studies be conducted that look at measures of bone density before, during, and after Depo-Provera use [20,39,40].

## Compliance

Compliance with diet and lifestyle changes may be difficult in premenopausal women because of their developmental stage and lack of firsthand knowledge of osteoporosis. Health care providers should begin with a concise but complete explanation of the risk factors and possible outcomes of osteoporosis. Awareness of the real possibility of fractures might persuade some individuals to follow prescribed treatments. The fact sheets "Osteoporosis in Young Women" and "Suggestions for Increasing Your Calcium Intake" (Table 31.3) may be reproduced and distributed to patients. Additionally, pictures of deformities caused by osteoporosis may also have some impact, especially with appearance-conscious young women. Athletes might be amenable to improving nutritional habits in order to increase physical performance. Adolescents may be motivated to practice habits that will enhance overall appearance and energy levels.

## Osteoporosis in Young Women

### What Is Osteoporosis?

Osteoporosis is a disease that weakens bones. As bones become more fragile, it is possible that they will break more easily and with less force than they would if they were strong and healthy. There is not one specific cause of osteoporosis, but there are many risk factors that increase the possibility that a person will get this disease. Some of the more important risk factors are female gender, having someone in your family with the disease, not getting enough calcium in your diet, not exercising regularly, and cigarette smoking. Osteoporosis usually only happens to women who are over 65 years old.

### Why Do I Have to Worry about Osteoporosis?

Another risk factor for osteoporosis is stopped or missed menstrual periods. At your age, your body should still be working on building strong bones. If your periods have stopped or are not regular each month, your body may not be doing this. This may put you at risk of breaking a bone now, or later in life. Osteoporosis can also cause curvature of the spine (hunchback) and joint deformities.

### How Would I Know If I Had Osteoporosis?

The first clue that someone has osteoporosis is usually a broken bone. By that time, the disease has caused the bones to be very weak and brittle. That is why osteoporosis can be a very dangerous disease.

### Is There a Cure for Osteoporosis?

There is no cure for this disease. There are some medications that may help to stop the disease from starting or to slow it down once it has started. Right now, the best treatment is to stop osteoporosis from starting.

### Is There Anything I Should Be Doing?

Your health care provider will discuss any treatment that you may need to help make your menstrual cycle regular. Once your cycle is regular, you won't have to worry too much about osteoporosis. However, it is always important for you to get enough calcium in your diet. Dairy foods have the most calcium, and there are many other foods that will give you this important mineral. Young women between the ages of 11 and 24 should get at least 1,200 mg of calcium each day. The recommendation for women over 24 is 1,000 mg per day. This sounds like a lot, but your health care provider can give you suggestions for increasing the amount of calcium you get in your diet. It is also a good idea for you to exercise for at least 20 to 30 minutes three days or more each week. The type of exercise that will protect you against osteoporosis is weight bearing exercise. Some examples are walking, aerobics classes, and jogging. Exercises that are not weight bearing are swimming and cycling. Finally, if you smoke cigarettes, you should try to quit. If you don't smoke, don't start. These suggestions will lower your risk of developing osteoporosis now and as you get older. They will also increase your overall health and energy levels.

Many individuals are more concerned with their current state of health than with the possibility of illness in the future and may not want to comply with prescribed treatments. Despite the best of efforts, some women may resist changing certain behaviors. Providers in such cases must be willing to accept that decision and to provide positive reinforcement for any changes that an individual is willing to make [2].

## Conclusion

An unknown number of female adolescents and young adults may be at risk of developing a very serious chronic disease. Osteoporosis affects every aspect in the lives of those who suffer from it. Chronic pain, bone deformities, and loss of mobility are very, possible outcomes, especially if the disease begins in early adulthood. Health care providers who work with females of childbearing age should be alert for the possibility of osteoporosis occurring in amenorrheic individuals. The time spent educating susceptible young women may make a difference that will last several decades.

*— by Carolyn McGee*

Carolyn McGee, MEd, RN, is a Lieutenant in the United States Navy Nurse Corps. She is a recent graduate of the Medical-Surgical Nursing program at the University of Maryland at Baltimore.

**Editor's Note:** The views expressed in this article are those of the author and do not reflect the official policy position of the Department of the Navy, Department of Defense, nor the U.S. Government.

## References

1.  Hergenroeder AC: Bone mineralization, hypothalamic amenorrhea, and sex steroid therapy in female adolescents and young adults. *J Pediatr* 1995;126(5 part 1):683-89.

2.  Ausenhus MK: Osteoporosis; Prevention during the adolescent and adult years. *Nurse Pract* 1988;13(9):42,45,48.

3.  Dempster DW, Lindsay R: Pathogenesis of osteoporosis. *Lancet* 1993; 341:797-801.

4. Recker RR, Davies KM, Hinders SM, et al: Bone gain in young adult women. *JAMA* 1992;268(17):2403-08.

5. Chesnut CH: Is osteoporosis a pediatric disease? Peak bone mass attainment in the adolescent female. *Public Health Rep* 1989;Suppl:50-54.

6. Khosla S, Riggs BL: Treatment options for osteoporosis. *Mayo Clin Proc* 1995;70(10):978-82.

7. Ulrich U, Pfeifer T, Buck G, et al: Osteopenia in primary and secondary amenorrhea. *Horm Metab Res* 1995;27(9):432-35.

8. Fruth SJ, Worrell TW: Factors associated with menstrual irregularities and decreased bone mineral density in female athletes. *J Orthop Sports Phys Ther* 1995;22(1):26-38.

9. Optimal calcium intake. *NIH Consens Statement* 1994;12(4):3-5.

10. Barrett-Connor E: The economic and human costs of osteoporotic fracture. *Am J Med* 1995;98(suppl 2A,): 3S- 11S.

11. Ribot C, Tremollieres F, Pouilles J: Can we detect women with low bone mass using clinical risk factors, *Am J Med* 1995;98(suppl 2A):52S-55S.

12. Mikhail BI: Reduction of risk factors for osteoporosis among adolescents and young adults. *Issues Compr Pediatr Nurs* 1992;15(4):271-80.

13. Arnaud CD: Osteoporosis: Using 'bone markers' for diagnosis and monitoring. *Geriatrics* 1996;51(4):24-30.

14. Prince RL, Smith M, Dick IM, et al: Prevention of postmenopausal osteoporosis: A comparative study of exercise, calcium supplementation, and hormone-replacement therapy. *N Engl J Med* 1991;325(17):1189-95.

15. Pernoll ML: Menstrual abnormalities and complications. In: Benson RC, Pernoll ML. *Handbook of Obstetrics and Gynecology, 9th ed.* New York: McGraw-Hill, Inc., 1994:609-26.

16. Kadel NJ, Teitz CC, Kronmal RA: Stress fractures in ballet dancers. *Am J Sports Med.* 1992;20(4):445-49.

17. Chikotas N: Secondary amenorrhea. *J Am Acad Nurse Pract* 1995;7(9):453-60.

18. Myburgh KH, Watkin VA, Noakes TD: Are risk factors for menstrual dysfunction cumulative? *Physician Sportsmed* 1992;20(4):114-25.

19. Yurth EF: Female athlete triad. *West J. Med* 1995;162(2):149-50.

20. Medroxyprogesterone acetate granted contraceptive indication in *U.S. Clin Pharm* 1993;12:92-93.

21. Cundy T, Evans M, Roberts H, et al: Bone density in women receiving depot medroxyprogesterone acetate for contraception. *BMJ* 1991;303(6793):13-16.

22. Kiningham RB, Apgar BS, Schwenk TL: Evaluation of amenorrhea. *Am Fam, Physician* 1996;53(4):1185-94.

23. Thein LA, Thein JM: The female athlete. *J Orthop Sports Phys Ther* 1996;23(2):134-48.

24. Horowitz IR, Gomella LG: Laboratory. tests and their Interpretation. In: Horowitz IR, Gomella LG. *Obstetrics and Gynecology on Call*, Norwalk, Conn: Appleton and Lange, 1993:293-337.

25. Jonnavithula S, Warren MP, Fox RP, et al: Bone density is compromised in amenorrheic women despite a return of menses: A two-year study. *Obstet Gynecol* 1993;81(5 part 1):669-74.

26. Robinson TL. Snow-Harter C. Taaffe DR, et al: Gymnasts exhibit higher bone mass than runners despite similar prevalence of amenorrhea and oligomenorrhea. *J Bone Miner Res* 1995;10(1):26-35.

27. Rigotti NA, Neer RM, Skates SJ, et al: The clinical course of osteoporosis in anorexia nervosa: A longitudinal study of critical bone mass. *JAMA* 1991:265(9);1133-38.

28. Bachrach LK, Guido D, Katzman D, et al: Decreased bone density in adolescent girls with anorexia nervosa. *Pediatrics* 1990;86(3):440-47.

29. Bachrach LK, Katzman DK, Litt IF, et al: Recovery from osteopenia in adolescent girls with anorexia nervosa. *J Clin Endocrinol Metab* 1991;72(3):602-06.

30. Cundy T, Cornish J, Evans MC, et al: Recovery of bone density in women who stop using medroxyprogesterone acetate. *BMJ* 1994;308(6923):241-48.

31. Szarewski A, Hollingworth B, Guillebaud J: Depot medroxyprogesterone acetate and osteoporosis. Monitor serum oestradiol concentration in users. *BMJ* 1994;308(6930):717.

32. Sharma JB, Newman MR, Smith RJ: Depot medroxyprogesterone acetate and osteoporosis. Smoking may explain findings. *BMJ* 1994;308(6930):717.

33. Mark S: Premenopausal bone loss and depot medroxyprogesterone acetate injection. *Int J Gynaecol Obstet* 1994;47(3):269-72.

34. Position of the American Dietetic Association and the Canadian Dietetic Association: Nutrition for physical fitness and athletic performance for adults. *J Am Diet Assoc* 1993;93(6):691-96.

34. Davis JR, Sherer K: Minerals: The unique workers/substances. In: Davis JR, Sherer K. *Applied Nutrition and Diet Therapy for Nurses, 2nd ed*. Philadelphia: Saunders, 1994: 221-51.

36. Kerstetter J, Markley E: Osteoporosis. In: Benardot D, ed. *Sports Nutrition: A Guide for the Professional Working with Active People, 2nd ed*. Chicago: American Dietetic Association, 1992:148-52.

37. Lorig K, Fries J: *The Arthritis Helpbook, revised ed*. Reading: Addison-Wesley Publishing, 1986:21.

38. Davis JR, Sherer K: *Nutrition support for mental health alterations*. In: Davis JR, Sherer K. Applied Nutrition and Diet Therapy for Nurses, 2nd ed. Philadelphia: Saunders, 1994:615-48.

39. Kaunitz AM: Long-acting injectable contraception with depot medroxyprogesterone acetate. *Am J Obstet Gynecol* 1994;170(5, part 2):1543-49.

40. Kaunitz AM Rosenfield A: Injectable contraception with depot medroxyprogesterone acetate. Current status. *Drugs* 1993;45(6):857-65.

# Chapter 32

# *Alcohol and Osteoporosis*

## *Alcohol and Hormones*

Hormones are chemical messengers that control and coordinate the functions of all tissues and organs. Each hormone is secreted from a particular gland and distributed throughout the body to act on tissues at different sites. Two areas of the brain, the hypothalamus and the pituitary, release hormones, as do glands in other parts of the body, such as the thyroid, adrenal glands, gonads, pancreas, and parathyroid. For hormones to function properly, their amount and the timing of their release must be finely coordinated, and the target tissues must be able to respond to them accurately. Alcohol can impair the functions of the hormone-releasing glands and of the target tissues, thereby causing serious medical consequences.

Hormones control four major areas of body function: production, utilization, and storage of energy; reproduction; maintenance of the internal environment (e.g., blood pressure and bone mass); and growth and development. This *Alcohol Alert* describes how, by interfering with hormone actions, alcohol can alter blood sugar levels and exacerbate or cause diabetes (1-4); impair reproductive functions (5,6); and interfere with calcium metabolism and bone structure, increasing the

National Institute on Alcohol Abuse and Alcoholism (NIAAA), *Alcohol Alert*, No. 26 PH 352 October 1994. Copies of this *Alcohol Alert* are available free of charge from the Scientific Communications Branch, Office of Scientific Affairs, NIAAA, Willco Building, Suite 409, 6000 Executive Boulevard, MSC 7003, Bethesda, MD 20892-7003. Telephone: 301-443-3860

261

risk of osteoporosis (7). Conversely, hormones also may affect alcohol consumption by influencing alcohol-seeking behavior.

## Alcohol Impairs Regulation of Blood Sugar Levels

The sugar glucose is the main energy source for all tissues. Glucose is derived from three sources: from food; from synthesis (manufacture) in the body; and from the breakdown of glycogen, a form of glucose that the body stores in the liver. Hormones help to maintain a constant concentration of glucose in the blood. This is especially important for the brain because it cannot make or store glucose but depends on glucose supplied by the blood. Even brief periods of low glucose levels (hypoglycemia) can cause brain damage.

Two hormones that are secreted by the pancreas and that regulate blood glucose levels are insulin and glucagon. Insulin lowers the glucose concentration in the blood; glucagon raises it. Because prevention of hypoglycemia is vital for the body, several hormones from the adrenal glands and pituitary back up glucagon function.

Alcohol consumption interferes with all three glucose sources and with the actions of the regulatory hormones. Chronic heavy drinkers often have insufficient dietary intake of glucose (8). Without eating, glycogen stores are exhausted in a few hours (1). In addition, the body's glucose production is inhibited while alcohol is being metabolized (2). The combination of these effects can cause severe hypoglycemia 6 to 36 hours after a binge-drinking episode (1).

Even in well-nourished people, alcohol can disturb blood sugar levels. Acute alcohol consumption, especially in combination with sugar, augments insulin secretion and causes temporary hypoglycemia (9). In addition, studies in healthy subjects (10) and insulin-dependent diabetics (3) have shown that acute alcohol consumption can impair the hormonal response to hypoglycemia.

Chronic heavy drinking, in contrast, has been associated with excessive blood glucose levels (hyperglycemia). Chronic alcohol abuse can reduce the body's responsiveness to insulin and cause glucose intolerance in both healthy individuals (11) and alcoholics with liver cirrhosis (12). In fact, 45 to 70 percent of patients with alcoholic liver disease are glucose intolerant or are frankly diabetic (1). In animals, chronic alcohol administration also increases secretion of glucagon and other hormones that raise blood glucose levels (13).

Alcohol consumption can be especially harmful in people with a predisposition to hypoglycemia, such as patients who are being treated for diabetes (3,4). Alcohol can interfere with the management of diabetes in different ways. Acute as well as chronic alcohol consumption can alter the effectiveness of hypoglycemic medications (14,15). Treatment of diabetes by tight control of blood glucose levels is difficult in alcoholics, and both hypoglycemic and hyperglycemic episodes are common (4). In a Japanese study, alcoholics with diabetes had a significantly lower survival rate than other alcoholics (16).

## Alcohol Impairs Reproductive Functions

The human reproductive system is regulated by many hormones. The most important are androgens (e.g., testosterone) and estrogens (e.g., estradiol). They are synthesized mainly by the testes and the ovaries and affect reproductive functions in various target tissues. Other reproductive hormones are synthesized in the hypothalamus and pituitary. Although men and women produce many of the same hormones, their relative concentrations and their functions vary.

In men, reproductive hormones are responsible for sexual maturation, sperm development and thus fertility, and various aspects of male sexual behavior. In women, hormones promote the development of secondary sexual characteristics, such as breast development and distribution of body hair; regulate the menstrual cycle; and are necessary to maintain pregnancy. Chronic heavy drinking can interfere with all these functions. Its most severe consequences in both men and women include inadequate functioning of the testes and ovaries, resulting in hormonal deficiencies, sexual dysfunction, and infertility (5,6).

Alcohol is directly toxic to the testes, causing reduced testosterone levels in men. In a study of normal healthy men who received alcohol for 4 weeks, testosterone levels declined after only 5 days and continued to fall throughout the study period (17). Prolonged testosterone deficiency may contribute to a "femininization" of male sexual characteristics, for example breast enlargement (18).

In addition, animal studies have shown that acute alcohol administration affects the release of hormones from the hypothalamus and pituitary (5). Even without a detectable reduction of testosterone levels, changes in these hormones can contribute to the impairment of male sexual and reproductive functions (19). Alcohol also may interfere with normal sperm structure and movement by inhibiting the metabolism of vitamin A (20), which is essential for sperm development.

In premenopausal women, chronic heavy drinking can contribute to a multitude of reproductive disorders. These include cessation of menstruation, irregular menstrual cycles, menstrual cycles without ovulation, early menopause, and increased risk of spontaneous abortions (6,21,22). These dysfunctions can be caused by alcohol's interfering directly with the hormonal regulation of the reproductive system or indirectly through other disorders associated with alcohol abuse, such as liver disease, pancreatic disease, malnutrition, or fetal abnormalities (6).

Although most of these reproductive problems were found in alcoholic women, some also were observed in women classified as social drinkers, who drank about three drinks per day during a 3-week study (23). A significant number of these women had abnormal menstrual cycles and a delay or lack of ovulation.

Alcohol also affects reproductive hormones in postmenopausal women. After menopause, estradiol levels decline drastically because the hormone is no longer synthesized in the ovaries, and only small amounts are derived from the conversion of testosterone in other tissues. This estradiol deficiency has been associated with an increased risk for cardiovascular disease and osteoporosis in postmenopausal women (24). Alcohol can increase the conversion of testosterone into estradiol (25). Accordingly, postmenopausal women who drank (24,26) were found to have higher estradiol levels than abstaining women. Studies have shown that in postmenopausal women, three to six drinks per week may reduce the risk of cardiovascular disease (27) without significantly impairing bone quality (24) or increasing the risk of alcoholic liver disease (28) or breast cancer (29).

### Alcohol Impairs Calcium Metabolism and Bone Structure

Calcium exists in two forms in the body. The main reservoirs are the bones and teeth, where the calcium content determines the strength and the stiffness of the bones. The rest of the body's calcium is dissolved in the body fluids. Calcium is important for many body functions, including communication between and within cells. The overall calcium levels depend on how much calcium is in the diet, how much is absorbed into the body, and how much is excreted. Calcium absorption, excretion, and distribution between bones and body fluids are regulated by several hormones, namely parathyroid hormone (PTH); vitamin D-derived hormones; and calcitonin, which is made by specific cells in the thyroid.

Alcohol can interfere with calcium and bone metabolism in several ways. Acute alcohol consumption can lead to a transient PTH deficiency and increased urinary calcium excretion, resulting in loss of calcium from the body (30). Chronic heavy drinking can disturb vitamin D metabolism, resulting in inadequate absorption of dietary calcium (31).

Studies in alcoholics also have shown that alcohol is directly toxic to bone-forming cells and inhibits their activity (32-34). In addition, chronic heavy drinking can adversely affect bone metabolism indirectly, for example by contributing to nutritional deficiencies of calcium or vitamin D (7). Liver disease and altered levels of reproductive hormones, both of which can be caused by alcohol, also affect bone metabolism (7).

Calcium deficiency can lead to bone diseases, such as osteoporosis. Osteoporosis is characterized by a substantial loss of bone mass and, consequently, increased risk of fractures. It affects 4 million to 6 million mainly older Americans, especially women after menopause. In alcoholics, the risk of osteoporosis is increased (35). Because many falls are related to alcohol use (36), adverse alcohol effects on bone metabolism pose a serious health problem.

Studies with abstinent alcoholics have found that alcohol-induced changes in bone metabolism, including toxic effects on bone-forming cells, are at least partially reversible after cessation of drinking (32,33,37,38).

## Hormones May Influence Alcohol-Seeking Behavior

The effects of alcohol on different hormonal pathways may in turn influence alcohol-seeking behavior. For example, in animals, alcohol-seeking behavior appears to be regulated in part through a system called the renin-angiotensin system, which controls blood pressure and salt concentrations in the blood. In rats, activation of this system through alcohol consumption caused the animals to reduce their alcohol intake (39). The mechanism and relevance of this effect are currently under investigation.

## Alcohol and Hormones—
## A Commentary by NIAAA Director Enoch Gordis, M.D.

Alcohol's wide-ranging effects on the hormone system present many practical clinical concerns. For example, managing diabetes, particularly with the current emphasis on stringent control of blood sugar, is complicated by alcohol's interference with blood sugar levels. In the emergency room, stupor in patients with alcohol on their breath often is not caused by alcohol intoxication, but by the hypoglycemia (low blood sugar) that is a complication of heavy drinking. Failure to treat the hypoglycemia could have life-threatening consequences. Heavy drinking has a major effect on the reproductive system, affecting libido, fertility, and pregnancy. Heavy drinking also places postmenopausal women at risk for fractures from falls due to their increased risk for osteoporosis from alcohol's effect on blood estrogen levels coupled with their increased risk of falling due to drinking. However, it is possible that moderate alcohol use may help protect postmenopausal women against osteoporosis by raising blood estrogen levels. Scientists are working to discover for which population this may be true and at what drinking levels. Finally, research on how alcohol's interactions with hormones may contribute to the pathological drive to consume alcohol is just beginning and may provide valuable insight into the mechanisms by which alcohol-seeking behavior can be controlled.

## *References*

1. Gordon, G.G., & Lieber, C.S. Alcohol, hormones, and metabolism. In: Lieber, C.S., ed. *Medical and Nutritional Complications of Alcoholism*. New York: Plenum Publishing Corp., 1992. pp. 55-90.

2. Sneyd, J.G.T. Interactions of ethanol and carbohydrate metabolism. In: Crow, K.E., and Batt, R.D., eds. *Human Metabolism of Alcohol, Vol. 3*. Boca Raton, FL: CRC Press, 1989. pp. 115-124.

3. Avogaro, A.; Beltramello, P.; Gnudi, L.; Maran, A.; Valerio, A.; Miola, M.; Marin, N.; Crepladi, C.; Confortin, L.; Costa, F.; MacDonald, I.; & Tiengo, A. Alcohol intake impairs glucose counter regulation during acute insulin-induced hypoglycemia in IDDM patients: Evidence for a critical role of free fatty acids. *Diabetes* 42(11):1626-1634, 1993.

4. Crane, M., & Sereny, G. Alcohol and diabetes. *British Journal of Addiction* 83(12):1357-1358, 1988.

5. Emanuele, M.A.; Halloran, M.M.; Uddin, S.; Tentler, J.J.; Emanuele, N.V.; Lawrence, A.M.; & Kelley, M.R. The effects of alcohol on the neuroendocrine control of reproduction. In: Zakhari, S., ed. *Alcohol and the Endocrine System*. National Institute on Alcohol Abuse and Alcoholism Research Monograph

No. 23. NIH Pub. No. 93-3533. Bethesda, MD: National Institutes of Health, 1993. pp. 89-116.

6.  Mello, N.K.; Mendelson, J.H.; & Teoh, S.K. An overview of the effects of alcohol on neuroendocrine function in women. In: Zakhari, S., ed. *Alcohol and the Endocrine System.* National Institute on Alcohol Abuse and Alcoholism Research Monograph No. 23. NIH Pub. No 93-3533. Bethesda, MD: National Institutes of Health, 1993. pp. 139-170.

7.  Laitinen, K., & Valimaki, M. Bone and the "comforts of life." *Annals of Medicine* 25(4):413-425, 1993.

8.  Palmer, T.N.; Cook, E.B.; & Drake, P.G. Alcohol abuse and fuel homeostasis. In: Palmer, T.N., ed. *Alcoholism: A Molecular Perspective.* NATO ASI Series. Series A, Life Sciences Vol. 206. New York: Plenum Press, 1991. pp. 223-235.

9.  O'Keefe, S.J., & Marks, V. Lunchtime gin and tonic a cause of reactive hypoglycemia. *Lancet* 1(8025):1286-1288, 1977.

10. Kolaczynski, J.W.; Ylikahri, R.; Harkonen, M.; & Koivisto, V.A. Acute effect of ethanol on counter-regulatory response and recovery from insulin-induced hypoglycemia. *Journal of Clinical Endocrinology and Metabolism* 67(2):384-388, 1988.

11. Shah, J.H. Alcohol decreases insulin sensitivity in healthy subjects. *Alcohol and Alcoholism* 23(2):103-109, 1988.

12. Letiexhe, M.R.; Scheen, A.J.; Gerard, P.L.; Bastens, B.H.; Pirotte, J.; Belaiche, J.; & Lefebvre, P.J. Insulin secretion, clearance, and action on glucose metabolism in cirrhotic patients. *Journal of Clinical Endocrinology and Metabolism* 77(5):1263-1268, 1993.

13. Adams, M.A., & Hirst, M. Adrenal and urinary catecholamines during and after severe ethanol intoxication in rats: A profile of changes. *Pharmacology, Biochemistry and Behavior* 21(1):125-131, 1984.

14. Lewis, H., & Kendall, M.J. Alcohol and treatment of diabetes. *Journal of Clinical Pharmacy and Therapeutics* 13:312-328, 1988.

15. Angelini, P.; Vendemiale, G.; & Altomare, E. Alcohol and diabetes mellitus. *Alcologia* 4(2):109-111, 1992.

16. Yokoyama, A.; Matsushita, S.; Ishii, H.; Takagi, T.; Maruyama, K.; & Tsuchiya, M. Impact of diabetes mellitus on the prognosis of alcoholics. *Alcohol and Alcoholism* 29(2)181-186, 1994.

17. Gordon, G.C.; Altman, K.; Southren, A.L.; Rubin, E.; & Lieber, C.S. The effects of alcohol (ethanol) administration on sex hormone metabolism in normal men. *New England Journal of Medicine* 295:793-797, 1976.

18. Bannister, P., & Lowosky, M.S. Ethanol and hypogonadism. *Alcohol and Alcoholism* 22(3):213-217, 1987.

19. Bartke, A. Chronic disturbances of the hypothalamic-pituitary-testicular axis: Effects on sexual behavior and fertility. In: Zakhari, S., ed. *Alcohol and the Endocrine System.* National Institute on Alcohol Abuse and Alcoholism Research Monograph No. 23. NIH Pub. No. 93-3533. Bethesda, MD: National Institutes of Health, 1993, pp. 69-87.

20. Leo, M.A., & Lieber, C.S. Hepatic vitamin A depletion in alcoholic liver injury. *New England Journal of Medicine* 307(10):597-601, 1982.

21. Alcohol and abortion. *New Zealand Medical Journal* 92:353, 1980.

22. Kline, J.; Levin, B.; Stein, Z.; Susser, M.; & Warburton, D. Epidemiologic detection of low dose effects on the developing fetus. *Environmental Health Perspectives* 42:119-126, 1981.

23. Mendelson, J.H., & Mello, N.K. Chronic alcohol effects on anterior pituitary and ovarian hormones in healthy women. *Journal of Pharmacological and Experimental Therapy* 245:407-412, 1988.

24. Gavaler, J.S., & Van Thiel, D.H. The association between moderate alcoholic beverage consumption and serum estradiol and testosterone levels in normal postmenopausal women: Relationship to the literature. *Alcoholism: Clinical and Experimental Research* 16(1):87-92, 1992.

25. Gordon, G.G.; Southren, A.L.; Vittek, J.; & Lieber, C.S. Effect of alcohol ingestion on hepatic aromatase activity and plasma steroid hormones in the rat. *Metabolism* 28(1):20-24, 1979.

26. Gavaler, J.S., & Van Thiel, D.H. Hormonal status of postmeno-pausal women with alcohol-induced cirrhosis: Further findings and a review of the literature. *Hepatology* 16(2):312-319, 1992.

27. Stampfer, M.J.; Colditz, G.A.; Willett, W.C.; Speizer, F.E.; & Hennekens, C.H. A prospective study of moderate alcohol con-sumption and the risk of coronary disease and stroke in women. *New England Journal of Medicine* 319:267-273, 1988.

28. Gavaler, J.S.; Kelly, R.H.; Wight, C.; Sanghvi, A.; Cauley, J.; Belle, S.; & Brandt, K. Does moderate alcoholic beverage con-sumption affect liver function/injury tests in postmenopausal women? *Alcoholism: Clinical and Experimental Research* 12(2):337, 1988.

29. Willett, W.C.; Stampfer, M.J.; Colditz, G.A.; Rosner, B.A.; Hennekens, C.H.; & Speizer, F.E. Moderate alcohol consump-tion and the risk of breast cancer. *New England Journal of Medicine* 316:1174-1180, 1987.

30. Laitinen, K.; Lamberg-Allardt, C.; Tunninen, R.; Karonen, S.L.; Tahetla, R.; Ylikahri, R.; & Valimaki, M. Transient hypo-parathyroidism during acute alcohol intoxication. *New En-gland Journal of Medicine* 324(11):721-727, 1991.

31. Bjorneboe, A.-E.A.; Bjorneboe, A.; Johnsen, J.; Skylv, N.; Oftebro, H.; Gautvik,K.M.; Hoiseth, A.; Morland, J.; & Drevon, C.A. Calcium status and calcium-regulating hor-mones in alcoholics. *Alcoholism: Clinical and Experimental Research* 12(2):229-232, 1988.

32. Jaouhari, J.; Schiele, F.; Pirollet, P.; Lecomte, E.; Paille, F.; & Artur, Y. Concentration and hydroxyapatite binding capacity of plasma osteocalcin in chronic alcoholic men: Effect of a three-week withdrawal therapy. *Bone and Mineral* 21(3):171-178, 1993.

33. Pepersack, T.; Fuss, M.; Otero, J.; Bergmann, P.; Valsamis, J.; & Corvilain, J. Longitudinal study of bone metabolism after ethanol withdrawal in alcoholic patients. *Journal of Bone and Mineral Research* 7(4):383-387, 1992.

34. Bikle, D.D.; Stesin, A.; Halloran, B.; Steibach, L.; & Recker, R. Alcohol-induced bone disease: Relationship to age and par-athyroid hormone levels. *Alcoholism: Clinical and Experimen-tal Research* 17(3)690-695, 1993.

35.  Rico, H. Alcohol and bone disease. *Alcohol and Alcoholism* 25(4):345-352, 1990.

36.  Hingson, R., & Howland, J. Alcohol as a risk factor for injury or death resulting from accidental falls: A review of the literature. *Journal of Studies on Alcohol* 48(3):212-219, 1987.

37.  Gonzalez-Calvin, J.L.; Garcia-Sanchez, A.; Bellot, V.; Munoz-Torres, M.; Raya-Alvarez, E.; & Salvatierra-Rios, D. Mineral metabolism, osteoblastic function and bone mass in chronic alcoholism. *Alcohol and Alcoholism* 28(5):571-579, 1993.

38.  Laitinen, K.; Lamberg-Allardt, C.; Tunninen, R.; Harkonen, M.; & Valimaki, M. Bone mineral density and abstention-induced changes in bone and mineral metabolism in noncirrhotic male alcoholics. *American Journal of Medicine* 93(6):642-650, 1992.

39.  Grupp, L.A. The renin-angiotensin system as a regulator of alcohol consumption: A review and some new insights. In: Zakhari, S., ed. *Alcohol and the Endocrine System.*

ACKNOWLEDGMENT: The National Institute on Alcohol Abuse and Alcoholism wishes to acknowledge the valuable contributions of Judith Fradkin, M.D., Chief, Endocrinology and Metabolic Diseases Program Branch, National Institute of Diabetes and Digestive and Kidney Diseases, to the development of this *Alcohol Alert.*

# Chapter 33

# *Smoking and Bone Health*

Many of the health consequences of tobacco use are well established. The Center for Disease Control reports that smoking-related illnesses result in nearly $50 billion in direct health care expenses each year. Cigarette smoking causes heart disease, lung and esophageal cancer, and chronic lung disease. What is less clear is the effect of tobacco use on bone density and fracture risk. While the majority of the research has implicated smoking as a risk factor for osteoporosis and fracture, some studies have failed to find an association. This chapter will explore the relationship between cigarette smoking and bone health.

## *Tobacco Use and Bone Density*

Cigarette smoking was first identified as a risk factor for osteoporosis more than 20 years ago. Subsequent studies have also demonstrated a direct relationship between tobacco use and decreased bone density. However, not all studies have supported this finding. Though the majority of research has focused on women, studies in men have also identified smoking as a risk factor for low bone density. In a study by Vogel and associates on Japanese-American men, bone loss was greatest at sites with the higher concentrations of cancellous bone. Significant bone loss has been found in postmenopausal women and older men with prolonged smoking exposure. Deficits ranging from 0.5 to 1.0 standard deviations have been identified in these groups. In addition, a relationship between cigarette smoking and low bone density in adolescence and early adulthood has been identified.

Analyzing the impact of cigarette smoking on the skeleton can be difficult for several reasons. It has been suggested that differences in bone density between smokers and non-smokers may be due to concomitant lifestyle factors. For example, smokers are often thinner than their non-smoking counterparts. Smokers also tend to have a higher consumption of alcohol, may be less physically active, often have nutritional deficiencies, and tend to have an earlier menopause than non-smokers. These characteristics place many smokers at an increased risk for osteoporosis apart from their tobacco consumption.

## Tobacco Use and Fracture

While the association between tobacco use and decreased bone density is fairly strong, the results are less consistent when fractures are considered. Most studies suggest at least a slight association between cigarette smoking and fracture, especially hip fracture and vertebral fracture. Not all studies have found such a relationship, however. Studies have yet to demonstrate an association between tobacco use and forearm fractures.

## Cigarette Smoking and Estrogen

In an arm of the Framingham study, Kiel and colleagues found that smoking use did not increase hip fracture risk in women. Importantly, the study also concluded that while estrogen replacement protected women from fracture, this protective effect was eliminated in women on estrogen replacement who smoked. Kiel's results support an anti-estrogenic effect of cigarette smoking that is consistent with the conclusions of other researchers. For example, smokers are less likely to develop uterine cancer, fibrocystic disease and fibroadenoma. Each of these conditions is believed to be related to estrogenic stimulation. Other reports have suggested that smokers have less effective absorption of calcium, opposite to the effect of estrogen, which is believed to enhance calcium absorption.

The anti-estrogen effect of tobacco use may help explain the increased risk for osteoporosis among female smokers. Postmenopausal smokers have lower estrogen levels than non-smokers and smokers tend to have an earlier menopause than their non-smoking counterparts.

This reduction in estrogen is likely to result in an increase in bone resorption, contributing to osteoporosis and fracture risk.

On a positive note, researchers have discovered that smoking cessation, even later in life, may help limit smoking-related bone loss.

For further information on smoking and bone health contact the Resource Center at 202-223-0344. The Resource Center publishes an annotated bibliography on smoking and osteoporosis. Free copies are available. Bibliographies can also be downloaded from the NIH ORBD—NRC web site.

National Institutes of Health
Osteoporosis and Related Bone Diseases—
National Resource Center
1150 17th St., NW, Suite 500, Washington, D.C. 20036
202-223-0344 or 800-624-BONE
Fax (202) 223-2237
TTY (202) 466-4315
E-Mail: orbdnrc@nof.org

The National Resource Center is supported by the National Institute of Arthritis and Musculoskeletal and Skin Diseases, with contributions from the National Institute of Child Health and Human Development, National Institute of Dental and Craniofacial Research, National Institute of Environmental Health Sciences, NIH Office of Research on Women's Health, Office of Women's Health, PHS, and the National Institute on Aging.

The Resource Center is operated by the National Osteoporosis Foundation, in collaboration with The Paget Foundation and the Osteogenesis Imperfecta Foundation.

Chapter 34

# Understanding the Female Athlete Triad: Eating Disorders, Amenorrhea, and Osteoporosis

**Abstract:** This article discusses the risk factors of eating disorders, amenorrhea, and osteoporosis, considered the triad of female athletes. Methods are offered for preventing the onset of these disorders and for identifying and treating these disorders once they occur.

## Introduction

Since passage of Title IX legislation in 1972, there has been a dramatic increase in the number of girls and women participating in organized sports. For most of these individuals, sport participation is a positive experience, providing improved physical fitness and better health.[1] Yet, for some the desire for athletic success, combined with the pressure to achieve a prescribed body weight, may lead to development of a triad of medical disorders—eating disorders, amenorrhea, and osteoporosis—known collectively as the female athlete triad, or the "Triad."[1-3] Alone or in combination, the disorders of the Triad can negatively affect health and impair athletic performance. Consequently, school personnel should have a working knowledge of the Triad components, their relationships, risk factors, and be prepared to develop procedures for identification, prevention, and treatment.

*Journal of School Health*, October 1999 Vol. 69, Issue 8, p. 337, © 1999 American School Health Association. Reprinted with permission. American School Health Association, Kent, Ohio.

## Triad Components

Pressure to achieve and maintain a particular body weight or body shape considered desirable in her chosen sport may place a female athlete at risk for developing disordered eating behaviors. The resulting energy restriction and pathogenic weight control behaviors predispose her to menstrual dysfunction, subsequent decreased bone mineral density, and premature osteoporosis.[1-9] Each individual disorder of the Triad poses a significant medical concern. When the three disorders of the Triad occur together, the potential health consequences become even more serious, and often life-threatening.[1,6]

### Disordered Eating

Disordered eating refers to the spectrum of abnormal and harmful eating patterns used in a misguided attempt to lose weight or maintain a lowered body weight.[2,10,11] Anorexia nervosa represents the extreme of restrictive eating behavior in which the individual feels terrified of gaining weight and views herself as overweight though she is significantly underweight (at least 15 percent below ideal body weight for age).[10] Bulimia nervosa is characterized by repeated cycles of uncontrolled bingeing and purging occurring a minimum of two times per week for at least three months.[10] Purging methods may include vomiting, excessive exercise, or use of laxatives, diuretics, or enemas. Individuals also may experience subclinical variations of anorexia and bulimia nervosa. These individuals do not meet diagnostic criteria of the clinical conditions,[10] yet they exhibit body image disturbances and pathogenic weight control behaviors that place them at risk for serious endocrine, metabolic, skeletal, and psychological disorders.[4,11]

Medical complications associated with disordered eating include, but are not limited to, depleted glycogen stores, decreased lean body mass, chronic fatigue, micronutrient deficiencies, dehydration, anemia, electrolyte and acid-base imbalances, gastrointestinal disorders, parotid gland enlargement, decreased bone density, and erosion of tooth enamel.[2,12-14] Psychological problems often accompany disordered eating, including decreased self-esteem, anxiety, depression, and death owing to suicide.[4,11]

### Amenorrhea

Amenorrhea is usually defined as the absence of three or more consecutive menstrual cycles.[2,9] Primary amenorrhea or delayed menarche is the absence of menstruation by age 16 in a girl with secondary sex characteristics.[2,15] Secondary amenorrhea is the absence of three or more consecutive menstrual cycles after menarche.[2,15] As with disordered eating, a continuum of menstrual dysfunction occurs in the female athlete, with complete cessation of menstruation at the extreme and periods of oligomenorrhea (menstrual cycles lasting longer than 36 days) falling at an intermediate point along the continuum.[1,15] Once considered a relatively benign and "normal" response to physical training, professionals now recognize menstrual dysfunction as a serious medical condition.[2,15] The primary medical concern from menstrual dysfunction includes decreased bone density and premature osteoporosis.[8,17,18]

## *Osteoporosis*

Osteoporosis in young female athletes refers to premature bone loss and inadequate bone formation resulting in low bone mineral density, microarchitectural deterioration, increased skeletal fragility, and increased risk of stress fractures to the extremities, hips, and spine. [1,3,7,19] Studies suggest that the bone mineral density lost as a result of amenorrhea may be completely or, at least partly, irreversible even with calcium supplementation, resumption of menses, and estrogen replacement therapy.[18,20]

## *Triad Risk Factors*

The American College of Sports Medicine considers all physically active females at risk for developing one or more of the components of the Triad.[2] However, the biological changes, peer pressure, societal drive for thinness, and body image preoccupation that occur during puberty may render adolescent girls the most vulnerable.[2]

Factors implicated in contributing to the development of disordered eating include societal pressures to be thin; chronic dieting; low self-esteem; family dysfunction; physical or sexual abuse; participation in sports that emphasize a low body weight or particular body shape such as figure skating, gymnastics, distance running, swimming, diving, tennis, volleyball and cheerleading; participation in individual sports versus team sports; elite or highly competitive versus recreational athlete; and traumatic life events such as personal or family illness or injury, a change of coach, or relationship problems.[2,21,22]

Risk factors implicated in the development of amenorrhea include disordered eating, low energy availability or chronic negative energy

**Table 34.1.** Warning Signs and Symptoms of the Female Athlete Triad

## Behavioral

- Excessive criticism of one's body weight or shape
- Noticeable weight loss or gain
- Preoccupation with food, calories and/or weight
- Compulsive, excessive exercise
- Mood swings
- Depression
- Secretly eating or stealing food
- Bathroom visits after eating
- Avoiding food-related social activities
- Excessive laxative, diuretic, and/or diet pill use
- Consumption of large amounts of food not consistent with the athlete's weight

## Physical

- Chronic fatigue
- Anemia
- Frequent gastrointestinal problems, such as excessive gas, abdominal bloating, constipation, ulcers
- Cold intolerance
- Lanugo
- Tooth erosion, excessive dental caries
- Callused fingers
- Irregular or absent menstrual cycles
- Frequent musculoskeletal injuries, particularly stress fractures
- Delayed/prolonged wound and/or injury healing

balance, and significant and abrupt increases in training volume or intensity.[5,10,23] The primary risk factor for the osteoporosis that occurs as part of the Triad is amenorrhea (and, perhaps, oligomenorrhea) and the resulting hypoestrogenemia.[8,18]

While female athletes represent the group most susceptible to developing the disorders of the Triad, physically active girls not competing in a specific sport, and even female nonathletes can be at risk.[2] In addition, male athletes, particularly those participating in sports with weight classifications such as wrestling, rowing, horse racing, weight lifting, and body building are at risk for developing disordered eating.[24,25]

## Prevention and Treatment

Prevention and treatment of athletes with eating disorders can be organized into three broad categories including primary, secondary, and tertiary prevention.[25] Primary prevention involves educational programs designed to prevent development of an eating disorder. Secondary prevention focuses on early identification and subsequent intervention. Tertiary prevention involves treating those who developed an eating disorder.[25] These same prevention categories can be readily adapted to include all the disorders of the Triad.

### Primary Prevention

For school health personnel, primary prevention may be viewed as a more manageable task to tackle versus treatment, due to the high failure rate of treatment and the irreversible nature of some of the disorders.[25] The goal of primary prevention is to inoculate athletes against the factors that may predispose them to developing these disorders.[25] Thus, primary prevention should focus on dispelling myths and misconceptions surrounding nutrition, dieting, body weight, and body composition and their effect on athletic performance, while stressing the role of sound nutrition in promoting health and optimal performance.

Because body weight concerns, dieting, and disordered eating tend to develop during junior high or high school, primary prevention should begin early in grade school as part of a coordinated school health program.[26-28] Effective prevention demands close cooperation among all school health personnel. Health educators can advance primary prevention efforts by including a nutrition unit in their curriculum. School counselors and school nurses can contribute to primary prevention by promoting acceptance of diverse body shapes and sizes and encouraging a healthful attitude about competition and performance. School food service staff can play an important role in primary prevention by providing a variety of healthy and appetizing food choices.

Primary prevention strategies also should be aimed at the athletic environment with the goal of changing prevailing attitudes and practices regarding body weight and performance that too often form an accepted part of sport. In certain sports, pathogenic weight loss measures and menstrual dysfunction have almost become an accepted part of the sport.[25] The athletic staff can play an important role in changing these attitudes and behaviors by being clear and direct about the acceptability of weight loss practices and training techniques. In addition, athletic support staff, especially males, need to understand that body weight, menstrual cycles, and eating habits can be sensitive issues for young women, and they should address these issues accordingly. While the athlete's behaviors need to be monitored, methods such as group weigh-ins or "constructive criticism" regarding body weight, size, and shape are counterproductive and potentially harmful, and they should be avoided.[25]

### Secondary Prevention

Secondary prevention involves early identification of athletes at risk for developing the disorders of the Triad with the goal of limiting the progression and shortening the duration of the disorders. To be successful, school health personnel should be familiar with the warning signs and symptoms of the Triad (Table 34.1). The National Collegiate Athletic Association (NCAA) published a list of warning signs for eating disorders. In addition, the American College of Sports Medicine developed a set of Triad educational materials available for purchase (see the list of female atlhete triad resources near the end of this chapter).[2]

Screening athletes for disorders of the Triad represents an effective method for early identification. The preparticipation physical exam provides the best opportunity to screen.[29] During the exam, clinicians should ask specific questions regarding menstrual irregularities, eating behaviors, weight loss attempts, and history of musculoskeletal injury.[1,2,30] Other issues such as life stressors, depressive symptoms, dissatisfaction with weight and body shape, training frequency and intensity, and other lifestyle behaviors may also be addressed at this time.[1,15,30,31] Johnson[30] and Tanner[31] provide a detailed description of components in the preparticipation exam.

## *Tertiary Prevention*

Treating the disorders of the Triad usually involves a treatment "team," including the athlete's physician, a psychologist or psychiatrist, a dietitian, and the athlete's parents. The decision regarding the most appropriate treatment is based on the severity of the disorder and the presence of medical complications or additional diagnoses such as substance abuse. Health professionals recommend that treatment programs include psychological counseling (behavioral, psychoeducational, psychodynamic group, and family therapy), medical and nutritional support, and in certain cases, medication.[25,32]

Depending on resources available to school districts, tertiary prevention may not be appropriate in the school setting. Consequently, school health personnel should maintain a list of local practitioners specializing in disorders of the Triad. Many national organizations provide information and resources that identify therapists, physicians, treatment programs, and hospitals specializing in treatment for disorders of the Triad (Table 34.2).

## Conclusion

Because of the serious, potentially life-threatening health consequences associated with disorders of the Triad, prevention and early identification are paramount. School health personnel must possess a working knowledge of the Triad components, be familiar with risk factors and warning signs of disordered eating and menstrual dysfunction, and maintain a list of referral sources for treatment. Likewise, athletes participating in school-sponsored sports programs should be required to undergo a pre-participation physical exam that includes screening for disorders of the Triad. Only through involvement and cooperation of all school health personnel can disorders of the Triad be detected early and prevented.

## Female Atlhete Triad Resources

### *American Anorexia and Bulimia Association, Inc.*
165W. 46th St. #1108
New York, NY 10036
212-575-6200
Fax: 212-278-0698
E-mail: info@aabainc.org
http://www.aabainc.org

***American College of Sports Medicine***
401 W. Michigan St.
Indianapolis, IN 46202
317-637-9200
www.acsm.org

***Anorexia Nervosa and Related Eating Disorders***
P.O. Box 5102
Eugene, OR 97405
503-344-1144
www.anred.com

***National Association of Anorexia Nervosa and Associated Disorders***
Box 7
Highland Park, IL 60035
847-831-3438
www.anad.org

***The National Collegiate Athletic Association***
700 W. Washington Ave.
P.O. Bos 6222
Indiana, IN 46206-6222
317-917-6222
Fax: 317-917-6888
E-mail: wrenfro@ncaa.org
http://www.ncaa.org

***National Eating Disorders Organization***
6655 S. Yale Ave.
Tulsa, OK 74136
918-481-4044
Fax: 918-481-4076
www.kidsource.com/nedo/nedointro.html

***Sports, Cardiovascular, and Wellness Nutritionists (SCAN)***
A practice group of the American Dietetic Association
90 S. Cascade Ave., Suite 1190
Colorado Springs, CO 80903
719-475-7751
www.nutrifit.org

# References

1. Nattiv A, Agostini R, Drinkwater BL, Yeager KK. The female athlete triad: the inter-relatedness of disordered eating, amenorrhea, and osteoporosis. *Clin Sports Med.* 1994:13(2):405-418.

2. American College of Sports Medicine Position Stand. The female athlete triad: disordered eating, amenorrhea, and osteoporosis. *Med Sci Sports Exerc.* 1997;29:i-ix.

3. Yeager KK, Agostini R, Nattiv A, Drinkwater BL. The female athlete triad: disordered eating, amenorrhea, osteoporosis [commentary]. *Med Sci Sports Exer.* 1993:25:775-777.

4. Beals KA, Manore MM. Prevalence and consequences of subclinical eating disorders in female athletes. *Int J Sport Nutr.* 1994;4:175-195.

5. Benson JE, Englebert-Fenton K, Eisenman PA. Nutritional aspects of amenorrhea in the female athlete triad. *Int J Sport Nutr.* 1996;6:134-145.

6. Constantini NW. Clinical consequences of athletic amenorrhea. *Sports Med.* 1994;17:213-223.

7. Lewis RD, Modlesky CM. Nutrition, physical activity, and bone health in women. *Int J Sport Nutr.* 1998;8:250-284.

8. Nattiv A, Armsey TD. Stress injury to bone in the female athlete. *Clin Sports Med.* 1997:16(2): 197-224.

9. Warren MP. Eating, body weight, and menstrual function. In: Brownell KD, Rodin J, Wilmore JH, eds. *Eating, Body Weight, and Performance: Disorders of Modern Society.* Philadelphia, Pa: Lea & Febiger; 1992:222-234.

10. American Psychiatric Association. *Diagnostic and Statistical Manual of Mental Disorders. 4th ed.* Washington, DC: American Psychological Association. 1994;539-550.

11. Beals KA, Manore MM. Subclinical eating disorders in physically active women. *Topics Clin Nutr.* 1999; 14:14-29.

12. Bachrach LK, Guido D, Katzman D, Marcus R. Decreased bone density in adolescent girls with anorexia nervosa. *Pediatrics.* 1990;86:440-447.

13. Brownell KD, Steen SN. Weight cycling in athletes; effects on behavior, physiology, and health. In Brownell KD, Rodin J, Wilmore JH, eds. *Eating, Body Weight, and Performance in Athletes: Disorders of Modern Society*. Philadelphia, Pa: Lea and Febiger; 1992:159-171.

14. Pomeroy C, Mitchell JE. Medical issues in the eating disorders. In Brownell KD, Rodin J, Wilmore JH, eds. *Eating, Body Weight, and Performance in Athletes: Disorders of Modern Society*. Philadelphia, Pa: Lea & Febiger; 1992:202-221.

15. Otis CL. Exercise associated amenorrhea. *Clin Sports Med*. 1992;11 (2):351-362.

16. Shangold M, Rebar RW, Wentz AC, Schiff I. Evaluation and management of menstrual dysfunction in athletes. *JAMA*. 1990;263:1665-1669.

17. Drinkwater BL, Nilson K, Chestnut CH III, Bremer WJ, Shainholtz S, Southworth MB. Bone mineral content of amenorrheic and eumenorrheic athletes. *N Engl J Med*. 1984;311:227-281.

18. Drinkwater BL. Amenorrhea, body weight, and osteoporosis. In Brownell KD, Rodin J, Wilmore JH, eds. *Eating, Body Weight, and Performance in Athletes: Disorders of Modern Society*. Philadelphia, Pa: Lea and Febiger; 1992:235-247.

19. Myburgh K, Jutchins J, Fataar AB, Low bone density is an etiological factor for stress fractures in athletes. *Ann Int Med*. 1990; 113:754-759.

20. Drinkwater BL, Nilson K, Orr S, Chestnut CH III. Bone mineral density after resumption of menses in amenorrheic athletes. *JAMA*. 1986;256:380-382.

21. Sundgot-Borgen J. Risk and trigger factors for the development of eating disorders in female elite athletes. *Med Sci Sports Exert*. 1994;26:414-419.

22. Wilson GT, Eldredge KL. Pathology and development of eating disorders: implications for athletes. In Brownell KD, Rodin J, Wilmore JH, eds. *Eating, Body Weight, and Performance: Disorders of Modern Society*. Philadelphia, Pa: Lea & Febiger: 1992:115-127.

23. Dueck CA, Manore MM, Matt KS. Role of energy balance in athletic menstrual dysfunction. *Int J Sport Nutr.* 1996:6:165-190.

24. Andersen AE. Eating disorders in males: A special case? In Brownell KD, Rodin J, Wilmore JH, eds. *Eating, Body Weight, and Performance in Athletes: Disorders of Modern Society.* Philadelphia, Pa: Lea and Febiger: 1992:172-190.

25. Thompson RA, Sherman RT. *Helping Athletes with Eating Disorders.* Champaign, Ill: Human Kinetics Publishers: 1993.

26. Allensworth D, Kolbe LJ. The comprehensive school health program: exploring an expanded concept. *J Sch Health.* 1987;57(10):409-412.

27. Marx E, Wooley SE, eds, with Northrop D. *Health is Academic: A Guide to Coordinated School Health Programs.* New York, NY: Teachers College Press, Columbia University; 1998.

28. Neumark-Sztainier D. School-based programs for preventing eating disturbances. *J Sch Health.* 1996;66(2):64-71.

29. Nattiv A, Lynch L. The female athlete triad: managing an acute risk to long-term health. *Phys Sportsmed.* 1994;22(1):60-68.

30. Johnson MD. Tailoring the preparticipation exam to the female athletes. *Phys Sportsmed.* 1992;20(7):61-72.

31. Tanner SM. Preparticipation examination targeted for the female athlete. *Clin Sports Med.* 1994;13(2):330-353.

32. Johnson C, Tobin D. The diagnosis and treatment of anorexia nervosa and bulimia among athletes. *JNATA.* 1991;26:119-128.

—by *Katherine A. Beals; Rebecca A. Brey; Julianna B. Gonyou.*

Katherine A. Beals, PhD, RD, Assistant Professor, Dept. of Family and Consumer Sciences;

Rebecca A. Brey, PhD, Assistant Professor: and Julianna B. Gonyou, Health Science Major, Dept. of Physiology and Health Science, Ball State University, Muncie, IN 47306.

This article was submitted April 19, 1999, and revised and accepted for publication August 20, 1999.

# Chapter 35

# *Weightlessness, Bed Rest, and Immobilization*

Researchers and clinicians who study osteoporosis have known for some time that weight-bearing exercise contributes to the development and maintenance of bone mass (e.g., Dalsky et al., 1988; Krall, 1994; Nelson et al., 1994). Conversely, studies as far back as 1892 by Wolff have shown that bone is negatively influenced by reduction of its load-carrying role. In fact, without gravitational or mechanical loading of the skeleton, there is a rapid and marked loss of bone.

Wolff's theory that bones become stronger in response to increased exercise is still accepted today (Drinkwater, 1994). Living bones adapt themselves, both in size and internal structure, to the mechanical forces applied to them, and the amount and strength of the bone are directly linked to the amount of activity that forces the bones to bear weight and move against resistance (Simkin, 1990).

Weight-bearing activity can be thought of as any activity that is done while upright, requiring the bones to fully support the body's weight against gravity (Bonnick, 1994). Impact-loading, weight-bearing activity, therefore, involves some impact or force being transmitted to the skeleton during weight bearing. Examples of impact-loading, weight-bearing exercise include: walking, jogging, stair climbing, dancing, weight training and cross-country skiing. Activities that involve less impact and less weight-bearing force include swimming and bicycling.

"Weightlessness, Bed Rest and Immobilization: Factors Contributing to Bone Loss," © 1997. Reprinted with permission of Osteoporosis and Related Bone Diseases—National Resource Center.

While weight bearing and impact loading stimulate the development of healthy bones, it must be remembered that for exercise to be effective, the mechanical stress placed on the bone by an activity must exceed the level to which the bone has adapted (i.e., short periods of intense loading can produce more new bone than long-term routine loading) (Frost, 1990). However, long-term routine loading is important in maintaining bone density. And although bone responds to mechanical loading, it is easier to lose bone through inactivity than to gain more through changes in functional loading. When weight-bearing exercise is not continued, bone mass reverts to pre-training levels (Daisky, 1988; Drinkwater, 1995).

People who cannot perform weight-bearing exercise may be especially at risk for bone loss. Prolonged bed rest (following fractures, surgery, spinal cord injuries, illness, stroke, or complications of pregnancy) or immobilization of some part of the body often result in significant bone loss. Exposure to reduced gravity during space travel has also been found to have a direct negative effect on bone. In fact, space travel has provided significant research data on the subject of weightlessness, immobility, and bone loss.

People who must stay in bed or immobile are not weightless, but their bones bear much less weight than when they are vertical. To understand this phenomenon, one must first have a basic understanding of bone metabolism.

Bone is a dynamic structure that is continuously remodeling itself through a closely balanced process of resorption and formation. During resorption, old bone tissue is broken down and removed by special cells called osteoclasts. Then bone formation begins and new bone tissue is laid down—by cells called osteoblasts—to replace the old.

There appears to be an acute increase in both bone resorption and bone formation during periods of bed rest and immobilization, although there is a higher relative increase in bone resorption, which leads to a net loss of bone mineral in the weight-bearing bones. Over several months the rates of bone resorption and bone formation gradually decrease, and the bones reach a new equilibrium, or "steady state," in response to the reduced load (Sinaki, 1995).

The precise mechanisms that cause the change in bone metabolism are being studied, although it is possible that the absence of weight-bearing alters bone cell function (Mundy, 1995). Other researchers speculate that bed rest triggers an increased recruitment of osteoclasts that continues until the end of the bed-rest period (Uebelhart, 1995).

When body weight is removed from the bones, the parts of the skeleton most affected are the lower extremities; those least affected are the upper extremities and the skull. This is because the higher a certain bone is positioned in the skeleton, the less body mass that bone must carry. Hence, the lower extremities and the spine are classified as weight-bearing bones, and the upper extremities as non-weight-bearing bones.

During bed rest, the body mass that usually presses on the bones in a top-to-bottom direction is loading the bones in a lateral direction, distributed over a larger area. This makes the bones experience considerably lower stress, resulting in a change of bone metabolism. Immobilization through casts and similar devices is usually accompanied by a reduction in loading of the bone, as well as a decrease in the force applied to bones by muscles. In space, there is a total removal of body weight from the skeleton due to micro-gravity (Hangartner, 1995).

## Trabecular and Cortical Bone

There are two types of bone in the body: cortical and trabecular. Cortical bone is dense and compact, and comprises 85 percent of the bone in the body. Trabecular bone has a spongy, honeycomb-like structure, and makes up the remaining 15 percent. The rate of remodeling is much faster in trabecular bone (e.g., the spine) than in cortical bone (e.g., the long bones and the hip) because remodeling takes place on the surface of bones, and trabecular bone tends to have greater surface area (Mundy, 1995).

The pattern of calcium imbalance' and bone loss due to disuse is similar in prolonged bed rest, immobilization, spinal cord injury, and space travel. Urinary calcium increases within days of the onset of disuse, and the body's calcium balance may become negative, reaching a peak at about five weeks[2] (Hangartner, 1995). However, there are differences in magnitude. In bed rest, the average urinary calcium loss at the peak is about -150 mg per day, which corresponds to 0.5 percent of total body calcium (Deitrick, 1948; Donaldson, 1970; Hangartner, 1995). Losses in bone density are greatest in weight-bearing bones with a large proportion of trabecular bone, such as the heel bone. The amount of bone loss in the spine is smaller and occurs later; in some studies, no significant bone loss was detectable in the spine (Hangartner, 1995; LeBlanc, 1987).

Studies of patients whose limbs were immobilized have shown that, if a weight-bearing bone is involved, immobilization leads to bone loss in that limb. The bone loss is more significant in trabecular bone than in cortical bone (Janes, 1993). Fortunately, these studies also suggest that there is a good chance to fully recover the lost bone if the immobilization period is limited to 5 to 10 weeks (Hangartner, 1995).

Spinal cord patients have the longest experience with disuse osteoporosis. In these patients, there is an immediate increase in urinary calcium, leading to a negative calcium balance of about -100 mg per day. The calcium balance usually reverts back to normal within 6-18 months, but by that time about one-third of cortical and one-half of trabecular bone may have been lost (Chantraine, 1979; Hangartner, 1994; Minaire, 1974).

Studies of bone atrophy during space travel indicate that urinary calcium levels increase immediately and the negative calcium balance peaks at about -200 mg per day (NASA, 1990). The calcium balance remained negative in flights up to 84 days. The most significant bone loss occurs in weight-bearing parts of the skeleton (NASA, 1990).

## Minimizing Bone Loss Caused by Disuse

In general, healthy people who undergo periods of bed rest or immobilization can regain bone density through the resumption of weight-bearing activities. It is not yet known whether bone lost in space travel is fully recovered upon return. The greatest concern is for patients who can never resume weight-bearing activities, because they typically do not regain lost bone density.

Numerous researchers have tested methods to minimize bone loss *during* the period of disuse. Methods studied include dietary changes, pharmaceutical agents, weight-bearing and strength training exercises when possible, and functional electrical stimulation (FES) of muscles.

Dietary changes, such as increased intake of calcium and/or vitamin D, have not proven effective at minimizing disuse bone loss (Sinaki, 1995). Research into the pharmacologic treatment of disuse osteoporosis has shown that several of the bisphosphonates may prove helpful in minimizing bone loss during periods of weightlessness or immobility.

There is some uncertainty as to whether physical activity can minimize bone loss during periods of disuse. Some early studies indicated that the stress on bones from any muscular activity (even in a supine position) can be beneficial (Wyse & Pattee, 1954; Abramson & Delagi, 1961). However, more recent research suggests that weight-bearing activity—through tilt-table exercises or periods of standing—is necessary to minimize disuse bone loss (Kaplan, 1981). Studies of physical countermeasures in space travel tend to support this latter conclusion (NASA, 1990).

Several studies have tried using FES with spinal cord-injured patients. Although some of these studies showed no positive effects, others showed that the rate of bone loss was less than expected. This illustrates the importance of assessing bone density data relative to expected losses rather than as absolute values. Even if an intervention does not fully halt or reverse bone loss, slowing down the loss may be a very positive result (Hangartner, 1995).

The search continues for new ways to minimize the bone loss that results during periods of disuse. As more accurate and sensitive techniques are developed to assess bone and connective tissue metabolism, more information will be available regarding bone loss in paralyzed and/or immobilized individuals. These techniques will definitely be helpful in orienting new therapeutic trials with drugs and/ or procedures intended to correct the loss of bone density resulting from bed rest, immobilization, or weightlessness.

## *The Bottom Line*

- A lifetime of weight-bearing exercise is important for everyone, to build and maintain bone mass, improve balance and coordination, and promote overall good health.

- Weight-bearing exercise should be resumed and maintained after a prolonged period of bed rest or immobilization to reverse bone loss during disuse.

- Those who cannot resume weight-bearing exercise are at significant risk for osteoporosis. Researchers are investigating alternative ways to protect bone mass among this population. Until scientific studies yield definitive results, the best advice is to reduce or eliminate other risk factors for osteoporosis.

### *Footnotes*

1. Negative calcium balance results when the body loses more calcium (through urine, sweat, feces) than is replaced by the diet each day.

2. Bone is the source of most of this excess calcium lost through the urine.

### *References*

Abramson, A.& Delagi, E. (1961). Influence of weight-bearing and muscle contraction on disuse osteoporosis. *Archives of Physical Medicine Rehabilitation, 42,* 147-151.

Bonnick, S.L. (1994). *The Osteoporosis Handbook*. Dallas: Taylor Publishing Company.

Dalsky, G., Stocke, K., Ehsani, A., et al. (1988). Weight-bearing exercise training and lumbar bone mineral content in postmenopausal women. *Annals of Internal Medicine, 108:824- 828*.

Chantraine, A., Heynen, G., & Franchimont, P. (1979). Bone metabolism, parathyroid hormone, and calcitonin in paraplegia. *Calcified Tissue International, 27, 199*.

Deitrick, J., Whedon, G., & Shorr, E. (1948). Effects of immobilization upon various metabolic and physiologic functions of normal men. *American Journal of Medicine, 4, 3*.

Donaldson, C., Hulley, S., Vogel, J., et al. (1970). Effect of prolonged bed rest on bone mineral. *Metabolism, 19, 1071*.

Drinkwater, B.L. (1994, Sept.). 1994 C.H. McCloy Research Lecture: Does physical activity play a role in preventing osteoporosis? *Research Quarterly for Exercise and Sport, 65(3),* 197-206.

Drinkwater, B.L. (1995, Aug.). Weight-bearing exercise and bone mass. In V. Matkovic (ed.), *Physical Medicine and Rehabilitation Clinics of North America: Osteoporosis,* 6(3), 567-578, Philadelphia: W.B. Saunders Company.

Frost, H.M. (1990). Skeletal structural adaptations to mechanical usage (SATMU)—Redefining Wolff's Law: The bone modeling problem. *The Anatomical Record,* 226, 403-413.

Hangartner, T.N. *(1995,* Aug.). Osteoporosis due to disuse. In V. Matkovic (ed.), *Physical Medicine and Rehabilitation Clinics of North America: Osteoporosis,* 6(3), 579-594, Philadelphia: W.B. Saunders Company.

Janes, G., Collopy, D., Price R., et al. (1993). Bone density after rigid plate fixation of tibial fractures. *Bone Joint Surgery, 75-B,* 914.

Kaplan, P., Roden, W., Gilbert, E., et al. (1981). Reduction of hypercalciuria in tetraplegia after weight-bearing and strengthening exercises. *Paraplegia, 19,* 289.

Krall, E., & Dawson-Hughes, B. (1994, Jan.). Walking is related to bone density and rates of bone loss. *American Journal of Medicine, 96,* 20-26.

LeBlanc, A., Schneider, V., Krebs, J. et al. (1987). Spinal bone mineral after five weeks of bed rest. *Calcified Tissue International, 41, 259.*

Minaire, P., Depassio, J., Berard, B. et al. (1987). Effects of clodronate on immobilization bone loss. *Bone, 8,* 63.

Minaire, P. Meunier, P., Edouard, C., Bernard, J., Courpron, P., & Bourret, J. (1974). Quantitative histological data on disuse osteoporosis: comparison with biological data. *Calcified Tissue Research*, 17, 57-73.

Mundy, G.R. *(1995). Bone remodeling and its disorders.* London: Martin Dunitz. National Aeronautics and Space Administration, National Institute~ of Health, & National Institute of Arthritis and Musculoskeletal and Skin Diseases~ (1990). The effects of space travel on the musculoskeletal system. Workshop held October 3 and 4, 1990. NIH Publication No. 93-3484.

Nelson, M.E., Fiatarone, M.A., et al. (1994). Effects of high-intensity strength training on multiple risk factors for osteoporotic fractures. *JAMA, 272(24),* 1909-19 14.

Rodan G. & Rodan, S. *(1995).* The cells of bone. In B.L. Riggs & L.J. Melton, III (eds.), *Osteoporosis: Etiology, Diagnosis, and Management,* 2nd ed., 1-39. Philadelphia: Lippincott-Raven Publishers.

Schneider, V. & McDonald, J. (1984). Skeletal calcium homeostasis and countermeasures to prevent disuse osteoporosis. *Calcified Tissue International,* 36, S151.

Simkin, A. & Ayalon, J. (1990). *Bone-loading: The new way to prevent and combat the thinning bones of osteoporosis.* London: Prion.

Sinaki, M. *(1995).* Musculoskeletal rehabilitation. In B.L. Riggs & L.J. Melton, III (eds)., *Osteoporosis: Etiology, Diagnosis, and Management,* 435-473. Philadelphia: Lippincott-Raven Publishers.

Uebelhart, D. Ct al. (1995, Nov.). Bone metabolism in spinal cord injured individuals and in other who have prolonged immobilization: A review. *Paraplegia, 33(11),* 669-673.

Vico, L. Chappard, D., Alexandre, C., et al. (1987). Effects of a 120-day period of bed rest on bone mass and bone cell activities in man: attempts at countermeasure. *Bone Mineral, 2,* 383.

Wolff, J., ed. (1892). *Das Gesetz der Transformation der Knochen.* Berlin: A Hirschwald. Wyse, D.& Pattee, C. *(1954).* Effect of the oscillating bed and tilt table on calcium, phosphorous and nitrogen metabolism in paraplegia. *American Journal of Medicine, 17,* 645-661.

# Chapter 36

# Calcium and Vitamin D Combination Reduces Bone Loss and Fracture Rate for Older People

Supplements of calcium and vitamin D can significantly reduce bone loss and the risk of fractures in older people, according to a new report from scientists at Tufts University. The research, the first to show that these supplements can help older men fight osteoporosis, also demonstrates that the benefits of these low cost and easily available supplements can be maintained over several years.

The findings by Bess Dawson-Hughes, M.D., and colleagues of the Jean Meyer U.S. Department of Agriculture Human Nutrition Research Center on Aging at Tufts University appear in the September 4, 1997, *The New England Journal of Medicine*. The research was funded by the National Institute on Aging (NIA) as part of its STOP/IT (Sites Testing Osteoporosis Prevention/Intervention Treatments) initiative.

"Older people can benefit from this therapy at essentially no risk and at low cost," said Dawson-Hughes. "Our research underscores the importance of calcium and vitamin D supplementation in helping healthy and active older people stay that way."

NIA scientists noted the importance of the finding for older men. "Until recently, osteoporosis has been considered to be a women's problem," said Sherry Sherman, Ph.D., Director, Clinical Endocrinology and Osteoporosis Research, NIA, and project officer for the study. "We know that older men do experience considerable bone loss over time.

NIH New Release, September 3, 1997, National Institutes of Health, National Institute on Aging.

With older people living longer than ever, increasing the intake of calcium and vitamin D can be an important lifelong strategy for both sexes."

The researchers chose a combination of calcium and vitamin D to take advantage of the vitamin's influence in helping the body absorb and utilize calcium. As people age, the absorption of calcium and, it is believed, vitamin D, declines, as does production of vitamin D by the skin. This reduced ability to absorb calcium contributes to bone loss as people age, and low bone density is an underlying cause of increased hip fracture among the elderly.

The amounts of calcium and vitamin D used in the study are in keeping with recent recommendations of a National Academy of Sciences (NAS) panel, which recommended changes in current dietary requirements for calcium and related nutrients. The NAS group suggested that people over 50 increase their daily intake of calcium to about 1,200 milligrams and found that about 400-600 International Units of vitamin D (cholecalciferol) would be adequate.

Dawson-Hughes followed 389 men and women age 65 and older for 3 years. The study participants kept to their usual diets, in which they were generally getting the old recommended dietary allowances of calcium and vitamin D. At bedtime, about half of the study participants took placebo pills of no nutritional value. The other half took two separate pills, one containing 500 milligrams of elemental calcium (calcium citrate malate) and the other 700 International Units of vitamin D. All participants visited Tufts every 6 months for measurements of bone mineral density and other tests. Researchers also noted the number of fractures that occurred during the study period.

Over the 3 years, the calcium/vitamin D group lost significantly less total body bone, and, in some areas, gained bone mineral density. In men, where the findings were more pronounced, those taking placebos lost about one percent of their bone density at the hip over 3 years. Men taking the calcium/vitamin D combination increased their bone density by about 1 percent. The benefit at the hip for men, therefore, totaled a 2 percent improvement in bone density for the supplemented group. For women, the positive effects were most notable in the total body bone density, with lesser effects at the hip and spine.

In addition, the supplements may be effective in maintaining the skeleton over the long term, Dawson-Hughes said. The researchers found that the supplements were beneficial to bone density at the hip, spine, and total body in the first year, and further improved bone density of the total body during the second and third years of the study. The initial effects of supplementation at the hip and spine during the first year held steady, but did not change appreciably, over the next two years.

Even small losses of bone mass each year are important, scientists say. The losses are cumulative and add up to significant decreases in bone mineral density over time. "If we could retard bone loss in older people, we could make a lot of headway in preventing the devastation of osteoporosis and the fractures that commonly come with it," said Sherman.

The group taking supplements did considerably better in avoiding fractures. Some 5.9 percent of the participants taking the calcium and vitamin D suffered fractures, compared with 12.9 percent who did not take the supplements. Most of the fractures occurred in women.

Some 28 million middle-aged and older people are at risk of osteoporosis, and hip fractures related to low bone mass are a leading cause of nursing home entry for the elderly.

The NIA leads the Federal effort conducting and funding basic, clinical, social, and behavioral research aimed at maintaining independence and improving lives of older people and their families. For more information on NIA and aging in general, visit the NIA website at http://www.nih.gov/nia. The public may also call the NIA's toll free information number at 1-800-222-2225 or TTY at 1-800-222-4225 for free consumer fact sheets on osteoporosis and other health issues of older people.

# Chapter 37

# *Lactose Intolerance and Bone Health*

## *The Scope of the Problem*

According to the National Institute of Diabetes and Digestive and Kidney Diseases (NIDDK), between 30 and 50 million Americans are lactose intolerant. Lactose intolerance is a condition that results from a deficit of lactase, an enzyme produced by the cells lining the small intestine. Lactase is necessary to digest lactose, the natural sugar found in milk. When sufficient lactase is not present, lactose is not properly broken down in the small bowel and travels through the intestines unchanged. In the intestines, undigested lactose has a laxative effect and stimulates the growth of bacteria that produce significant amounts of gas. Within 30 minutes to two hours after ingesting lactose, abdominal cramping and diarrhea often occur. These symptoms are essential to a diagnosis of lactose intolerance.

In most individuals, intestinal lactase levels are highest during infancy and early childhood, when milk is the primary source of nutrition. After weaning, there is a gradual decline in intestinal lactase activity in more than 70 percent of the population. In less than 30 percent of the population, especially in those of northern European descent, high lactase levels continue until adulthood. For this reason individuals of northern European ancestry are least commonly affected by lactose intolerance. Lactase activity decreases with age among individuals in select ethnic and racial groups. According to NIDDK, up to 75 percent of all adult African Americans and Native Americans and 90 percent of Asian Americans are considered to be lactose intolerant.

## Lactose Maldigestion

Some experts have proposed that the prevalence of lactose intolerance has been exaggerated. The National Dairy Council suggests that many people who report being lactose intolerant may actually have lactose maldigestion. Individuals with lactose maldigestion have insufficient lactase to break down lactose completely, but they do not develop the severe gastrointestinal symptoms as those who are lactose intolerant. Unlike men and women who are lactose intolerant, individuals with lactose maldigestion tend to produce enough lactose to permit consumption of small portions of dairy products without developing symptoms. The key with these individuals is to consume small amounts of dairy products at a time so that there are sufficient amounts of intestinal lactase available to digest the lactose load. When the lactose is sufficiently digested, symptoms do not develop.

## The Impact on Bone Health

Since dairy products are a major source of dietary calcium, it might be argued that individuals with lactase deficiency might avoid dairy products, be calcium deficient, and at increased risk for osteoporosis. However, research exploring the role of lactose intolerance on calcium intake and bone health has produced conflicting results. Studies involving perimenopausal Finnish women and postmenopausal Italian women found that lactase deficiency negatively impacted bone mineral density. Other studies, however, have not shown such an association. For example, Slemenda and associates found no evidence that lactase deficiency impacted bone density in pre- or postmenopausal women. This finding was supported in other studies involving postmenopausal women.

Perhaps one reason that women with lactose deficiency may not be at increased risk for osteoporosis, is that such women may not avoid milk and other dairy products. This contention was supported by an analysis of NHANES and NHANES II data that showed that the presence of lactase deficiency in certain ethnic groups was not predictive of milk consumption practices. This analysis, by Looker and associates, also demonstrated the importance of other dietary sources of calcium in various ethnic groups, such as corn tortillas for Mexican Americans, and pizza and rice for Cuban Americans and Puerto Ricans.

Studies have shown that in people who have at least some intestinal lactase, tolerance to lactose can be increased when dairy products are gradually introduced into the diet. Also, certain sources of dairy products may be easier for people with lactase deficiency to digest. For example, ripened cheese may contain up to 95 percent less lactose than whole milk. Yogurt containing active cultures also lessens gastrointestinal symptoms. A variety of lactose-reduced dairy products—including milk, cottage cheese, and processed cheese slices—are available, as are lactase replacement pills or liquid.

### *Resources on Lactose Intolerance Are Available from the Following Organizations:*

National Digestive Diseases Information Clearinghouse produces a fact sheet *Lactose Intolerance*. Single copies are available by writing 2 Information Way, Bethesda Maryland, 20892-3570. Information can also be obtained at the NIDDK web site.

National Fluid Milk Processor Promotion Board produces a brochure *The Lowdown on Lactose Intolerance*. Single copies are available by calling 1-800-WHY-MILK. Information can also be obtained at the Why Milk website.

ORBD—NRC is supported by the National Institute of Arthritis and Musculoskeletal and Skin Diseases, National Institutes of Health Osteoporosis and Related Bone Diseases—National Resource Center 1150 17th St., NW, Suite 500, Washington, D.C. 20036
202-223-0344 or 800-624-BONE
TTY (202) 466-4315
E-Mail: orbdnrc@nof.org

# Chapter 38

# *Depression Linked to Bone Loss*

Depression may increase a woman's risk for broken bones, suggests a study by scientists at the National Institute of Mental Health (NIMH). The hip bone mineral density of women with a history of major depression was found to be 10 to 15 percent lower than normal for their age—so low that their risk of hip fracture increased by 40 percent over 10 years.

"Although further research is required to determine the underlying mechanisms, our findings underscore the fact that depression is not only a psychological problem, but also a biological syndrome," said NIMH researcher David Michelson, M.D., first author of the study, published in the Oct. 17th issue of *The New England Journal of Medicine*. "Bone mineral density, once lost, is not easily regained. Thus, losses that may occur during recurrent episodes of depression could be additive."

"Since depression affects 5 to 9 percent of women, providing early treatment could have significant public health implications by reducing the risk of fracture," added Philip Gold, M.D., chief of the NIMH Clinical Neuroendocrinology Branch, where the research was conducted. "The affected women in this study, average age 41, had bone loss equivalent to that of 70-year-old women. More than a third faced a markedly increased risk of fracture."

The researchers measured bone mineral density in the spine, hip and radius (forearm) of 24 women with past or current major

NIH Press Release, October 16, 1996, National Institutes of Health, National Institute of Mental Health.

depression and also 24 control subjects, matched for age, body mass and menstrual status. They also measured indicators of bone metabolism and stress hormones.

Compared to established norms for their age, women who had experienced depression, as a group, showed bone density reductions of 6.5 percent at the spine, and 10 to 15 percent in the upper leg and hip. They also showed moderately reduced bone metabolism and moderate increases in the stress hormone cortisol.

Excess cortisol secretion, a common feature of some forms of depression, is known to cause bone loss and could account for some of the observed deficits, say the researchers. They saw little relationship with other possible factors, such as antidepressant medications, physical activity levels and appetite.

Other NIMH researchers participating in the study were: Lauren Hill and Elise Galliven. Also participating were: James Reynold, M.D., NIH Clinical Center, and Constantine Stratakis, M.D., Ph.D., and George Chrousos, M.D., National Institute of Child Health and Human Development.

The National Institute of Mental Health is a component of the NIH, an agency of the U.S. Public Health Service, part of the U.S. Department of Health and Human Services.

# Chapter 39

# *Corticosteroid-Induced Osteoporosis*

**Abstract:** Corticosteroid drugs, although powerful and effective uninflammable, can cause a loss of bone mineral density that can increase the risk of fracture. Long-term use of drugs, such as prednisone, can lead to osteoporosis and broken bones. These medications cause a loss of bone density, and may alter bone deposition. Biphosphonates, hormone replacement therapy, and other drugs can reduce the loss of healthy bone and protect some women from fractures.

By far the commonest form of osteoporosis is that due to postmenopausal hormonal changes. However, the disorder is also commonly an adverse effect of corticosteroid therapy. The use of oral corticosteroids has long been recognized to increase the risk of fractures. [1] The introduction of techniques for the precise measurement of bone density has enabled the detailed study of the effect of corticosteroid use on bone loss and subsequent fractures. Bone loss is most rapid during the first year of therapy, [2] but it can persist with longer use. [3] Corticosteroids not only reduce bone density, but they may also cause a qualitative bone defect since fractures among corticosteroid users occur at bone-mineral densities higher than those found with other forms of osteoporosis. [4] How corticosteroids induce bone loss is not fully understood. However, there is a clear decrease in bone formation, which reduces the thickness of the walls of trabecular bone packets, and

Stevenson, J.C., "Management of Corticosteroid-Induced Osteoporosis," in *The Lancet*, October 24, 1998, p. 1327(1), © 1998 Lancet Ltd. Reprinted with permission of *The Lancet*.

an increase in the activation frequency of bone-remodelling cycles. [5] There is also evidence of increased bone resorption, perhaps due in part to corticosteroid-induced malabsorption of calcium and in part to a reduction in concentrations of gonadal steroid hormones. Hence, therapies that either increase bone formation or reduce bone resorption could theoretically be useful in the prevention of corticosteroid-induced bone loss. One of the problems in the assessment of the efficacy of such therapies is that certain disorders for which corticosteroids are given may themselves produce abnormalities in bone metabolism. Because the effect of preventive treatments may thus vary according to the disorder for which corticosteroids are given, the findings of studies of therapeutic measures to prevent corticosteroid-induced bone loss in patients with rheumatoid arthritis, for instance, may not necessarily be applicable to those with asthma. Furthermore, there are still few studies of sufficient size and duration to provide satisfactory evidence of efficacy of various treatment options. Thus, since corticosteroid osteoporosis cannot be ignored, its management commonly has to be intuitive rather than evidence-based.

The strategy for the management of corticosteroid-induced bone loss may be primary prevention therapy initiated at the start of corticosteroid therapy to preserve bone density, or secondary prevention to reduce fracture risk among those with established corticosteroid-induced bone loss. [6] Most published studies of primary and secondary prevention have used antiresorptive agents or vitamin D preparations, usually given for only 1-2 years.

The first obvious step in the overall management of corticosteroid-induced bone loss is to give the minimum dose necessary and, where possible, to avoid oral steroids. An oral dose of prednisolone above 7.5 mg daily has long been thought to be necessary to induce bone loss, but clinical practice indicates that there is substantial variation among individuals in the effect of corticosteroid dose on bone loss. Another possible step is to choose those glucocorticoids with the least detrimental skeletal effects, but there is still a paucity of evidence to show their advantage. Certain groups of patients may lend themselves to specific therapies. For example, hormone-replacement therapy (HRT) prevents postmenopausal bone loss, and its use in postmenopausal women receiving corticosteroids seems logical. Yet there have been no prospective studies of HRT as a primary-prevention measure for corticosteroid-induced osteoporosis, and only one as a secondary prevention measure. [7] Similarly, testosterone replacement seems logical in men on corticosteroids who are hypogonadal, yet there is only one published secondary-prevention study. Moreover, the number of patients was small and the study was short. [8]

Bisphosphonates have been used as antiresorptive agents for both primary and secondary prevention of corticosteroid-induced bone loss. Two prospective primary-prevention studies of satisfactory size showed efficacy of cyclically administered oral etidronate. [9,10] Secondary prevention studies with the same agent have also shown positive results but numbers of patients were small. All studies, whether of primary or secondary prevention, have been short. Two studies have shown a positive effect of oral alendronate for primary [11] and secondary [12] prevention. Other therapies, such as calcium and vitamin D, calcitriol, calcitonin, and fluoride, have been evaluated in a few studies, but numbers have been small and results inconsistent.

What conclusion can be drawn in order to provide recommendations for the management of corticosteroid-induced bone loss? Guidelines need to be developed locally by clinicians commonly prescribing corticosteroids, such as rheumatologists, respiratory physicians, and oncologists. Consensus guidelines [6] should be valuable in this respect. Either primary or secondary prevention should be considered in patients taking more than 7.5 mg prednisolone daily for 6 months or longer, although bone-density measurements are of great assistance for decision-making for individuals. Patients with normal bone density and low rates of bone loss can be spared additional therapy. Despite the paucity of evidence, the use of HRT seems very logical in postmenopausal women and perhaps in hypogonadal men. Oral bisphosphonates seem to be effective in the prevention and treatment of corticosteroid-induced bone loss and could be considered for use in both men and premenopausal women. Follow-up bone-density measurements for monitoring the effect of therapy should be considered, with measurements being repeated after 1-2 years, depending on the initial degree of bone loss.

Much more research is needed into the management of corticosteroid-induced bone loss. Therapeutic regimens need to be tested in properly controlled prospective studies in different disorders requiring corticosteroid treatment. The use of bone biochemical markers to assess therapeutic responses, as an adjunct or an alternative to bone-density measurements, needs to be evaluated. Finally, a means of predicting which individuals will be at risk of corticosteroid-induced osteoporosis would enable targeting of primary preventive therapy, but this approach still seems a long way off.

*—by J C Stevenson*

Rosen Laboratories of the Wynn Institute, Endocrinology and Metabolic Medicine, Imperial College School of Medicine, St Mary's Hospital, London W2 1PG, UK

1. Adinoff AD, Hollister JR. Steroid-induced fractures and bone loss in patients with asthma. *N Engl J Med* 1983; 309: 265-68.

2. Sambrook P, Birmingham J, Kempler S, et al. Corticosteroid effects on proximal femur bone loss. *J Bone Miner Res* 1990; 5: 1211-16.

3. Saito JK, Davis JW, Wasnich RD, Ross PD. Users of low-dose glucocorticoids have increased bone loss rates: a longitudinal study. *Calcif Tissue Int* 1995; 57: 115-19.

4. Luengo M, Picado C, Rio LD, Guanabens N, Montserrat JM, Setoain J. Vertebral fractures in steroid dependent asthma and involutional osteoporosis: a comparative study. *Thorax* 1991; 46: 803-06.

5. Dempster DW, Arlot MA, Meunier PJ. Mean wall thickness and formation periods of trabecular bone packets in corticosteroid-induced osteoporosis. *Calcif Tissue Int* 1983; 35: 410-17.

6. Eastell R, Reid DM, Compston J, et al. A UK Consensus Group on management of glucocorticoid-induced osteoporosis: an update. *J Intern Med* 1998: 244: 271-92.

7. Hall GM, Daniels M, Doyle DV, Spector TD. Effect of hormone replacement therapy on bone mass in rheumatoid arthritis patients treated with and without steroids. *Arthritis Rheum* 1994; 37: 1499-505.

8. Reid IR, Wattie DJ, Evans MC, Stapleton JP. Testosterone therapy in glucocorticoid-treated men. *Arch Intern Med* 1996; 156: 1373-77.

9. Adachi JD, Bensen WG, Brown J, et al. Intermittent etidronate therapy to prevent corticosteroid-induced osteoporosis. *N Engl J Med* 1997; 337: 382-87.

10. Roux C, Oriente P, Laan R, et al. Randomized trial of effect of cyclical etidronate in the prevention of corticosteroid-induced bone loss. *J Clin Endocrinol Metab* 1998; 83: 1128-33.

11.  Gonnelli S, Rottoli P, Cepollaro C, et al. Prevention of corticos-
     teroid-induced osteoporosis with alendronate in sarcoid pa-
     tients. *Calcif Tissue Int* 1997; 61: 382-85.

12.  Saag KG, Emkey R, Schnitzer TJ et al. Alendronate for the
     prevention and treatment of glucocorticoid-induced osteoporo-
     sis. *N Engl J Med* 1998; 339: 292-29.

# Chapter 40

# Asthma Medicine and Bone Health

## Inhaled Steroids and Bone Density

Steroids are wonder drugs. They can work miracles against inflammation—including the inflammation that is a part of asthma. But steroids can cause problems with bone density, and that's why doctors are often reluctant to use steroids on a long term basis.

Inhaled steroids are frequently an important part of the treatment asthma, especially in children. A recent study found that inhaled steroid use for three to six years didn't affect the total body calcium, the amount of calcium in the bones, and the height of children. And it helped to control their asthma.

The researchers concluded that long term inhaled steroid use doesn't "adversely affect statural growth when the dose is tailored to the severity of the disease." *American Journal of Respiratory Critical Care Medicine*, 157[1]: 178-83, 1998.

## Inhaled Budesonide and Bone Formation in Children

Anti-inflammatory medicines such as inhaled corticosteroids have been shown to be effective in treating asthma. Nevertheless, many

This chapter contains two articles: "Inhaled Steroids and Bone Density" from *Pediatrics for Parents*, November 1998, p. 2(1), © 1998 Pediatrics for Parents, Inc. Reprinted with permission. And, "Inhaled Budesonide and Bone Formation in Children," by Terrence J. Joyce from *American Family Physician*, June 1998, Vol. 57, No. 11, 2819(1), © 1998 American Academy of Family Physicians. Reprinted with permission.

311

physicians hesitate to prescribe inhaled corticosteroids for children because of possible adverse effects on bone growth and formation. Agertoft and Pedersen evaluated the long-term effects of inhaled budesonide on total-body bone mineral density, total-body bone mineral capacity, total-body bone calcium and body composition in children with asthma.

A total of 268 children participated in the controlled, prospective clinical study. The study group included 157 children who were treated with inhaled budesonide at a mean dosage of 504 [micro] g (range: 189 to 1,322 [micro] g) for an average of three to six years. This group was matched by age, weight, height and sex with a control group of 111 children with asthma. Members of the control group had never received inhaled corticosteroids for more than two weeks per year. Exclusion criteria for participation in the study included use of systemic steroids for more than 14 days, use of topical steroids over more than 25 percent of the body (after two years of age) and use of nasal corticosteroids for more than one month per year. The dosage of inhaled steroid in the study group was chosen for a level that controlled clinical symptoms while maintaining the minimum dosage to relieve symptoms. Dual energy photon absorptiometry (DEXA scan) was used to compare the bone mineral density, bone mineral capacity, bone calcium and body composition of children treated with budesonide and children in the control group.

No statistically significant difference was found between the children receiving budesonide and the control subjects with regard to bone mineral density, bone mineral capacity or bone calcium. No correlation was found between these parameters and duration of treatment or cumulative dosage received by the study group.

The authors conclude that treating children with inhaled budesonide for an average of 4.5 years at a mean daily dosage of 504 [micro] g has no detectable effect on the total bone mineral density; total bone mineral capacity, total bone calcium or body composition of children with asthma. The dosage, however, must be tailored to the severity of, disease. They caution that this data should not be extrapolated to include other inhaled corticosteroids or higher dosages of budesonide, which may have long-term adverse effects in children.

Agertoft L, Pedersen S. Bone mineral density in children with asthma receiving long-term treatment with inhaled budesonide. Am J Respir Crit Care Med January 1998;157:178-83.

*—by Terrence J. Joyce*

# Chapter 41

# *Bone Builders:*
# *Support Your Bones with*
# *Healthy Habits*

## Bone Information

Unearthed skeletons from ancient times testify to the durability of bone long after other bodily tissue turns to dust. Living bone in the body, however, can lose mineral and fracture easily if neglected—a disorder called osteoporosis, or porous bones. One in two women and one in eight men over 50 suffer such fractures, including sometimes life-threatening hip fractures.

But during your preteen and teenage years, you can reduce your risk of fractured bones later in life with calcium-rich foods and physical activity.

### *Bone Behavior*

Your body's 206 living bones continually undergo a buildup, breakdown process called remodeling.

The body starts to form most of its bone mass before puberty, the beginning of sexual development, building 75 to 85 percent of the skeleton during adolescence. Women reach their peak bone mass by around age 25 to 30, while men build bone until about age 30 to 35. The amount of peak bone mass you reach depends largely on your genes. Then gradually, with age, the breakdown outpaces the buildup, and in late middle age bone density lessens when needed calcium is

U.S. Food and Drug Administration (FDA), *FDA Consumer* magazine (September-October 1997).

withdrawn from bone for such tasks as blood clotting and muscle contractions, including beating by the heart.

"You can't do anything about the genes you're dealt," says Mona Calvo, Ph.D., a calcium expert for the Food and Drug Administration. "As a teenager, though, you can make the most of things you do control that can build your bones and help reduce the risk of fractures when you are older."

Supporting the skeleton with healthful habits now so it can support you later in life is especially important if you have an increased risk of osteoporosis—for example, if you're female or have a thin, small-boned frame. These habits are proper diet, exercise, and avoiding bone risks—lifestyle choices that are bad for bone, like smoking.

### *Eat Your Way to Strong Bones*

The main mineral in bones is calcium, one of whose functions is to add strength and stiffness to bones, which they need to support the body. To lengthen long bones during growth, the body builds a scaffold of protein and fills this in with calcium-rich mineral. From the time you're 11 until you're 24, you need about 1,200 milligrams (mg) of calcium each day.

Adolescent bodies are tailor-made to "bone up" on calcium. Calvo says that with the start of puberty, "your body is at a higher capacity to absorb and retain calcium."

Bone also needs vitamin D, to move calcium from the intestine to the bloodstream and into bone. You can get vitamin D from short, normal day-to-day exposure of your arms and legs to sun and from foods fortified with the vitamin. Also needed are vitamin A, vitamin C, magnesium and zinc, as well as protein for the growing bone scaffold.

Mother Nature provides many foods with these nutrients. One stands out, however, as "almost a perfect package," according to Calvo. "Milk is rich in calcium and high-quality protein. Nearly all U.S. milk has vitamins D and A added. And it has magnesium and zinc."

Still, as excellent as milk is for bones, it and other dairy products are not the only foods that contain calcium. All groups in the Food Guide Pyramid, in fact, offer calcium sources—from the pyramid's grain-based foods that you need the most of, to the produce and high-protein groups in the middle, and even to the fats and sweets "use sparingly" group at the top. The importance of choosing calcium sources from the different food groups is that each group offers its unique package of other nutrients as well.

To learn how much calcium is in a food, you can read the food label's Nutrition Facts panel. Look for the "percent Daily Value" (percent DV) set by FDA for calcium. The calcium DV is 1,000 mg. But if you are 11 to 24 years old, your growing bones need more—the recommended 1,200 mg. So, each day's calcium percent DVs in the foods you eat should add up to 120 percent.

Because many foods are now fortified with calcium, your investigation of labels may turn up surprising sources. To identify foods with at least 10 percent DV of calcium per serving, FDA allows these terms on their labels:

- 20 percent DV or more: "High in Calcium," "Rich in Calcium," "Excellent Source of Calcium"

- 10 percent to 19 percent DV: "Contains Calcium," "Provides Calcium," "Good Source of Calcium"

- 10 percent DV calcium or more added: "Calcium-Enriched," "Calcium-Fortified," "More Calcium."

An easy daily plan is to drink a calcium source at every meal and eat one calcium food as a snack, says Ruth Welch, a registered dietitian with FDA.

If the lactose sugar in dairy products causes problems like gas, bloating or diarrhea, try lactose-reduced or lactose-free milk. When fortified, these products can have up to 50 percent DV for calcium in one serving. Also available are lactase drops and tablets, which can help you digest dairy products like ice milk, yogurt, and cheese.

### *Get Enough Weight-Bearing Exercise*

Growing bone is especially sensitive to the impact of weight and pull of muscle during exercise, and responds by building stronger, denser bones. That's why it's especially important when you're growing a lot to be physically active on a regular basis.

And as far as bone is concerned, Calvo says impact activity like jumping up and down appears to be the best. "But the important thing is to get off the couch and get moving at some activity. It really is a matter of 'Use it now, or lose it later'."

Such activities include sports and exercise, including football, basketball, baseball, jogging, dancing, jumping rope, inline skating, skateboarding, bicycling, ballet, hiking, skiing, karate, swimming, rowing a canoe, bowling, and weight-training. And when your parents make you mow the lawn, rake leaves, or wash and wax the car, they're doing your muscles and bones a favor.

FDA's Welch adds, "Day-to-day activities that start in the teen years, like walking the dog or using stairs instead of elevators, can become life-long habits for healthy bones."

### Avoid Bone Risks

Some habits in the teenage years can steal calcium from your bones or increase the need for it, weakening the skeleton for life.

Skipping meals is risky for bone, Welch says. In our three-meal-a-day society, skipping a meal may reduce by a third your chance of getting your 120 percent DV for calcium—simply by eliminating one occasion to eat.

Replacing milk with nondairy drinks like soda pop or fruit-flavored teas or drinks is another eating habit that prevents bones from getting the calcium and other nutrients they need.

In a survey comparing 1994 daily beverage intakes with those in the late 1970s, the U.S. Department of Agriculture found a switch from milk to other drinks among young people:

- Milk drinkers among teenagers dropped from three-fourths to little more than half.

- Two to three times more children and teenagers drank non-citrus fruit juices.

- Teenage boys nearly tripled their intake of soft drinks, three-fourths of them drinking about 34 ounces; two-thirds of teenage girls drank 23 ounces.

Alcohol abuse and cigarette smoking can hurt bone. Calvo says, "Alcohol abuse can cause loss of calcium, magnesium and zinc in the urine. Many who abuse alcohol also have poor diets and malnourished, weaker bones." Cigarette smoke is also toxic to bone and can influence how much exercise you get because it affects your stamina, she says.

Eating disorders can weaken bone. The repeated vomiting in bulimia and extreme dieting in the appetite disorder anorexia can upset the body's balance of calcium and important hormones like bone-protective estrogen, decreasing bone density. And extreme exercising by young women with or without eating disorders can postpone or stop menstruation, when blood levels of estrogen are reduced.

## Small Changes for Big Benefits

As a disorder of aging, osteoporosis may seem far away for worry when you're 15. But, small changes today for better bones tomorrow may be more important than you might guess.

Laura Bacharach, M.D., of Stanford University, wrote in *Nutrition & the M.D.* last year that adolescents who make "even a 5 percent gain in bone mass can reduce the risk of osteoporosis by 40 percent." And this is in addition to "immediate benefits of feeling stronger and more fit now with these changes!"

# "Calcium! Do You Get it?"

Unlike boys, growing girls typically have low calcium intakes. Concerned about the low intakes, the Food and Drug Administration recently developed a pilot education program, funded by the agency's Office of Women's Health, just for girls ages 11 to 14. "Calcium! Do You Get It?" encourages girls to get enough calcium and exercise for healthy bones and to carry these healthy behaviors throughout life. This chapter includes much of the information in the program.

### Girls Don't Get Enough Calcium

Between the ages 11 and 24, people need at least 1,200 milligrams (mg) of calcium every day. A 1995 survey by the U.S. Department of Agriculture, however, found that girls and young women 12 to 19 got only 777 mg of the mineral daily, overall. Intake by boys and young men in the same age group was 1,176 mg daily.

Daily calcium intake by preteen girls was far short of the recommended level also in 1990-1992 and fell with age, wrote Ann Albertson, M.S., R.D., and others recently in the *Journal of Adolescent Health*. Calcium consumption was only 781 mg at ages 11 to 12, 751 at ages 13 to 14, and a mere 602 mg—barely half what it should be—at ages 15 to 18.

*Why is calcium intake in girls and young women so low?*

USDA's Agricultural Economic Report No. 746 gives some clues. Compared with other children, female adolescents:

- drink the least amount of fluid milk

- have the highest tendency to skip morning meals, which offer the most calcium because of milk and cereals

- have the highest share of calories from fast-food places, which have a calcium density much lower than foods prepared at home, schools or restaurants.

### *Eat Enough Calcium and a Balanced Diet, Too*

To get enough calcium for growing bones, each day you need to eat foods whose percent Daily Value for calcium adds up to 120 percent. Because the amount of calcium in foods can vary, read the food label check the percent DV for calcium in what you eat.

So your body will have all the other nutrients it needs, too, be sure to eat the recommended number of servings from the food groups that make up the Food Guide Pyramid:

- **Grain Products Group:** 6-11 servings
- **Vegetables Group:** 3-5 servings
- **Fruits Group:** 2-4 servings
- **Milk Products Group:** 2-3 servings
- **Meat and Bean Group:** 2-3 servings
- **Fats, Oils, and Sweets:** Use sparingly

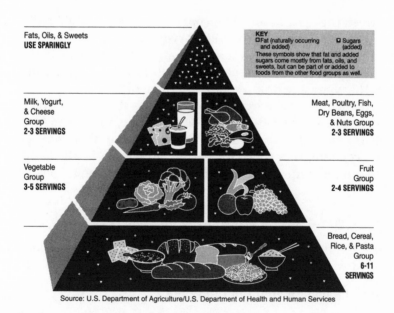

Source: U.S. Department of Agriculture/U.S. Department of Health and Human Services

***Figure 41.1.*** *Food Pyramid*

As shown in Table 41.1 [beginning on the next page], each group includes foods that provide calcium. The food examples are listed by their serving size and percent DV for calcium.

## Want More Information?

### *Dairy Council of California*
1101 National Drive, Suite B
Sacramento, CA 95834
In California: 888-868-3133
Outside California: 888-868-3083
http://www.dairycouncilofca.org

### *National Osteoporosis Foundation (NOF)*
has information for health professionals and the public. Contact:
NOF
1232 22nd Street, N.W.
Washington, D.C. 20036-4603
202-223-2226
E-mail: communications@nof.org
http://www.nof.org

### *Osteoporosis and Related Bone Diseases—National Resource Center (ORBD)*
1232 22nd St., NW,
Washington, D.C. 20037-1292
202-223-0344 or 800-624-BONE
TTY (202) 466-4315
Fax: 202-293-2356
E-mail orbdnrc@nof.org
http://www.osteo.org

National Resource Center on Osteoporosis and Related Bone Diseases is a national clearinghouse with information on the risks, prevention, and treatment of osteoporosis. For more information call: 1-800-624-BONE

*—by Dixie Farley*

Dixie Farley is a staff writer for FDA Consumer.

**Table 41.1.** Food Examples and Calcium Content

| Food | Serving Size | Percent DV |
|---|---|---|
| **Grain Products** | | |
| waffles(4-inch square) | 2 waffles | 20 percent DV |
| pancakes (5-inch) | 3 pancakes | 20 percent DV |
| calcium-fortified cereal | 1 cup | 15 percent DV |
| calcium-fortified bread | 1 slice | 8 percent DV |
| corn tortilla | 3 tortillas | 8 percent DV |
| bread | 1 slice | 4 percent DV |
| **Vegetables** | | |
| collards | 1/2 cup | 20 percent DV |
| turnip greens | 2/3 cup | 15 percent DV |
| kale | 2/3 cup | 10 percent DV |
| bok choy | 1/2 cup | 10 percent DV |
| broccoli | 1 stalk | 6 percent DV |
| carrot | 1 medium carrot | 2 percent DV |
| **Fruits** | | |
| calcium-fortified orange juice | 1 cup | 30 percent DV |
| dried figs | 2 figs | 6 percent DV |
| orange | 1 orange | 4 percent DV |
| kiwi | 2 kiwis | 4 percent DV |
| strawberries | 8 berries | 2 percent DV |
| **Milk Products** | | |
| nonfat milk, calcium-fortified | 1 cup | 40 percent DV |
| yogurt | 1 cup | 35 percent DV |
| milk, whole, 2 percent, 1 percent, skim | 1 cup | 30 percent DV |
| cheese | 1 ounce | 20 percent DV |
| cheese spread | 2 Tbsp. | 15 percent DV |
| pudding | 1/2 cup | 10 percent DV |
| frozen yogurt | 1/2 cup | 10 percent DV |
| cottage cheese | 1/2 cup | 6 percent DV |

**Table 41.1.** Food Examples and Calcium Content, continued.

| Food | Serving Size | Percent DV |
|---|---|---|
| **Meat and Beans** | | |
| calcium-processed tofu | 3 oz. | 60 percent DV |
| dry-roasted almonds | 1/4 cup | 10 percent DV |
| scrambled eggs | 2 eggs | 8 percent DV |
| baked beans with sauce | 1/2 cup | 8 percent DV |
| black-eyed peas | 1/2 cup | 2 percent DV |
| **Fats, Oils and Sweets** | | |
| milk chocolate | 1.5-ounce bar | 8 percent DV |
| **Mixed Dishes** | | |
| cheese pizza (12-inch) | 1/4 pizza | 25 percent DV |
| macaroni and cheese | 1 cup | 25 percent DV |
| grilled cheese sandwich | 1 sandwich | 25 percent DV |
| lasagna | 1 cup | 25 percent DV |
| soups prepared with milk | 1 cup | 15 percent DV |
| chili con carne with beans | 1 cup | 10 percent DV |
| taco with cheese | 1 taco | 10 percent DV |
| tuna salad sandwich | 1 sandwich | 8 percent DV |
| chicken noodle soup | 1 cup | 2 percent DV |

(Source: "Calcium! Do You Get It?" pilot education program funded by FDA's Office of Women's Health)

# Chapter 42

# Hormone Replacement Therapy: Should You Take It?

Menopause is the stage in a woman's life when menstruation stops and she can no longer bear children. During menopause, the body makes less of the female hormones, estrogen and progesterone. After menopause, the lower hormone levels free a woman from concerns about monthly menstrual periods and getting pregnant. But they can also cause troublesome symptoms, such as hot flashes (a sudden flush or warmth, often followed by sweating) and sleep problems. Sometimes women have other physical problems, such as vaginal dryness. While many women have little or no trouble with menopause, others have moderate to severe discomfort. Estrogen loss also raises a woman's risk for other serious health problems. They include heart disease and stroke, leading causes of death for women over the age of 50. Estrogen loss also can lead to bone loss.

Some bone loss is normal as people age. However, a more serious condition called osteoporosis weakens bones and lets them break easily. It affects 24 million people in this country. Women have a higher risk than men.

Doctors sometimes prescribe hormones to replace those lost during menopause. This treatment, called hormone replacement therapy (HRT), can ease symptoms of menopause and protect against risks of heart disease, stroke, and osteoporosis. Although millions of women take HRT, this may not be the right choice for everyone.

Administration on Aging (AoA) and National Institute on Aging (NIA), updated July 31, 1995.

## What Can You Do?

Doctors usually prescribe HRT combining estrogen and another female hormone, progestin. They usually prescribe estrogen without progestin for women who have had their uterus removed (hysterectomy). Estrogen can be used in pill or tablet form, vaginal creams, or shots. There are also patches that attach to the skin and release estrogen through the skin. The form of estrogen your doctor chooses may depend on your symptoms. For instance, creams are used for vaginal dryness, while pills or patches are used to ease different menopause symptoms, such as hot flashes, or to prevent bone loss. Progestin usually is taken in pill form.

Doctors may prescribe different schedules for taking HRT. Some women take estrogen for a set number of days, add progestin for a set number of days, and then stop taking one or both for a specific period of time. They repeat the same pattern every month. This pattern often causes regular monthly bleeding like a menstrual period. Some women take HRT every day of the month without any break. This pattern usually stops regular monthly bleeding. Talk with your doctors about the system that is best for you.

## Who Should Take HRT

Many experts believe that the benefits of HRT may be greater than the risks. but scientists do not yet fully know the risks of long-term HRT. Before you decide about HRT, discuss the possible benefits, risks, and side effects with your doctor.

## Risk Factors for Osteoporosis

Women who are at high risk of getting osteoporosis may want to think about taking HRT to prevent it. Risk factors include:

- Having early menopause (natural or due to surgery)
- Being White or Asian
- Being physically inactive
- Taking corticosteriod medicines (prescribed for arthritis or other inflammatory diseases)
- Having a slight build
- Getting too little calcium from diet
- Smoking cigarettes

- Drinking more than a moderate amount of alcohol
- Having thyroid or kidney disease

Your doctor may warn against HRT if you have high blood pressure, diabetes, liver disease, blood clots, seizures, migraine headaches, gall-bladder disease, or a history of cancer. Also, daughters of mothers who took DES (diethylstilbestrol) during pregnancy may have changes to their reproductive system that make HRT dangerous.

## Side Effects and Risks of HRT

Some women may have side effects from HRT, such as unwanted vaginal bleeding, headaches, nausea, vaginal discharge, fluid retention, swollen breasts, or weight gain. Other health concerns for women taking HRT include:

**Cancer of the uterus (endometrial cancer)**. Research shows that women who have their uterus and use estrogen alone are at risk for endometrial cancer. But today, most doctors prescribe the combination of estrogen and progestin. Progestin protects against endometrial cancer. If a woman who still has a uterus takes estrogen alone, her doctor should take sample tissue from her uterus (endometrial biopsy) to check for cancer every year. Women without a uterus have no risk of endometrial cancer.

**Breast cancer.** Today, many scientists are studying the possible link between HRT and breast cancer. Some studies have shown that HRT increases the risk of breast cancer.

**Heart disease.** Estrogen alone or combined with progestin reduces the risk of heart disease. Scientists recently have shown that estrogen lowers risks of heart disease and stroke in women over the age of 50, when they are most at risk for heart disease and stroke.

**Abnormal vaginal bleeding**. Women taking HRT are more likely than other women to have abnormal vaginal bleeding. When this happens, the doctor may perform a "D and C" (dilation and curettage) to find the cause of bleeding. In more serious cases, the doctor may suggest removing the uterus.

Scientists are still studying the risks of taking estrogen alone or in combination with progestin over a long period of time. Women who have their uterus, are at low risk for stroke, heart disease, or serious bone disease, and have no major menopause symptoms may choose to avoid HRT.

## Medical Checkups

If you are taking hormones, you should have regular medical check-ups. The American College of Obstetricians and Gynecologists recommends that all women taking HRT get a medical checkup every year. At that time, the doctor or nurse should read your blood pressure, give you pelvic and breast exams, and take an x-ray picture of your breasts (mammogram) to check for breast cancer.

## If You Don't Take HRT

If you decide against HRT, there are other ways to deal with the symptoms of menopause. There are drugs that can reduce hot flashes, and you can apply water soluble surgical jelly (**not** petroleum jelly) to the vagina to reduce dryness. Simply lowering the room temperature may help you sleep better and ease uncomfortable hot flashes.

To strengthen your bones, good health habits can help, even if you don't start until later in life. Experts suggest that all adult women have 1,000 mg of calcium each day; after menopause, women not using HRT should have 1,500 mg each day. Low-fat milk and dairy foods such as cheese and yogurt are good sources for calcium. If you find it hard to get that amount from your diet, you can take calcium supplements.

Your body also needs vitamin D to absorb calcium. Most people get enough vitamin D just by being out in the sun for at least a short time every day. Supplements or milk fortified with vitamin D are also good sources for this vitamin.

Weight-bearing exercises, which make your muscles work against gravity, help strengthen bones and prevent osteoporosis. Walking, jogging, and playing tennis are all good weight-bearing exercises.

You may also want to ask your doctor about a new drug to treat osteoporosis in women past menopause. The new treatment is safe and effective in increasing bone mass.

## Resources

You can get more information on this topic by contacting the organizations listed below.

**The American College of Obstetricians and Gynecologists (ACOG)** offers the following pamphlets, *Hormone Replacement Therapy, Preventing Osteoporosis, and The Menopause Years*. To obtain copies, send a self-addressed envelope to:
ACOG
P.O. Box 96920
409 12th Street, S.W.
Washington, D.C. 20024-2188

**American Association of Retired Persons (AARP) Women's Initiative** has a fact sheet, *Hormone Replacement Therapy: Facts to Help You Decide*. To obtain a copy, write:
AARP
601 E Street, N.W.
Washington, D.C. 20049
1-800-424-3410

**The National Osteoporosis Foundation (NOF)** has information for health professionals and the public. Contact:
NOF
1232 22nd Street, N.W., Suite 500
Washington, D.C. 20036-4603
202-223-2226

**The National Resource Center on Osteoporosis and Related Bone Diseases** is a national clearinghouse with information on the risks, prevention, and treatment of osteoporosis. For more information call: 1-800-624-BONE

**The North American Menopause Society (NAMS)** answers written requests for information. Write:
NAMS
P.O. Box 94527
Cleveland, Ohio 44101-4527
440-442-7550

**The National Women's Health Network** distributes educational materials on a variety of women's health topics. Contact:
National Women's Health Network
514 10th Street, N.W.
Washington, D.C. 20004
202-347-1140

**The Older Women's League (OWL)** educates the public about problems and issues of concern to middle age and older women. Contact:
666 11th Street, N.W., Suite 700
Washington, D.C. 20001
202-783-6686

**The National Cancer Institute (NCI),** part of NIH, funds cancer research and offers information for health professionals and the public. For more information about cancer risks and other related issues, call: 1-800-4-CANCER

**The National Heart, Lung, and Blood Institute,** part of NIH, carries out research and provides educational information on heart disease, stroke, and other related topics. For more information call: 301-251-1222

**National Institute on Aging Information Center** has information on menopause, osteoporosis, and a variety of other topics related to health and aging. Contact:
Building 31, Room 5C27
31 Center Drive, MSC 2292
Bethesda, MD 20892
1-800-222-2225
1-800-222-4225 (TTY)

# Chapter 43

# *Estrogen to Prevent Osteoporosis*

## *The Estrogen Decision: Are Lower Doses Good Enough?*

Can a little bit of estrogen go a long way? For some women, less may indeed be more—or at least adequate to the tasks at hand. That's good news for women who would like to step down from the standard dose.

But as per usual in the confusing world of hormone-replacement therapy (HRT), there are caveats and unanswered questions, thanks to a lack of long-term data.

## *Stamp of Approval*

In the one-size-fits-all approach to HRT, the dogma has been that 0.625 milligrams (mg) of conjugated equine estrogens (Premarin) is the dose needed to prevent osteoporosis. That's no longer true now that a low-dose estrogen preparation has received an osteoporosis indication.

Although the product—a 0.3-mg formulation of Estratab—has been on the market for years, this is the first time that the U.S. Food and Drug Administration has recognized any low-dose estrogen formulation for its bone-building benefits.

---

"Estrogen," from *Women's Health Advocate Newsletter*, July 1998, Vol. 5, No. 5, © 1998. Reprinted with permission from *Women's Health Advocate Newsletter*.

In a study of more than 400 postmenopausal women, low-dose Estratab (which comprises several different estrogens) increased bone mineral density at the spine and hip over a two-year period, researchers reported late last year in the *Archives of Internal Medicine.*

Moreover, low-dose Estratab also produced positive changes in the women's lipid levels—decreases in low-density lipoprotein (LDL) and increases in high-density lipoprotein (HDL)—and helped ease hot flashes, night sweats, and painful inter-course. (Estrogen's ability to prevent coronary heart disease is commonly assumed but not absolutely proven.)

The use of low-dose estrogen isn't a brand-new concept. Many— but not all—physicians have been willing to prescribe low-dose estrogens for some time.

"We've prescribed them for women who couldn't take more, didn't need more, or wouldn't take more," says Robert Rebar, M.D., professor and chair of the department of obstetrics[1] and gynecology at the University of Cincinnati College of Medicine and a member of the Estratab/Osteoporosis study group. "But we didn't have the data that said if a woman is unwilling to take a large dose of estrogen, giving her just a little may be just as good."

For most medications, the rule of thumb is to take the least amount required for the benefit desired. It stands to reason that smaller doses of estrogen would be less likely to cause many of the side effects that lead so many women to discontinue therapy.

However, the question that bedevils many women—is a lower dose less likely to increase the risk of breast cancer?—remains to be answered.

An unexpected finding of the Estratab study was that the 0.3-mg dose didn't induce endometrial hyperplasia, an overgrowth of the uterine lining that can lead to endometrial cancer. The various doses of estrogen given in the study–0.3, 0.625, and 1.25 mg—were all given unopposed, without a progestin, in order to better evaluate the effects of estrogen alone.

"To our surprise, the 0.3-mg dose offered bone and lipid benefits with-out increasing the risk of endometrial hyperplasia over two years," Dr. Rebar says. "That's not to say that the risk wouldn't have been increased at three years; it might well have been."

He adds that while he doesn't recommend that estrogen be used unopposed in women with a uterus, physicians do, on occasion, prescribe estrogen by itself, under close monitoring, for women who simply can't tolerate progestins.

## Nagging Questions

Low-dose Estratab joins alendronate (Fosamax), raloxifene (Evista), and a variety of higher-dose estrogens as prevention and treatment options for osteoporosis. None is perfect, and questions remain about each approach:

- Will lower-dose estrogens be less likely to increase a woman's risk of breast cancer? (With traditional estrogen regimens, breast cancer risk doesn't appear to rise until after 8 or 10 years of use.)

- Will long-term use of alendronate adversely affect bone? Dr. Rebar points out that the drug is absorbed into bone, where it has a half-life of several years. No one knows what effect taking alendronate for more than several years will have on a woman's bones.

- What are the long-term effects of taking raloxifene? "Raloxifene and tamoxifen are birds of a feather," Dr. Rebar notes. "Data now indicate that taking tamoxifen (for breast cancer) for more than five years begins to negate its benefits, Will the same be true for raloxifene? We don't have any long-term data."

As researchers continue to study these issues, there may come a time when women won't be faced with an either/or proposition. For instance, one alternative scenario for treating osteoporosis might be that women start out on low-dose estrogen for 8 to 10 years, followed by a switch to raloxifene for 5 years, and then alendronate after that.

"My belief is that we'll be using all three classes of drugs. What we haven't sorted out is when to use each one," Dr. Rebar says. "It's really an issue of who is the most appropriate candidate for each drug and when the drugs should be used. The answers will be evolving over our lifetime."

In the meantime, he says, "Estrogens remain the primary modality for the prevention and treatment of osteoporosis. That is a fact. And estrogen is still the only one of the agents that will relieve menopausal signs and symptoms and that has a clearly beneficial effect on lipids."

## Rating Raloxifene

A drug that builds bone, benefits the heart, and prevents breast cancer—what more do we need? For starters, how about more long-term data and head-to-head comparisons?

331

Although raloxifene (Evista) holds great promise, there's much that we don't know about the drug. Here's a brief rundown of some findings:

**Bone.** A study published in the Dec. 4, 1997 *New England Journal of Medicine* reported that raloxifene increased bone density in the hip and spine by 2 percent to 3 percent over a two-year period.

Its effect on the spine doesn't appear to be as strong as that of estrogen or alendronate, but its effects on the hip and total body are more comparable. It remains to be determined whether raloxifene can reduce the risk of fractures, as estrogen and alendronate can.

**Heart.** A study published in the May 13 *Journal of the American Medical Association* compared raloxifene to conventional HRT (0.625 mg Premarin plus 2.5 mg medroxyprogesterone). Both regimens produced similar reductions in LDL levels; however, the estrogen-progestin combination did a better job at raising HDL cholesterol and lowering lipoprotein(a).

Eli Lilly and Co., raloxifene's maker, reportedly is beginning to recruit women at high risk of coronary heart disease (CHD) to evaluate the drug's ability to prevent CHD.

**Breast.** Preliminary findings released at the American Society of Clinical Oncology meeting in May 1998 suggest that raloxifene may be able to prevent breast cancer. However, the findings have not been published. Moreover, a head-to-head comparison between tamoxifen (Nolvadex) and raloxifene is urgently needed; such a study is planned and could begin as early as this fall.

**Brain.** There's no information available on raloxifene's effects on memory or mood. In comparison, some evidence suggests that estrogen can maintain memory—and possibly prevent Alzheimer's disease—and enhance mood.

# Chapter 44

# *Optimal Calcium Intake*

NIH Consensus Statements are prepared by a non-advocate, non-Federal panel of experts, based on (1) presentations by investigators working in areas relevant to the consensus questions during a 2-day public session; (2) questions and statements from conference attendees during open discussion periods that are part of the public session; and (3) closed deliberations by the panel during the remainder of the second day and morning of the third. This statement is an independent report of the consensus panel and is not a policy statement of the NIH or the Federal Government.

## *Abstract*

The National Institutes of Health Consensus Development Conference on Optimal Calcium Intake brought together experts from many different fields including osteoporosis and bone and dental health, nursing, dietetics, epidemiology, endocrinology, gastroenterology, nephrology, rheumatology, oncology, hypertension, nutrition and public education, and biostatistics, as well as the public to address the following questions: (1) What is the optimal amount of calcium intake? (2) What are the important cofactors for achieving optimal calcium intake? (3) What are the risks associated with increased levels

National Institutes of Health (NIH) Consensus Development Program, *Optimal Calcium Intake*. NIH Consensus Statement Online, June 6-8, 1994; 12(4)1-31. Available at http://odp.od.nih.gov/consensus/cons/097/ 097_statement.htm.

of calcium intake? (4) What are the best ways to attain optimal calcium intake? (5) What public health strategies are available and needed to implement optimal calcium intake recommendations? and (6) What are the recommendations for future research on calcium intake?

The consensus panel concluded that

- A large percentage of Americans fail to meet currently recommended guidelines for optimal calcium intake.

- On the basis of the most current information available, optimal calcium intake is estimated to be 400 mg/day (birth-6 months) to 600 mg/day (6-12 months) in infants; 800 mg/day in young children (1-5 years) and 800-1,200 mg/day for older children (6-10 years); 1,200-1,500 mg/day for adolescents and young adults (11-24 years); 1,000 mg/day for women between 25 and 50 years; 1,200-1,500 mg/day for pregnant or lactating women; and 1,000 mg/day for postmenopausal women on estrogen replacement therapy and 1,500 mg/day for postmenopausal women not on estrogen therapy. Recommended daily intake for men is 1,000 mg/day (25-65 years). For all women and men over 65, daily intake is recommended to be 1,500 mg/day, although further research is needed in this age group. These guidelines are based on calcium from the diet plus any calcium taken in supplemental form.

- Adequate vitamin D is essential for optimal calcium absorption. Dietary constituents, hormones, drugs, age, and genetic factors influence the amount of calcium required for optimal skeletal health.

- Calcium intake, up to a total intake of 2,000 mg/day, appears to be safe in most individuals.

- The preferred source of calcium is through calcium-rich foods such as dairy products. Calcium-fortified foods and calcium supplements are other means by which optimal calcium intake can be reached in those who cannot meet this need by ingesting conventional foods.

- A unified public health strategy is needed to ensure optimal calcium intake in the American population.

The full text of the consensus panel's statement follows.

## Introduction

It has been a decade since the 1984 Consensus Development Conference on Osteoporosis first suggested that increased intake of calcium might help prevent osteoporosis. Osteoporosis affects more than 25 million people in the United States and is the major underlying cause of bone fractures in postmenopausal women and the elderly. Previous surveys have revealed that the U.S. population experiences more than 1.5 million fractures annually at a cost in excess of $10 billion per year to the health care system. Two important factors that influence the occurrence of osteoporosis are optimal peak bone mass attained in the first two to three decades of life and the rate at which bone is lost in later years. Adequate calcium intake is critical to achieving optimal peak bone mass and modifies the rate of bone loss associated with aging. A number of publications have addressed the possible role of calcium intake in the prevention of disorders other than osteoporosis, including other bone diseases, oral bone loss, colon cancer, hypertension, and preeclampsia, a hypertensive disorder of pregnancy. The results of recent research investigating these issues indicate that the optimal amount of calcium intake may be greater than the amount consumed by most Americans. At the same time, the general public and scientists have been exposed to a body of information emphasizing the value of ensuring adequate calcium intake throughout life.

Calcium is an essential nutrient. Optimal calcium intake may vary according to a person's age, sex, and ethnicity. Other factors play a role in calcium intake, including vitamin D, which is needed for adequate calcium absorption. Many factors can negatively influence calcium availability, such as certain medications or food components. Optimal calcium intake may be achieved through diet, calcium-fortified foods, calcium supplements, or various combinations of these.

In view of the great public interest in nutrition and disease prevention, the scientific community has an obligation to integrate new data and to provide health care practitioners and the public with guidance, even though all of the necessary long-term studies may not have been completed. In some cases, the new data, however exciting, point to the need for further research rather than to specific recommendations. Future investigations in this rapidly expanding area of research will lead undoubtedly to more definitive information, which will provide the basis for new recommendations.

To address issues related to optimal calcium intake, the National Institute of Arthritis and Musculoskeletal and Skin Diseases together with the Office of Medical Applications of Research of the National

Institutes of Health, convened a Consensus Development Conference on Optimal Calcium Intake on June 6-8, 1994. The conference was cosponsored by the Office of Research on Women's Health, Office of the Director; the National Institute on Aging; the National Cancer Institute; the National Institute of Child Health and Human Development; the National Institute of Diabetes and Digestive and Kidney Diseases; the National Heart, Lung, and Blood Institute; and the National Institute of Dental Research, all of the National Institutes of Health. Conference participants included experts from many different fields, including osteoporosis and bone and dental health, nursing, dietetics, epidemiology, endocrinology, gastroenterology, nephrology, rheumatology, oncology, hypertension, nutrition and public education, and biostatistics, as well as representatives from the public.

After 1-1/2 days of presentations by experts in the relevant fields and audience discussion, an independent, non-Federal consensus panel weighed the scientific evidence and formulated a consensus statement in response to the following six questions:

1. What is the optimal amount of calcium intake?

2. What are the important cofactors for achieving optimal calcium intake?

3. What are the risks associated with increased levels of calcium intake?

4. What are the best ways to attain optimal calcium intake?

5. What public health strategies are available and needed to implement optimal calcium intake recommendations?

6. What are the recommendations for future research on calcium intake?

The consensus panel prepared a draft report summarizing the evidence pertinent to the key issues regarding optimal calcium intake.

## What Is the Optimal Amount of Calcium Intake?

Calcium is a major component of mineralized tissues and is required for normal growth and development of the skeleton and teeth. Optimal calcium intake refers to the levels of consumption that are necessary for an individual (a) to maximize peak adult bone mass, (b) to maintain adult bone mass, and (c) to minimize bone loss in the later years.

Calcium requirements vary throughout an individual's lifetime, with greater needs during the periods of rapid growth in childhood and adolescence, during pregnancy and lactation, and in later adult life (see Table 44.1). Because 99 percent of total body calcium is found in bone, the need for calcium is largely determined by skeletal requirements. Most studies examining the efficacy of calcium intake on bone mass have used measures of external calcium balance and bone densitometry as primary outcomes. The results of balance studies suggest a threshold effect for calcium intake: Body retention of calcium increases with increasing calcium intake up to a threshold, beyond which further calcium intake causes no additional increment in calcium retention.

A great deal of recent data related to calcium intake and its effects on calcium balance, bone mass, and the prevention of osteoporosis was

**Table 44.1.** Optimal Calcium Requirements

| Group | Optimal Daily Intake (in mg of calcium) |
|---|---|
| **Infant** | |
| Birth -6months | 400 |
| 6 months-1 year | 600 |
| **Children** | |
| 1-5 years | 800 |
| 6-10 years | 800-1200 |
| **Adolescents/Young Adults** | |
| 11-24 | 1200-1500 |
| **Men** | |
| 25-65 years | 1000 |
| Over 65 years | 1500 |
| **Women** | |
| 25-50 years | |
| Over 50 years (postmenopausal) | 1500 |
| On estrogens | 1000 |
| Not on estrogens | 1500 |
| Over 65 years | 1500 |
| Pregnant and nursing | 1200-1500 |

reviewed, with attention given to the calcium requirements over the life cycle. The current *Recommended Dietary Allowances*(RDA) (10th edition, 1989) for calcium intake were considered as reference levels and used as guidelines to determine optimal calcium intake in light of new data on calcium-related disorders.

## Infants (Birth-12 Months) and Young Children (1-10 Years)

Calcium intake of exclusively breast-fed infants during the first 6 months of life is in the range of 250-330 mg/day, with a fractional calcium absorption between 55 and 60 percent. A lower fractional absorption of 40 percent is found with cow milk-based formulas. These formulas contain nearly twice the calcium content of human milk; this results in comparable calcium retentions of 150-200 mg/day from both formula and breast milk. Net calcium absorption from soy-based formulas is comparable to, or higher than, that of breast milk or cow milk formulas because of its considerably higher calcium content. For infants between the ages of 6 and 12 months, calcium intake ranges from 400 to 700 mg/day. On the basis of balance data, the current RDAs for calcium, 400 mg/day for infants from birth to 6 months and 600 mg/day for those from 6 to 12 months, seem sufficient to provide optimal calcium intake. However, special circumstances such as low birth weight may require higher calcium intake.

Limited data from one recent study suggest that in children 6-10 years old, intake above 800 mg/day may lead to increased rates of bone accumulation. Coupled with calcium balance data, this suggests that an intake of greater than 800 mg/day may be optimal for this age group. It should also be noted that poor calcium nutrition in childhood may be related to development of enamel hypoplasia and accelerated dental caries.

## Children and Young Adults (11-24 Years)

Calcium accumulation in bone during preadolescence is between 140 and 165 mg/day and may be as high as 400-500 mg/day in the pubertal period. Fractional intestinal absorption is very efficient and estimated to be approximately 40 percent. Peak adult bone mass, depending on the skeletal site examined, is largely achieved by 20 years of age, although important additional bone mass may accumulate through the third decade of life. Furthermore, cross-sectional studies reveal a small but positive association between life-long calcium intake and adult bone mass. Therefore, optimal calcium intake

338

in childhood and young adulthood is critical to achieving peak adult bone mass.

Recent evidence suggests that adding 500-1,000 mg/day to current calcium intake may, at least temporarily, increase bone accretion rates in preadolescent boys and girls. With this supplementation, total calcium intake in these studies exceeded the current RDA of 1,200 mg/day; however, it is unclear whether the effect on bone accretion rates persists beyond the reported 18-month to 3-year periods of treatment and whether these increased rates of bone formation translate into higher peak adult bone mass. Recent balance studies in adolescents indicate a calcium intake threshold in the range of 1,200-1,500 mg/day.

Collectively, these data suggest that calcium intake in the range of 1,200-1,500 mg/day might result in higher peak adult bone mass. Additional research is necessary, particularly longitudinal, long-term dose-ranging studies of the effects of varying calcium intake on bone mass, to more precisely define optimal calcium intake for this age group. Importantly, population surveys of girls and young women 12-19 years of age show their average calcium intake to be less than 900 mg/day, which is well below the calcium intake threshold. The consequences of low calcium intake during this crucial period of rapid skeletal accrual raise concerns that achievement of optimal peak adult peak bone mass may be seriously compromised. Special education and public measures aimed at improving dietary calcium intake in this age group are essential.

*Calcium Intake in Adults (25-65 Years of Age)*

Once peak adult bone mass is reached, bone turnover is stable in men and women such that bone formation and bone resorption are balanced. In women, resorption rates increase and bone mass declines beginning with the fall in estrogen production that is associated with the onset of menopause. The decline in circulating 17-beta-estradiol is the predominant factor in the accelerated bone loss that begins after the onset of menopause and continues for 6-8 years. Unlike hormone replacement therapy, supplemental calcium during this initial phase will not slow the decline in bone mass due to estrogen deficiency. Although the effects of calcium can be shown more clearly in postmenopausal women after the period when the effects of estrogen deficiency are no longer dominant (approximately 10 years after menopause), it is likely that the early postmenopausal years are also an important time to ensure optimal calcium intake. Between 25 and 50 years of age, women who are otherwise healthy should maintain a calcium intake of 1,000 mg/day (Osteoporosis. NIH Consensus Statement 1984 Apr 2-4;5(3):1-6). For postmenopausal women who are receiving estrogen replacement therapy, a calcium intake of 1,000 mg/day is recommended to maintain calcium balance and stabilize bone mass. For postmenopausal women who do not take estrogen, it is estimated that a calcium intake of 1,500 mg/day may limit loss of bone mass, but should not be considered a replacement for estrogen. Therefore, recommended calcium intake for postmenopausal women up to 65 years of age is 1,000 mg/day in conjunction with hormonal replacement and 1,500 mg/day in the absence of estrogen replacement.

Adult men also sustain fractures of the hip and vertebrae, although at a lower frequency than women. In several prospective and cross-sectional studies, hip fracture risk in men has been found to be inversely correlated with calcium intake. Although the data are less extensive in men than in women, the evidence in men suggests that inadequate calcium intake is associated with reduced bone mass and increased fracture risk. Available data, although sparse, indicate an optimal calcium intake among adult men similar to women, namely 1,000 mg/day.

*Calcium Intake in Adults (Older than 65 Years)*

In men and women 65 years of age and older, calcium intake of less than 600 mg/day is common. Furthermore, intestinal calcium absorption is often reduced because of the effects of estrogen deficiency in women and the age-related reduction in renal 1,25-dihydroxy vitamin D production. Calcium insufficiency due to low calcium intake and reduced absorption can translate into an accelerated rate of age-related bone loss in older individuals. Among the homebound elderly and persons residing in long-term care facilities, vitamin D insufficiency has been detected and may contribute to reduced calcium absorption. Calcium intake among women later in the menopause, in the range of 1,500 mg/day, may reduce the rates of bone loss in selected sites of the skeleton such as the femoral neck. (These findings also indicate that the calcium threshold for reducing bone loss may vary for different regions of the skeleton.)

The physiology of calcium homeostasis in aging men over 65 is similar to that of women with respect to the rate of bone loss, calcium absorption efficiency, declining vitamin D levels, and changes in markers of bone metabolism. It seems reasonable, therefore, to conclude that in aging men, as in aging women, prevailing calcium intakes are insufficient to prevent calcium-related erosion of bone mass.

Thus, in women and in men over 65, calcium intake of 1,500 mg/day seems prudent.

## Pregnant and Lactating Women

The current RDA for calcium intake during pregnancy and lactation is 1,200 mg/day. Pregnancy represents a significant physiological stress on maternal skeletal homeostasis. A full-term infant accumulates approximately 30 grams of calcium during gestation, most of which is assimilated into the fetal skeleton during the third trimester. Available data suggest that, with pregnancy, no permanent decline in body calcium occurs if recommended levels of dietary calcium intake are maintained. There is no association between parity and bone mass. Furthermore, there is no evidence to support changing the current recommendation of calcium intake for well-nourished pregnant women. There is, however, a large population of pregnant women who are not ingesting sufficient calcium, especially those who are undernourished. These women need to be identified, and appropriate adjustments in their calcium intake should be made. Data are not available regarding the calcium requirement for pregnant women at the extremes of reproductive years, for those who experience non-singleton births, and for those with closely spaced pregnancies.

During lactation, 160-300 mg/day of maternal calcium is lost through production of breast milk. Longitudinal studies in otherwise healthy women demonstrate acute bone loss during lactation that is followed by rapid restoration of bone mass with weaning and the resumption of menses. Women who are lactating should ingest at least 1,200 mg of calcium per day. Lactating adolescents and young adults should ingest up to 1,500 mg of calcium per day.

## Diseases Other than Osteoporosis

Low calcium intake has been implicated as a determinant of preeclampsia and several other chronic conditions including colon cancer and hypertension. Data regarding the role of supplemental calcium in reducing preeclampsia are conflicting. A large multicenter trial to evaluate this question is under way; the results, which will be available in 1996, should provide the information needed to judge the utility of increased calcium for preeclampsia.

In some recent epidemiological studies, higher calcium intake has been associated with a lower risk for the development of colon cancer. However, the findings are inconsistent, and the number of reports addressing this relationship are limited. Results of short-term clinical trials of the effect of increased calcium intake on rectal mucosal cell proliferation have been mixed and suffer from considerable methodological constraints. Currently, there are insufficient data to establish the role of calcium in colon cancer risk; therefore, a recommendation for increased calcium intake for colon cancer prevention is not warranted at this time.

There are considerable epidemiological and clinical trial data on the relationship between blood pressure levels and calcium intake. Although a number of epidemiological studies suggest an inverse association between blood pressure and calcium intake, most of these studies have been of cross-sectional design, and few prospective studies are available to confirm this association. Results of randomized controlled trials of calcium supplementation on blood pressure have been equivocal. Pooled analyses indicate a small reduction in systolic blood pressure and no effect on diastolic blood pressure. There is speculation that only a subgroup of individuals respond to calcium supplementation; however, randomized trial data are currently not available. A recommendation for increased calcium intake for prevention of hypertension is not warranted at this time, but additional information is needed to identify subpopulations that may benefit from this treatment.

## What are the Important Cofactors for Achieving Optimal Calcium Intake?

Several cofactors modify calcium balance and influence bone mass. These include dietary constituents, hormones, drugs, and the level of physical activity. Unique host characteristics may also modify the effects of dietary calcium on bone health. These include the individual's age and ethnic and genetic background, the presence of gastrointestinal disorders such as malabsorption and the postgastrectomy syndrome, and the presence of liver and renal disease. Interactions among these diverse cofactors may affect calcium balance in either a positive or negative manner and thus alter the optimal levels of calcium intake.

### Cofactors That Enhance Calcium Absorption

Vitamin D metabolites enhance calcium absorption. 1,25-Dihydroxy vitamin D, the major metabolite, stimulates active transport of calcium in the small intestine and colon. Deficiency of 1,25-dihydroxy vitamin

D, caused by inadequate dietary vitamin D, inadequate exposure to sunlight, impaired activation of vitamin D, or acquired resistance to vitamin D, results in reduced calcium absorption. In the absence of 1,25-dihydroxy vitamin D, less than 10 percent of dietary calcium may be absorbed. Vitamin D deficiency is associated with an increased risk of fractures. Elderly patients are at particular risk for vitamin D deficiency because of insufficient vitamin D intake from their diet, impaired renal synthesis of 1,25-dihydroxy vitamin D, and inadequate sunlight exposure, which is normally the major stimulus for endogenous vitamin D synthesis. This is especially evident in homebound or institutionalized individuals. Supplementation of vitamin D intake to provide 600-800 IU/day has been shown to improve calcium balance and reduce fracture risk in these individuals. Sufficient vitamin D should be ensured for all individuals, especially the elderly who are at greater risk for development of a deficiency. Sources of vitamin D, besides supplements, include sunlight, vitamin D-fortified liquid dairy products, cod liver oil, and fatty fish. Calcium and vitamin D need not be taken together to be effective. Excessive doses of vitamin D may introduce risks such as hypercalciuria and hypercalcemia and should be avoided. Anticonvulsant medications may alter both vitamin D and bone mineral metabolism, particularly in certain disorders, in the institutionalized, and in the elderly. Although symptomatic skeletal disease is uncommon in non-institutionalized settings, optimal calcium intake is advised for persons using anticonvulsants.

Sex hormone deficiency is associated with excessive bone resorption in women and men. Low calcium intake can exacerbate the deleterious consequences of sex hormone deficiency. One study suggested that calcium supplementation can decrease the minimum estrogen dosage required to maintain bone mass in postmenopausal women. However, oral calcium alone does not prevent the postmenopausal bone loss resulting from estrogen deficiency. In addition to estrogen, other endogenous cofactors that could enhance net calcium absorption include growth hormone, insulin-like growth factor-I, and parathyroid hormone.

An interrelationship between physical activity and calcium balance has not been established conclusively. In a single study, increased physical activity enhanced the beneficial effect of oral calcium supplementation on bone mass in young adults. Thus far, studies of elderly individuals and perimenopausal women have failed to establish a positive interaction between calcium intake and exercise to increase bone mass. Therefore, the positive effects of exercise on skeletal health are not likely to be related to calcium intake.

Immobilization has been shown to produce a rapid decrease in bone mass. This loss has been well documented in individuals placed on bed rest and in individuals with regional forms of immobilization such as that seen in para- and quadriplegia. Under these circumstances, the rate of bone loss may be rapid, which is in part related to an increase in bone resorption accompanied by a decrease in bone formation. There is concern that increased calcium intake may increase the risk of hypercalcemia, ectopic calcification, ectopic ossification, and nephrolithiasis in these individuals. Thus, any recommendations for increasing calcium intake are tempered in these individuals by the potential for undesirable consequences.

*Factors That Decrease Calcium Availability*

Calcium intake, intestinal absorption, urinary excretion, and endogenous fecal loss influence calcium balance. Intake and absorption account for only 25 percent of the variance in calcium balance, whereas urinary loss accounts for approximately 50 percent. The typical American diet consists of high amounts of sodium and animal protein, both of which can significantly increase urinary calcium excretion. High oxalate and phytate in a limited number of foods can reduce the availability of calcium in these foods. With the exception of large amounts of wheat bran, fiber has not been found to affect calcium absorption significantly. Other dietary components, including fat, phosphate, magnesium, and caffeine, have not been found to affect calcium absorption or excretion significantly. Aluminum in the form of antacid medication, when taken in excess, may significantly increase urinary calcium loss.

Glucocorticoids decrease calcium absorption. States of glucocorticoid excess are associated with negative calcium balance and a marked increase in fracture risk. In a recent study, oral calcium supplements plus 1,25-dihydroxy vitamin D decreased glucocorticoid-associated bone loss. On the basis of these observations and other studies, oral calcium supplements should be considered in all patients who are receiving exogenous glucocorticoids. The specific disease for which the glucocorticoid therapy is used (e.g., rheumatoid arthritis, inflammatory bowel disease, asthma) can be a determining factor in the occurrence and degree of bone loss.

Genetic and ethnic factors significantly influence many aspects of calcium and skeletal metabolism. Twin studies indicate a significant influence of genetic factors on peak bone mass. However, environmental factors appear to be more important in determining rates of bone loss in postmenopausal women. Racial and ethnic differences in bone mass and fracture incidence have been described, but these are not accounted for by differences in calcium intake. Whether there are genetic and ethnic differences in optimal calcium requirements needs to be determined.

## What Are the Risks Associated with Increased Levels of Calcium Intake?

High levels of calcium intake have several potential adverse effects. The efficiency of calcium absorption decreases as intake increases, thereby providing a protective mechanism to lessen the chances of calcium intoxication. This adaptive mechanism can, however, be overcome by a calcium intake of greater than approximately 4 g/day. It is well known that calcium toxicity, with high blood calcium levels, severe renal damage, and ectopic calcium deposition (milk-alkali syndrome), can be produced by overuse of calcium carbonate, encountered clinically in the form of antacid abuse. Even at intake levels less than 4 g/day, certain otherwise healthy persons may be more susceptible to developing hypercalcemia or hypercalciuria. Likewise, subjects with mild or subclinical illnesses marked by dysregulation of 1,25-dihydroxy vitamin D synthesis (e.g., primary hyperparathyroidism, sarcoidosis) may be at increased risk from higher calcium intakes. Nevertheless, in intervention studies (albeit of relatively short duration—less than 4 years), no adverse renal effects of moderate supplementation up to 1,500 mg/day have been reported. Furthermore, one large study suggested that within the current ranges of calcium intake in the population, a higher calcium intake in men is associated with a decreased risk of stone formation. However, a dose-response relationship was not detected. Caution must be used, however, in supplementing individuals who have a history of kidney stones, because high calcium intakes can increase urinary calcium excretion and might increase the risk of stone formation in these patients.

The strategy of increasing calcium intake by increasing dairy products could tend to increase the intake of saturated fat. These potential problems can be averted by the use of low-fat dairy products. Reduced-fat or no-fat dairy products contain as much calcium per serving size as high-fat dairy products. The use of dairy products to increase calcium intake could increase side effects in people who are sensitive to milk products. Nondairy alternative sources are indicated in these individuals.

Concern has been raised that increased calcium intake might interfere with absorption of other nutrients. Iron absorption can be decreased by as much as 50 percent by many forms of calcium supplements or milk ingestion, but not by forms that contain citrate and ascorbic acid, which enhance iron absorption. Thus, increased intakes of specific sources of calcium might induce iron deficiency in individuals with marginal iron status. Population studies suggest that this is not a common or severe problem, but more study is needed. Whether calcium supplements interfere with absorption of other nutrients has not been thoroughly studied. Calcium may also interfere with absorption of certain medications, such as tetracycline.

Gastrointestinal side effects of calcium supplements have been observed, usually at relatively high dosages. A variable effect on the incidence of constipation has been reported in controlled studies of calcium supplements. The calcium ion stimulates gastrin secretion and gastric acid secretion, which can produce a "rebound hyperacidity" when calcium carbonate is used as an antacid. These side effects should not be major problems with a modest increase in calcium intake.

Certain preparations of calcium (e.g., bone meal and dolomite) can have significant contamination with lead and other heavy metals. However, most commercial calcium preparations are tested to ensure that they do not contain significant heavy metal contamination.

In conclusion, a modest increase in calcium intake should be safe for most people. Practices that might encourage total calcium intake to approach or exceed 2,000 mg/day seem more likely to produce adverse effects and should be monitored closely.

## *What Are the Best Ways to Attain Optimal Calcium Intake?*

The preferred approach to attaining optimal calcium intake is through dietary sources. Additional strategies include the consumption of calcium-fortified foods and calcium supplements. For many Americans, dairy products are the major contributors of dietary calcium because of their high calcium content (e.g., approximately 250-300 mg/8 oz milk) and frequency of consumption. It may be necessary for individuals with lactose intolerance to limit or exclude liquid dairy foods, but adequate calcium intake can be achieved through the use of low-lactose-containing dairy products (solid dairy food) or through milk rendered lactose deficient. Vegans who voluntarily limit their intake of dairy products can obtain dietary calcium through other sources. Other good food sources of calcium include some green vegetables (e.g., broccoli, kale, turnip greens, Chinese cabbage), calcium-set tofu, some legumes, canned fish, seeds, nuts, and certain fortified food products. Breads and cereals, while relatively low in calcium, contribute significantly to calcium intake because of their frequency of consumption.

Recommended calcium intake levels are based on the total calcium content of the food. To maximize calcium absorption, food selection decisions should include information on their bioavailability. Bioavailability (absorption) of calcium from food depends on the food's total calcium content and the presence of components that enhance or inhibit absorption. As mentioned previously, oxalic acid, which is present at high levels in some vegetables (e.g., spinach), has been found to depress absorption of the calcium present in the food but not of calcium in coingested dairy or other calcium-containing foods. Phytic acid also depresses calcium absorption but to a lesser extent. Dietary fiber, except for wheat bran, has little effect on calcium absorption. When present in high concentration, wheat bran has been found to depress calcium absorption from milk.

A number of calcium-fortified food products are currently available, including fortified juices, fruit drinks, breads, and cereals. Although some of these foods provide multiple nutrients and may be frequently consumed, their quantitative contribution and role in the total diet are not currently defined.

For some individuals, calcium supplements may be the preferred way to attain optimal calcium intake. Calcium supplements are available as various salts, and most preparations are well absorbed except when manufactured such that they do not disintegrate during oral ingestion. Absorption of calcium supplements is most efficient at individual doses of 500 mg or less and when taken between meals. Ingesting calcium supplements between meals supports calcium bioavailability, since food may contain certain compounds that reduce calcium absorption (e.g., oxalates). However, absorption of one form of calcium supplementation, calcium carbonate, is impaired in fasted individuals who have an absence of gastric acid. Absorption of calcium carbonate can be improved in these individuals when it is taken with certain food. The potential for calcium supplementation to interfere with iron absorption is an important consideration when it is ingested with meals. Alternatively, calcium supplementation in the form of calcium citrate does not require gastric acid for optimal absorption and thus could be considered in older individuals with reduced gastric acid production. In individuals with adequate gastric acid production, it is preferable to ingest calcium supplements between meals.

Maintenance of optimal bone health depends on an adequate supply of calcium and other essential nutrients. Current dietary intake data indicate that calcium intake is below recommended levels in most individuals. To attain the optimal calcium levels proposed, a change in dietary habits, including increased frequency of consumption of dairy products and/or calcium-rich vegetable sources, is needed. This approach of recommending the consumption of calcium-rich foods is consistent with current dietary guidelines (the U.S. Department of Agriculture (USDA) Food Guide Pyramid), which includes 2-3 servings per day of dairy products and 3-5 servings of vegetables. Recommendations for supplements should be made in the context of the total diet since recommendations are for calcium from all sources. The task for individuals to meet calcium requirements on a continuing daily basis is a formidable challenge.

## What Public Health Strategies Are Available and Needed to Implement Optimal Calcium Intake Recommendations?

Optimizing the calcium intake of Americans is of critical importance. Recent improvements in calcium intake have been reported for most age groups (phase 1 of the Third National Health and Nutrition Examination Survey, 1988-1991—NHANES III). However, contemporary 6- to 11-year-old children showed a decrease in calcium intake, as compared with those a decade earlier (NHANES II, 1976-1980). NHANES III also documents that a large percentage of Americans still fail to meet currently recommended guidelines for calcium intake. The impact of suboptimal calcium intake on the health of Americans and the health care cost to the American public is a vital concern. It is thus appropriate that increasing calcium intake is a national health promotion and disease prevention objective in the *Healthy People 2000* agenda (Department of Health and Human Services Publication Number 91.50212). Public health strategies to promote optimal calcium intake should have a broad outreach and should involve educators, health professionals, and the private and public sectors.

### Public Education

A public education program is needed to do the following:

- Disseminate consensus recommendations to the public.

- Convene meetings of public leaders and representatives of national groups to disseminate information on optimal calcium intake for the general population and high-risk groups and to develop action plans for public education.

348

- Develop health education materials and programs to address the diverse linguistic and cultural needs of the multiethnic American population.

- Work with existing national organizations and the mass media to distribute information, decrease consumer confusion, and encourage consumers, including children, adolescent girls, postmenopausal women, and older Americans, to adopt health-promoting changes in their daily calcium intake.

*Health Professionals*

Primary care physicians, dentists, and other health professionals should play a strong role in educating their patients about bone health and calcium intake. An educational program to support this work of health professionals would:

- Disseminate consensus recommendations to health professionals.

- Develop and distribute educational materials, by serving as a clearinghouse for information on calcium-related research, and developing curricula for health professional training programs.

- Distribute educational materials through health professional organizations at their national and regional meetings.

- Initiate sessions at national meetings of health professionals focusing on promoting optimal calcium intake or initiating national meetings focusing specifically on calcium-related research.

*Private Sector*

The private sector can play an active part in promoting optimal calcium intake.

Manufacturers and producers of food products should continue to develop and market a wide variety of calcium-rich foods to meet the needs and tastes of our multiethnic population.

Restaurants, grocery stores, and other food outlets should increase the accessibility and visibility of calcium-rich products for the consumer.

Biotechnology research groups should develop accessible cost-effective technologies to screen for populations who are at high risk of fracture and who would be candidates for increased calcium intake.

*Public Sector*

The Federal Government should take the following actions:

- The Government should ensure that guidelines for calcium intake across all agencies, departments, and institutions are consistent and that these guidelines reflect the current state of scientific knowledge.

- The National Center for Health Statistics and the USDA should widely disseminate their data on nutrient intakes and food consumption patterns, with respect to calcium, as well as their information on relevant trends in these nutrient intakes and food consumption patterns. To maximize educational, programmatic, and policy efforts, these data should be specific to age, gender, ethnic group, region, and socioeconomic status where possible.

- Existing Federal food and food subsidy programs and federally regulated facilities for infants, children, low-income populations, and the elderly in the Department of Health and Human Services, the Veterans Administration, the Department of Defense and other agencies should ensure achievement of optimal calcium intake for program recipients.

- The USDA should direct school food services to promote calcium intake by serving calcium-rich foods and to urge that calcium be included in all nutrition education efforts within public schools.

- Government cafeterias should serve as models to promote optimal calcium intake by serving calcium-rich foods, labeling calcium content in single servings of those foods, and distributing brochures about the relationship between dietary calcium needs and good health to their customers.

- Address, within health care reform, the need for financial coverage of calcium supplements for those who cannot reach optimal calcium intake through foods alone and financial support for screening of target populations to identify individuals who are at high risk of fracture and who would be likely to benefit from increased calcium intake.

## *What are the Recommendations for Future Research on Calcium Intake?*

- Prospective longitudinal studies to investigate long-term effects of calcium intake on regional (e.g., spine, hip, forearm) changes in bone mass and on fracture incidence in postmenopausal women and in older men.

- Prospective longitudinal studies of adolescent girls and boys to investigate the long-term effects of different levels of calcium intake on the achievement of peak bone mass.

- Studies to determine optimal calcium intake in the decade before the menopause and the potential role of declining estrogen levels during this time.

- Evaluation of the long-term effects of calcium intake on bone remodeling.

- Investigation of interactions between calcium supplementation and the absorption of other nutrients.

- Evaluation of dose-response relationships between calcium intake and estrogen replacement therapy.

- Determination of optimal calcium requirements in different ethnic populations.

- Evaluation of the effect of long-term calcium supplementation on the development or prevention of kidney stones.

- Studies on the effect of dietary calcium on bone mass and fracture incidence.

- Evaluation of the role of vitamin D metabolites in optimizing calcium balance.

- Development of a cost-effective means by which calcium-deficient individuals can be identified at all ages.

- Development of effective health-promoting programs to change population behavior with respect to calcium intakes that are tailored to specific age, sex, ethnic, socioeconomic status, and regional needs.

351

- Improved methods to achieve and maintain optimal dietary intake of calcium by both nutritional and supplemental means.

## Conclusions

- A large percentage of Americans fail to meet currently recommended guidelines for optimal calcium intake.

- On the basis of the most current information available, optimal calcium intake is estimated to be 400 mg/day (birth-6 months) to 600 mg/day (6-12 months) in infants, 800 mg/day in young children (1-5 years) and 800-1,200 mg/day for older children (6-10 years), 1,200-1,500 mg/day for adolescents and young adults (11-24 years), 1,000 mg/day for women between 25 and 50 years, 1,200 mg for pregnant or lactating women, and 1,000 mg/day for postmenopausal women on estrogen replacement therapy and 1,500 mg/day for postmenopausal women not on estrogen therapy. Recommended daily intake for men is 1,000 mg/day (25-65 years). For all women and men over 65, daily intake is recommended to be 1,500 mg/day, although further research is needed in this age group. These guidelines are based upon calcium from the diet plus any calcium taken in supplemental form.

- Adequate vitamin D is essential for optimal calcium absorption. Dietary constituents, hormones, drugs, age, and genetic factors influence the amount of calcium required for optimal skeletal health.

- Calcium intake, up to a total intake of 2,000 mg/day, appears to be safe in most individuals.

- The preferred source of calcium is through calcium-rich foods such as dairy products. Calcium-fortified foods and calcium supplements are other means by which optimal calcium intake can be reached in those who cannot meet this need by ingesting conventional foods.

- A unified public health strategy is needed to ensure optimal calcium intake in the American population.

# Chapter 45

# *Fluoride Plus Calcium Prevents Bone Fractures*

## *The Effect of Sodium Monofluorophosphate plus Calcium on Vertebral Fracture Rate in Postmenopausal Women with Moderate Osteoporosis: A Randomized, Controlled Trial*

From University of Liege, Liege, Belgium; Georgetown University Medical Center, Washington, D.C.; Rotta Research Laboratorium, Monza, Italy; and Klinik der Fürstenhof, Bad Pyrmont, Germany. For current author addresses, see end of text.

**Background:** Fluoride is effective in increasing trabecular bone mineral density (BMD) in the spine, but its efficacy in reducing vertebral fracture rates and its effect on BMD at cortical sites are controversial.

**Objective:** To study the effect of low-dose fluoride (sodium monofluorophosphate [MFP]) plus a calcium supplement over 4 years on vertebral fractures and BMD at the lumbar spine and total hip in postmenopausal women with moderately low BMD of the spine.

Reginster et al, "The Effect of Sodium Monofluorophosphate Plus Calcium on Vertebral Fracture Rate in Postmenopausal Women with Moderate Osteoporosis," from *Annals of Internal Medicine*, 1998, Vol. 129, p. 1-9, © 1998. Reprinted with permission of American College of Physicians—American Society of Internal Medicine.

**Design:** Randomized, double-blind, controlled clinical trial.

**Setting:** Outpatient clinic for osteoporosis at a university medical center.

**Patients:** 200 postmenopausal women with osteoporosis (according to the World Health Organization definition) and a T-score less than -2.5 for BMD of the spine.

**Intervention:** Women were randomly assigned (100 patients per group) to continuous daily treatment for 4 years with 1) oral MFP (20 mg of equivalent fluoride) plus 1000 mg of calcium (as calcium carbonate) or 2) calcium only.

**Measurements:** Lateral spine radiographs were taken at enrollment and at each year of follow-up for detection of new vertebral fractures (defined as a reduction greater than or equal to 20% and greater than or equal to 4 mm from baseline in any of the heights of a vertebral body). Nonvertebral fractures were also recorded. All analyses were done with the intention-to-treat approach.

**Results:** Radiologic follow-up was possible for 164 of 200 patients (82%). The rate of new vertebral fractures during the 4 years of the study was lower in the MFP-plus-calcium group (2 of 84 patients; 2.4% [95% CI, 0.3% to 8.3%]) than in the calcium-only group (8 of 80 patients; 10% [CI, 4.4% to 18.8%]). The difference between the groups was 7.6 percentage points (CI, 0.3 to 15 percentage points) (P = 0.05). A moderate but progressive increase in BMD of the spine (10.0% ± 1.5% at 4 years) was found for MFP plus calcium compared with calcium only (P < 0.001), whereas the more modest increase in BMD of the total hip seen with MFP plus calcium (1.8% ± 0.6%) did not differ from the increase seen with calcium only.

**Conclusions:** Low-dose fluoride (20 mg/d) given continuously with calcium for prolonged periods can decrease vertebral fracture rates compared with calcium alone in patients with mild to moderate osteoporosis.

## Full Text

During the past 30 years, fluoride salts have been studied as agents for the treatment of osteoporosis in postmenopausal women with the expectation that stimulation of osteoblastic proliferation and activity and the subsequent increase in bone formation would be followed by a significant decrease in fracture rates (1-3). It is widely accepted that fluoride is effective in increasing trabecular bone mass in the spine (4). However, discrepant results have been obtained from studies evaluating the effects of fluoride salts on cortical bone mass and, more important, on the quality of the newly synthesized bone and on vertebral and nonvertebral fracture rates (5-9). These differences are probably related to differences in fluoride dose, formulation, and regimen; duration of therapy; and treated populations. Because bone-forming agents such as fluoride are expected to work mainly by increasing bone mineral content without restoring disrupted bone tissue integrity, they may be particularly useful in patients with mild to moderate osteoporosis in whom the microarchitecture of the skeleton is not excessively damaged. To test this hypothesis, we studied the effect of low-dose fluoride (sodium monofluorophosphate [MFP]) plus calcium in a 4-year, randomized, double-blind, controlled clinical trial in postmenopausal women with moderately low bone mineral density (BMD) of the spine.

## Methods

### Patients

Our study included white postmenopausal women with lumbar (L2 to L4) BMD of the spine below the 90th percentile of the distribution of BMD of the spine seen in Belgian women with osteoporosis (10, 11). This degree of bone loss corresponded to a T-score of -2.5, in accordance with the operational definition of osteoporosis recently proposed by a World Health Organization study group (12). Patients were included in the study regardless of whether they had previously had vertebral or nonvertebral fractures; most of the patients were thought to be free of vertebral fractures at enrollment. Previous hip fracture was an exclusion criterion. All patients were free of other causes of osteoporosis, such as diseases or medications known to interfere with bone metabolism; none had been treated with any drug for postmenopausal osteoporosis; and no such treatment was allowed during the study. Hormone replacement therapy was continued, for ethical reasons, in women for whom it had been prescribed before enrollment for purposes other than bone therapy. Randomization was not stratified with respect to hormone replacement therapy. Patients with bone diseases other

355

than osteoporosis, renal insufficiency, hypochlorhydria, or severe chronic disorders that could have interfered with the study were excluded.

*Study Design*

Patients were randomly assigned in a blinded manner to one of two therapeutic groups. Every day for 4 years, they received either two chewable tablets that each contained 76 mg of MFP (10 mg of equivalent fluoride [fluoride ion]) and 1250 mg of calcium carbonate (500 mg of equivalent calcium) or two chewable tablets that each contained 1250 mg of calcium carbonate alone and were similar in appearance to the MFP-plus-calcium tablets. Total daily dosages, therefore, were 20 mg of equivalent fluoride plus 1000 mg of calcium in the MFP-plus-calcium group and 1000 mg of calcium in the calcium-only group.

The two tablets were taken at different meals. We determined compliance at each study visit by asking each patient for the number of days on which she had not taken the tablets and by counting the unused tablets. Compliance was expressed as the percentage of tablets taken (100% if the patient had taken all of the tablets).

Patients received randomization numbers sequentially. Randomization was computer generated in blocks of four according to a strict standard operating procedure by persons who had no contact with the persons in the center who assigned patients to study groups. The randomization code was kept at the study sponsor's facility under secure conditions that were detailed in writing. The clinical research center was given opaque, sealed envelopes, each of which contained the code for one patient. Treatment assignment and other relevant information were thus concealed and were to be revealed only in the case of a medical emergency.

Blinding was achieved by using the following procedures. First, the persons who did the visual readings of the spine radiographs saw the codes only after the results were analyzed. Second, the data were analyzed under blinded conditions: that is, a first analysis was done with groups "A" and "B"; the analysts did not know which group had received which treatment.

*Efficacy Evaluation Criteria*

The primary end point was the number of patients with new vertebral fractures during the 4-year treatment period, in accordance with recently published guidelines for the evaluation of drugs to be registered in Europe for the prevention or treatment of osteoporosis (13).

Standardized lateral radiographs of the thoracic and lumbar spine were obtained at enrollment and at each year of follow-up, for up to 4 years, in a single radiology center. The radiographs were sent to an independent assessor. Films were digitized, and the anterior, middle, and posterior heights of each vertebral body from the fourth thoracic (T4) to the fifth lumbar (L5) were determined (accuracy of the digitizer, 0.025 mm) by a computer program. This was done by persons with no knowledge of treatment assignment or film sequence. A new vertebral fracture (incident fracture) was defined as a reduction of at least 20% and an absolute decrease of at least 4 mm in any height of at least one vertebral body between enrollment and the latest follow-up film. All fractures, including borderline cases, were confirmed by visual reading. This definition was applied to vertebrae that were not fractured at enrollment, whereas fractures present at enrollment were determined on the digitized enrollment radiographs by using the Melton-Riggs 25% unadjusted algorithm (14). The possible progression of such baseline lesions was assessed with the Vertebral Deformity Index obtained for each vertebra (T5 through L5); these were then summed to obtain the Spine Deformity Index, a continuous measure of vertebral deformities (15). The Spine Deformity Index was also used as a secondary variable in patients with incident or progressing vertebral deformities, in whom it was expressed as the mean change between the last observed value and baseline. Bone mineral density was measured by using dual-energy x-ray absorptiometry on the same densitometer (Hologic QDR 1000, Waltham, Massachusetts) at 6-month intervals at the lumbar spine (L2 to L4) and the nondominant hip (total hip) after previously described and validated procedures were performed (11, 16). In our hands, the long-term coefficients of variation of dual-energy x-ray absorptiometry are 0.8% for BMD of the spine and 1.1% for BMD of the total hip (17).

Biochemical determinations of bone remodeling were made at 6-month intervals. Bone formation was assessed by radioimmunoassay of serum bone-specific alkaline phosphatase (Ostase, Hybritech, San Diego, California). For bone resorption, we measured the ratio of urinary hydroxyproline to creatinine on the second fasting urine spot (2-hour morning urine) (Hypronostikon kit, Organon Technika, Oss Boxtel, the Netherlands).

All peripheral (nonvertebral) fractures that occurred during the study were recorded independently of the nature and severity of the trauma that may have determined them.

*Statistical Analysis*

All analyses were done according to the intention-to-treat approach: that is, all patients who had at least one valid measurement after randomization were considered in the analysis, whether they were still taking the study drug or not. In the case of drop-out and, thus, discontinuation of therapy with the study medication, the patient was invited to return to the clinic at annual intervals (for 4 years, if possible) so that the radiography necessary to record outcome could be done.

An exact-significance chi-square test was done to compare the number of patients with new vertebral fractures in the two groups. We calculated 95% CIs for vertebral fracture rates in each study group and for the difference in rates between the two groups, along with the point estimates of these rates. These rates were also expressed in terms of the number needed to treat for 4 years to prevent one fracture, including values for the lower and upper bounds of the 95% CIs. Changes in the Spine Deformity Index in patients with incident or progressing vertebral deformities were compared by analysis of variance.

Analysis of variance for repeated measurements was used to compare the absolute values for BMD of the spine over the course of the study in the two groups. Analysis of variance for repeated measurements was also done to compare BMD of the total hip and percentage changes in biochemical markers of bone remodeling throughout the study. All P values are two-tailed.

All statistical analyses were done with the SPSS/WIN 6.2 statistical package (SPSS, Inc., Chicago, Illinois).

*Role of Study Sponsor*

The trial was approved by the Ethical Committee of Liege University (registration no. 90/43-1262 of 14 May 1990), and all patients gave full informed consent before inclusion. The Rotta Research Group, which markets MFP and calcium combinations in Germany, Italy, and other countries, provided the drugs and funding for the study. Scientists from the Rotta Research Group were directly involved in the design, monitoring, and data management of the study and agreed to be listed as authors. However, the Rotta Research Group as a corporate entity had no control over the decision to approve or submit the manuscript for publication.

## Results

Two hundred patients were enrolled in the study. The characteristics of the entire patient sample (100 patients were assigned to each group) at enrollment are shown in Table 45.1.

The two groups were similar with regard to demographic data, baseline BMD of the spine, and biochemical markers of bone remodeling,

**Table 45.1.** Baseline Characteristics of Patients Who Could and Could Not be Evaluated in the Vertebral Fracture Analysis

|  | Evaluable Patients | | Nonevaluable Patients | |
| --- | --- | --- | --- | --- |
| Variable | Calcium Only (n=80) | MFP plus Calcium (n=84) | Calcium Only (n=20) | MFP plus Calcium (n=16) |
| Mean age ±SE, y | 63±1 | 64±1 | 63±2 | 63±2 |
| Mean age at menopause ±SE, y | 48±1 | 49±1 | 47±1 | 47±1 |
| Mean height ±SE, cm | 158±1 | 157±1 | 158±2 | 157±2 |
| Mean weight ± SE, kg | 62±1 | 62±1 | 61±3 | 61±1 |
| Smoker, n(%) | 14 (17.5) | 17 (20.2) | 7 (35.0) | 4 (25.0) |
| Physically active, n(%) | | | | |
|    Little Activity, n(%) | 10 (12.5) | 6 (7.2) | (1 (5.0) | 0 (0.0) |
|    Moderate Activity, n(%) | 52 (65.0) | 61 (72.6) | 13 (65.0) | 14 (87.5) |
|    Intense Activity, n(%) | 18 (22.5) | 17 (20.2) | 6 (30.0) | 2 (12.5) |
| Ovariectomized, n(%) | 20 (25.0) | 15 (17.9) | 5 (25.0) | 6 (37.5) |
| Vertebral fractures at enrollment, n(%) | 1 (1.3) | 3 (3.6) | 2 (10.0)1 (6.3) | |
| Receiving HRT, n(%) | 11 (13.8) | 12(14.3) | 0 (0.0) | 1 (6.3) |
| Mean BMD ± SE, g/cm$^2$ | | | | |
|    Lumbar spine | 0.795±0.010 | 0.796±0.008 | 0.796±0.017 | 0.793±0.022 |
|    Total hip | 0.756±0.011 | 0.755±0.010 | 0.733±0.026 | 0.734±0.028 |
| Mean bone alkaline phosphatase ± SD, ng/ml | 11.5±3.3 | 10.8±3.6 | 11.7±3.9 | 10.6±3.2 |
| Mean ratio of hydroxyproline to creatinine, mg:g | 15.4:7.2 | 15.1:6.4 | 14.6:4.6 | 14.7:6.1 |

and no differences were seen between the evaluable and the nonevaluable subpopulations. About 10% of patients in each group received hormone replacement therapy during the study; the overall proportion of patients who had had ovariectomy was 20% to 25% at enrollment. The following estrogen products and daily doses were used: 0.625 mg of oral conjugated estrogens, 50 mg of transdermal estradiol, 1.5 g of percutaneous estradiol, or 1 to 2 mg of oral estradiol valerate. In women with an intact uterus, a progestin was also used; no differences between groups or patients were seen in type and dosage of drug. The duration of hormone use in individual patients in the two groups is shown in Table 45.2.

**Table 45.2.** Duration of the Use of Hormone Replacement Therapy

| Duration of Use | Patients Receiving Calcium Only | Patients Receiving MFP plus Calcium |
|---|---|---|
| 6 months | 1 | 4 |
| 12 months | 2 | 0 |
| 18 months | 0 | 1 |
| 24 months | 3 | 1 |
| 30 months | 0 | 1 |
| 36 months | 1 | 1 |
| 42 months | 1 | 1 |
| 48 months | 3 | 4 |

The average duration of hormone replacement therapy did not differ between the two groups. The study sample consisted mainly of patients without vertebral fractures because only 4 patients in the MFP-plus-calcium group and 3 patients in the calcium-only group had a single vertebral fracture at enrollment. Compliance with study medication was good and was identical in the two groups throughout the study; on average, evaluable patients in both groups took 87% of their tablets. It was not necessary to open the sealed envelopes that contained the randomization codes, and no envelopes were opened accidentally; this was verified at the end of the study and several times during the monitoring procedures. Therefore, the persons who actually conducted the intervention never had access to the randomization codes during the study. This was also true for those who read the dual-energy x-ray absorptiometry results and those who did the biochemical analyses.

Vertebral fracture rates were evaluated on the basis of analysis of the radiographs from 164 of the 200 patients (82%): 80 in the calcium-only group and 84 in the MFP-plus-calcium group. Overall, 36 patients were not included in the fracture rate analysis because of early drop out and no possibility of radiologic follow-up (30 patients) or because their radiographs could not be evaluated (6 patients). Fewer patients in the MFP-plus-calcium group (2 of 84; 2.4% [95% CI, 0.3% to 8.3%]) than in the calcium-only group (8 of 80; 10% [CI, 4.4% to 18.8%]) had new vertebral fractures (P = 0.05). The difference between the rates was 7.6 percentage points (CI, 0.3 to 15.0 percentage points), and the number needed to treat for 4 years to prevent one fracture was 13 (CI, 7 to 356).

Two patients receiving hormone replacement therapy (1 in the calcium-only group had been receiving it for <12 months and 1 in the MFP-plus-calcium group had been receiving it for <6 months) were among those who had a new vertebral fracture during the study. When patients receiving hormone replacement therapy were excluded from analysis, fewer patients in the MFP-plus-calcium group (2 of 71; 2.8% [CI, 0.4% to 9.8%]) than in the calcium-only group (8 of 69; 11.6% [CI, 5.2% to 21.6%]) had a new vertebral fracture. The difference between the rates was 8.78 percentage points (CI, 0.3 to 17.3 percentage points), and the number needed to treat for 4 years to prevent one fracture was 11 (CI, 6 to 334).

Patients had only single vertebral fractures, with the exception of one patient in the calcium-only group who had fractures of two different vertebrae at the same time point and one patient in the MFP-plus-calcium group who had two sequential reports of new fractures.

New vertebral fractures were identified in the calcium-only group after 12 months (5 fractures), 24 months (1 fracture), 36 months (1 fracture), and 48 months (1 fracture). In the MFP-plus-calcium group, these patients were identified after 24 months (1 fracture) and 48 months (1 fracture). However, the patient in the MFP-plus-calcium group who had the fracture after 48 months had discontinued treatment with MFP plus calcium after 24 months. All patients with new fractures had no fractures at baseline; no further fractures occurred in the few patients who had had one vertebral fracture at enrollment. The Vertebral Deformity Index/Spine Deformity Index analysis outlined no progression of prevalent fractures in these patients. Overall, the evaluable mean change in the Spine Deformity Index in patients with incident or progressing vertebral deformities throughout the study showed a nonsignificant (P = 0.14) difference between the two groups (0.1 ± 0.03 with MFP plus calcium compared with 0.2 ± 0.04 with calcium only in 28.6% and 33.3% of patients, respectively).

Patients receiving MFP plus calcium had a progressive increase in BMD of the spine to 10.0% ± 1.5% above baseline at the end of the study; the calcium-only group had a change of -0.4% ± 0.7% below baseline (P < 0.001). For BMD of the total hip, the final increase with MFP plus calcium was 1.8% ± 0.06%; this was not statistically significantly different from the increase seen with calcium only (0.7% ± 0.7%) (P = 0.07).

**Table 45.3.** Nonvertebral Fractures during the 4-Year Trial

| Variable | Patients Receiving Calcium Only (n=100) | Patients Receiving MFP plus Calcium (n=100) |
|---|---|---|
| Patients with peripheral fractures, n | 11 | 12 |
| Rate per person-years (95% CI), %* | 3.4 (1.7-6.0) | 3.6 (1.9-6.2) |
| Fractures, n | 13 | 15 |
| Rate per person-years (95% CI), %* | 4.0 (2.2-6.8) | 4.5 (2.5-7.3) |
| Patients per site of fractures, n | | |
| Hip | 1 | 1 |
| Leg or patella | 1 | 2 |
| Ankle, foot, or toe | 5 | 4 |
| Upper arm | 1 | 0 |
| Wrist | 3 | 5 |
| Rib | 1 | 2 |
| Sternum | 0 | 1 |
| Face | 1 | 0 |

*Based on 335 patient-years of follow-up in the calcium-only group and 324 patient-years of follow-up in the sodium-monofluorophosphate-plus-calcium group*

Serum bone-specific alkaline phosphatase significantly increased throughout the study in the MFP-plus-calcium group (to 11.5% ± 4.2% over baseline) and nonsignificantly decreased in the calcium-only group (change, -16.1% ± 2.7%) at 1 year, decreasing to -2.3% ± 4.0% at the end of the study (P = 0.002). Changes in the ratio of urinary hydroxyproline to creatinine varied and were not statistically significant in either group.

Peripheral fractures (Table 45.3) occurred with a similar incidence in the two groups. Of the 100 patients randomly assigned to receive calcium only, 11 had a total of 13 fractures during 324 patient-years of follow-up. Twelve patients receiving MFP plus calcium had a total of 15 fractures during 335 patient-years of follow-up. The difference between the groups was not significant. Hip fracture occurred in only one patient in each group.

Table 45.4 shows the number of and the reasons for drop out in the entire patient sample, including the early drop outs that accounted for most of the nonevaluable patients. The proportion of patients who discontinued treatment with the study drug was nearly identical in the two groups, and reasons for drop out were similar. The pattern of reasons for drop out did not differ in the patients who could not be

**Table 45.4.** Premature Discontinuations during the 4-year Trial

| Variable | Patients Receiving Calcium Only (n=100) | Patients Receiving MFP plus Calcium (n=100) |
|---|---|---|
| Adverse events | 15 | 12 |
| Medical reasons unrelated to study | 6 | 6 |
| Free Choice | 9 | 8 |
| Lost to follow-up | 6 | 6 |
| No compliance or no acceptance | 1 | 5 |
| Never started treatment | 0 | 1 |
| **Total** | **40** | **38** |

included in the fracture rate analysis compared with the evaluable patient sample (data not shown).

Gastrointestinal problems were the most frequently reported adverse reaction in both groups. No differences were seen between the MFP-plus-calcium group and the calcium-only group with regard to the incidence, type, or severity of any adverse event. Lower limb pain was reported by 4.7% of patients receiving calcium only and 3% of patients receiving MFP plus calcium.

## Discussion

Our study shows a statistically significant reduction in the number of women with moderately low BMD of the spine who acquire new vertebral fractures when they receive continuous low-dosage (20 mg/d) fluoride, given as MFP, plus a calcium supplement. Similar results were previously reported (7) when 22.6 mg of fluoride per day, given as 50 mg of enteric-coated sodium fluoride, was compared with the therapies usually prescribed in France in women with at least one vertebral crush fracture.

More recently, 50 mg of slow-release sodium fluoride per day, given for 14-month cycles (12 months of sodium fluoride therapy followed by 2 months of no therapy), significantly reduced individual fracture rates, increased the fracture-free interval, and increased the time to new fracture in women with prevalent nontraumatic fractures (6).

In contrast, Riggs and colleagues (5) reported that 75 mg of plain sodium fluoride per day increased cancellous BMD but decreased cortical BMD at some skeletal sites without significant effects on fracture rates. Later, these results were reevaluated on the basis of the dose of sodium fluoride actually taken (and, therefore, the amount of fluoride absorbed). A bimodal effect of sodium fluoride was suggested, with low doses reducing fracture rates and higher doses (>60 mg/d) having a deleterious effect on bone structural resistance (18). It should also be emphasized that the bioavailability of the plain sodium fluoride used by Riggs and colleagues (5) was 60% higher than that of the enteric-coated sodium fluoride used in the French study (7), with high plasma peaks of fluoride ion (3). In another trial that was done in parallel using a similar study design, Kleerekoper and coworkers (9) concluded that sodium fluoride (75 mg/d) was no more effective than calcium only in retarding the progression of spinal osteoporosis.

In a recent study by the Fluoride and Vertebral Osteoporosis (FAVOS) study group (8), osteoporotic women treated with a regimen of fluoride, calcium, and vitamin D (800 U/d) had no reduction in vertebral fracture rates compared with women who received only calcium and vitamin D, a significant increase in BMD of the spine notwithstanding. However, the duration of treatment was shorter in this study (2 years) than in our trial. Stimulation of bone formation and secondary mineralization of recently synthesized matrix may require a prolonged period to ensure optimal biomechanical resistance, despite a rapid increase in BMD. Therefore, a significant reduction in fracture rate might be expected only after 3 to 4 years of treatment. The FAVOS study also targeted women whose osteoporosis was more severe (women with prevalent fractures) than that of the women in our study. Severe osteoporosis is related not only to a decrease in bone mineral content (which might be partly reversed by bone-forming agents) but also to a deterioration of bone microarchitecture (loss of structural integrity), which would not be expected to respond to such substances as fluoride (19). Bone-forming agents might be particularly efficient in the presence of relatively mild to moderate osteoporosis, when the major damage to be corrected is related to a decrease in bone mineral. The FAVOS study also compared three different fluoride regimens—50 mg of enteric-coated sodium fluoride per day, 150 mg of MFP per day, and 200 mg of MFP per day—but was underpowered to separately evaluate the antifracture effects of each regimen.

The MFP formulation used in our trial was previously shown to be a highly soluble fluoride salt readily absorbed in the duodenum and the small intestine (20). Skeletal uptake of fluoride after ingestion of MFP seems to be similar to or greater than that after ingestion of sodium fluoride (20, 21), and MFP has also been shown to be better tolerated by the gastric mucosa than sodium fluoride (22). Furthermore, and in contrast to sodium fluoride, MFP is compatible not only with calcium salts but also with meals (23). Thus, when it is given with meals, as it was in our study, bioavailability is not impaired but plasma concentrations are low and persistent (23). This avoids the high peaks seen with plain sodium fluoride (3).

The low dosage of fluoride (20 mg/d) used in our protocol resulted in a moderate but steady increase in BMD of the spine (10% after 4 years), which paralleled the pattern of increase in serum bone-specific alkaline phosphatase (11.5% after 4 years) and is consistent with the known action of fluoride on bone formation. We suggest that such a slow but progressive increase in bone synthesis and bone density maximizes the chance that newly synthesized bone has the biochemical and structural properties needed to prevent further fractures.

This pattern of response may also prevent the secondary hyperparathyroidism, related to calcium deficiency, that has been reported to occur despite calcium supplementation in patients who had a rapid, fluoride-dependent increase in BMD of the spine (24). We did not record any deleterious effect of MFP plus calcium on BMD of the hip; this is consistent with the results of other studies that used low-dose fluoride formulations (6-8) but not with the results of a trial of high-dose fluoride (5). Finally, general tolerance to the drug and pain in the lower limbs were similar in the two treated groups.

Certain limitations of our trial should be acknowledged, including a possible confounding effect of hormone replacement therapy and the implications of the drop-out rate. However, the number of drop outs and the reasons for these drop outs were similar in the two groups, minimizing the likelihood of bias. Most drop outs occurred early (within the first months of the study), and they were primarily responsible for the 36 patients who could not be evaluated in the fracture rate analysis. Moreover, the remaining drop outs (those that occurred in the remaining 3 years of the 4-year trial) were reasonable (<30%) for such a long-term study, and these patients were included in the intention-to-treat analysis. Therefore, the drop-out rate is unlikely to have influenced the implementation of this regimen in practice because the difficulties encountered during the trial are similar to those likely to be found with any long-term treatment in current clinical practice. Finally, the small number of outcome events limits the strength of the inference about vertebral fractures, which makes it difficult to assess the effect of potential confounders and to draw meaningful conclusions about hip fracture rates.

When these limitations are taken into account, our data suggest that fluoride, given as MFP, plus a calcium supplement decreases the incidence of vertebral fractures compared with calcium alone in postmenopausal women with mild to moderate osteoporosis when it is given continuously in low dosages for a prolonged period.

**Acknowledgments:** The authors thank T. Bruckner and G. Leidig-Bruckner, Heidelberg, Germany, for their contribution to the analysis of the study radiographs.

**Grant Support:** In part by the Rotta Research Group, Monza, Italy.

**Requests for Reprints:** Professor J.Y. Reginster, CHU Centre Ville, Quai Godefroid Kurth 45, Bâtiment K1, B4020 Liege, Belgium.

**Current Author Addresses:** Drs. Reginster, Meurmans, Zegels, Taquet, Collette, and Gosset: Bone and Cartilage Metabolism Unit,

CHU Centre Ville, Quai Godefroid Kurth 45, B4020 Liege, Belgium. Dr. Minne: Klinik der Fürstenhof, Center of Endocrinology, Gust. Pommer e.v. Am Hylligen Born 7, D31812 Bad Pyrmont, Germany. Drs. Rovati, Giacovelli, and Setnikar: Rotta Research Laboratorium, via Valosa di Sopra 7/9, 20052 Monza, Italy.

### References

1. Farley JR, Wergedal JE, Baylink DJ. Fluoride directly stimulates proliferation and alkaline phosphatase activity of bone-forming cells. *Science*. 1983;222:330-2.

2. Reed BY, Zerwekh JE, Antich PP, Pak CY. Fluoride-stimulated 913H 93thymidine uptake in a human osteoblastic osteosarcoma cell line is dependent on transforming growth factor b. *J Bone Miner Res*. 1993;8:19-25.

3. Kanis JA. Treatment of symptomatic osteoporosis with fluoride. *Am J Med*. 1993;95:S53-S61.

4. Heaney RP, Baylink DJ, Johnston CC Jr, Melton LJ 3d, Meunier PJ, Murray TM, et al. Fluoride therapy for the vertebral crush fracture syndrome. A status report. *Ann Intern Med*. 1989;111:678-80.

5. Riggs BL, Hodgson SF, O'Fallon WM, Chao EY, Wahner HW, Muhs JM, et al. Effect of fluoride treatment on the fracture rate in postmenopausal women with osteoporosis. *N Engl J Med*. 1990;322:802-9.

6. Pak CY, Sakhaee K, Adams-Huet B, Piziak V, Peterson RD, Poindexter JR. Treatment of postmenopausal osteoporosis with slow-release sodium fluoride. Final report of a randomized controlled trial. *Ann Intern Med*. 1995;123:401-8.

7. Mamelle N, Meunier PJ, Dusan R, Guillaume M, Martin JL, Gaucher A, et al. Risk-benefit ratio of sodium fluoride treatment in primary vertebral osteoporosis. *Lancet*. 1988;2:361-5.

8. Meunier PJ, Sebert JL, Reginster JY, Briancon D, Appelboom P, Netter G, et al. Fluoride salts are no better prevention at preventing new vertebral fractures than calcium-vitamin D in postmenopausal osteoporosis: the FAVOS study. *Osteoporosis Int*. 1998;8:4-12.

9. Kleerekoper M, Peterson EL, Nelson DA, Phillips E, Schork MA, Tilley BC, et al. A randomized trial of sodium fluoride as a treatment for postmenopausal osteoporosis. *Osteoporosis Int.* 1991;1:155-61.

10. Riggs BL, Wahner HW, Dunn WL, Mazess RB, Oxford KP, Melton LJ 3d. Differential changes in bone mineral density of the appendicular and axial skeleton with aging: relationship to spinal osteoporosis. *J Clin Invest.* 1981;67:328-35.

11. Reginster JY, Janssen C, Deroisy R, Zegels B, Albert A, Franchimont P. Bone mineral density of the spine and the hip measured with dual energy x-ray absorptiometry: normal range and fracture threshold for western European (Belgian) postmenopausal females. *Clin Rheum.* 1995;14:68-75.

12. Assessment of Fracture Risk and Its Application to Screening for Postmenopausal Osteoporosis. Report of a World Health Organization Study Group. Geneva: World Health Organization; 1994.

13. Reginster JY, Compston JE, Jones EA, Kaufman JM, Audran M, Bouvenot G, et al. Recommendations for the registration of new chemical entities used in the prevention and treatment of osteoporosis [Editorial]. *Calcif Tissue Int.* 1995;57:247-50.

14. Melton LJ 3d, Kan SH, Frye KM, Wahner HW, O'Fallon WM, Riggs BL. Epidemiology of vertebral fractures in women. *Am J Epidemiol.* 1989;129:1000-11.

15. Minne HW, Leidig G, Wuster C, Siromachkostov L, Baldauf G, Bickel R, et al. A newly developed spine deformity index (SDI) to quantitate vertebral crush fractures in patients with osteoporosis. *Bone Miner.* 1988;3:335-49.

16. Stein JA, Lazewatski JL, Hochberg AM. Dual-energy x-ray bone densitometer incorporating an internal reference system [Abstract]. *Radiology.* 1987;165P:313.

17. Reginster JY. *Osteoporose Postménopausique: Traitement Prophylactique.* Paris: Masson; 1993.

18. Riggs BL, O'Fallon W, Hodgson S, Chao E, Wahner H, Muhs J, et al. Clinical trial of fluoride in osteoporotic women: extended observation and additional analyses [Abstract]. *Bone Miner.* 1992;17:S74.

19. Parfitt AM. Bone remodelling: relationship to the amount and structure of bone and the pathogenesis and prevention of fractures. In: Riggs BL, Melton LJ 3d, eds. *Osteoporosis: Etiology, Diagnosis, and Management*. New York: Raven; 1988:45-93.

20. Delmas PD, Dupuis J, Duboeuf F, Chapuy MC, Meunier PJ. Treatment of vertebral osteoporosis with disodium monofluorophosphate: comparison with sodium fluoride. *J Bone Miner Res*. 1990;5(Suppl):S143-7.

21. Ericsson Y. Monofluorophosphate physiology: general considerations. *Caries Res*. 1983;17:S46-S55.

22. Muller P, Schmid K, Warnecke G, Setnikar I, Simon B. Sodium fluoride-induced gastric mucosal lesions: comparison with sodium monofluorophosphate. *Z Gastroenterol*. 1992;30:252-4.

23. Warneke G, Setnikar I. Effects of meal on the pharmacokinetics of fluoride from oral monofluorophosphate. *Arzneimittelforschung*. 1993;43:592-5.

24. Dure-Smith BA, Farley SM, Linkhart SG, Farley JR, Baylink DJ. Calcium deficiency in fluoride-treated osteoporotic patients despite calcium supplementation. *J Clin docrinol Metab*. 1996;81:269-75.

# Chapter 46

# *Taking Supplements for Osteoporosis*

## *Yes, but Which Calcium Supplement?*

**Abstract:** Calcium supplements are a good way for people to ensure they ingest enough calcium to reduce their risk of developing osteoporosis later in life. However, the nutritional benefits and costs of the supplements vary greatly. Calcium citrate supplements are absorbed better but are not packaged well.

Guidelines issued by the National Institutes of Health indicate that adults need from 1,000 to 1,500 milligrams of calcium a day, but surveys show that they consume, on average, only 500 to 600 milligrams. Over time, this calcium deficit is a significant risk factor for thinning bones that are prone to fracture.

Experts agree that increasing the intake of calcium-rich foods is the best way to tackle the calcium shortfall. Calcium in food comes packaged with a host of other nutrients essential for a healthful diet. But some people may find it difficult to meet their needs from foods alone. A 70-year-old, for example, would need to drink 5 cups of milk—or the equivalent—to achieve the recommended daily intake of 1,500 milligrams for men and women 65 and older.

"Yes, But Which Calcium Supplement?" from *Tufts University Health and Nutrition Letter*, February 1997, Vol. 14, No. 12, p. 4(2), © 1997. Reprinted with permission, Tufts University Health and Nutrition Letter, telephone: 1-800-274-7581.

Fortunately, the vast majority of people absorb and utilize supplemental calcium as well as the calcium found in food. When it comes to choosing a supplement, however, consumers may be met by a dizzying array. When we visited Boston-area drugstores to survey calcium supplements, one store alone boasted 36 different choices.

Ask the following questions while sorting through the options to find a supplement that is right for you.

1. What is the form of calcium in the supplement? Supplemental calcium always comes chemically partnered with another substance. Available forms include calcium carbonate, calcium citrate, calcium phosphate, calcium lactate, and calcium gluconate.

   • **Calcium carbonate** is by far the most common form on the market, found in at least 90 percent of calcium pills as well as in antacids such as Rolaids and Tums. It is also a highly concentrated form. Single tablets can contain 600 milligrams of the mineral, providing a distinct advantage to consumers who want to take as few pills as possible to fill their calcium gap.

   Common sources of calcium carbonate include ground limestone (specified on labels simply as "calcium carbonate") or ground oyster shell. Unless it is purified, calcium carbonate from oyster shell may contain heavy metal contaminants, such as lead. Thus, we recommend avoiding it.

   Note that for 1 out of 5 people over 60 and 2 out of 5 over 80, calcium carbonate taken on an empty stomach will not break down properly for absorption. That's because those people have a condition known as atrophic gastritis, which is a deficiency of stomach acid. Only when they have just eaten and the stomach has secreted acidic juices will enough acid be present to break down a calcium carbonate tablet.

   The solution is simple: just take a calcium carbonate pill right after eating. Bess Dawson-Hughes, MD, chief of the Calcium and Bone Metabolism Laboratory at Tufts's USDA Human Nutrition Research Center on Aging, recommends that all people, whether or not they have atrophic gastritis, take their calcium supplements with meals. The presence of food slows the emptying of the stomach, allowing more time for the calcium tablet to be broken down and for the mineral to be absorbed by the body.

- **Calcium citrate** is the best absorbed form of supplemental calcium. And unlike calcium carbonate, it will be property utilized by anybody who takes it, whether between or with meals.

  That might make it sound as though calcium citrate is a better choice than calcium carbonate. But calcium citrate is hard to pack into a pill. As the chart shows, to get at least 500 milligrams of calcium, a consumer would have to swallow 2 or 3 calcium citrate tablets. Even the slight advantage in absorption that calcium citrate has over other forms doesn't justify all that pill popping.

- **Calcium phosphate**, like calcium carbonate, is a highly concentrated form of supplemental calcium. But it is especially difficult for the body to break down and therefore should be avoided, according to Ralph Shangraw, PhD, a Professor Emeritus of the University of Maryland's School of Pharmacy who has studied calcium supplements extensively.

- **Calcium lactate and calcium gluconate** are best skipped, too. As with calcium citrate, too many pills—6 in the case of Osco's calcium lactate—are needed just to reach 500 milligrams. We could not even find a single calcium gluconate preparation at the 3 drug stores, health food store, or K-Mart we visited or at several supermarket chains.

2. How much does the supplement cost? For as little as 5 cents, you can get 500 milligrams of calcium carbonate. Compare that, for instance, to AARP's Formula 687 calcium citrate, at 18 cents for the same amount. Over a year's time, that comes to a difference of $47.

Note that there's no need to pay more for supplements with any of the following claims: "no starch"; "no sugar"; "no preservatives"; "recommended by pharmacists"; "high potency"; "premium quality"; "free of milk"; "free of yeast"; "physician recommended"; "natural"; and "proven release." Most of these claims actually can be made for any calcium supplement.

3. How many milligrams of calcium are in each tablet? Consumers looking to supplement their dietary calcium with only a small amount of the mineral can turn to lower-dose preparations, such as Rolaids or Walgreens Chewables. However, those who want to add 500 to 1,000 milligrams should choose a higher-dose pill, like AARP Formula 314 or Sundown Calcium 600, so they can take fewer tablets each day.

   Dr. Dawson-Hughes recommends taking no more than 500 to 600 milligrams of calcium at a time. The body may not be able to absorb larger doses all at once. If your supplement is calcium carbonate, splitting the daily dosage over 2 or 3 meals also cuts down on the possibility of constipation, a problem for some calcium carbonate takers.

   **Note:** While some manufacturers clearly list the milligrams of calcium in each tablet, others list the contents of the whole pill—calcium plus carbonate, for example—requiring you to do a bit of math to figure out the actual amount of calcium. For the products in the chart, we have done the arithmetic for you.

4. Does the supplement contain "extras," such as vitamin D, magnesium, or zinc? For the most part, extra vitamins and minerals in calcium supplements are not necessary The exception in some cases is vitamin D, which is essential for the body's proper utilization of calcium. Research indicates that older women need from 400 to 800 International Units of vitamin D a day, but people not getting a fair amount of sun or drinking several cups of milk a day (each cup has 100 units) might not be getting that much. In such cases, a calcium/vitamin D preparation like Caltrate 600 + D can be useful.

5. How well does the supplement dissolve? If a label has the letters "USP," the supplement meets the U.S. Pharmacopeia's strict standard for dissolution. Most calcium pills without the USP designation also dissolve well. But when we tested the products in the chart without the USP mark, we did find 2 clinkers: Schiff Super Calcium '1200' and Twinlab Calcium Citrate Caps.

**Table 46.1.** A Bare-Bones Look at Calcium Supplements, continued on next page.

The 27 calcium supplements listed came from Boston-area pharmacies, a health food store, K-Mart, and Safeway and Kroger supermarkets. Others came by mail order from the American Association for Retired Persons (AARP).

| Product | Calcium per Tablet in mg | Cost per Tablet | Cost per 500 mg* | Cost per 30 Days† | Form of Calcium | % DV Vit. D** | Comments |
|---|---|---|---|---|---|---|---|
| **AARP Formula 314 Calcium** | 600 | 5¢ | 5¢ | $1.50 | Carbonate | — | "No starch" claim superfluous |
| **AARP Formula 564 Calcium with Vitamin D** | 600 | 5¢ | 5¢ | $1.50 | Carbonate | 50 | "No sugar" claim superfluous; even chewable pills have very little sugar |
| **AARP Formula 687 Calcium Citrate** | 200 | 6¢ | 18¢ | $5.40 | Citrate | — | Label claim of 950 mg refers to calcium and citrate combined |
| **Caltrate Plus** | 600 | 12¢ | 12¢ | $3.60 | Carbonate | 50 | — |
| **Caltrate Plus Chewables** | 600 | 12¢ | 12¢ | $3.60 | Carbonate | 50 | Chew well to help dissolution |
| **Caltrate 600 + D** | 600 | 12¢ | 12¢ | $3.60 | Carbonate | 50 | "More calcium for your bones than any leading brand" claim not true |

375

**Table 46.1.** A Bare-Bones Look at Calcium Supplements, from previous page, continued on next page.

| Product | Calcium per Tablet in mg | Cost per Tablet | Cost per 500 mg* | Cost per 30 Days† | Form of Calcium | % DV Vit. D** | Comments |
|---|---|---|---|---|---|---|---|
| Citracal Calcium Citrate Liquitab | 500 | 6¢ | 6¢ | $1.80 | Citrate | — | Dissolves in water like Alka-Seltzer |
| Citracal Calcium Citrate Ultradense Caplets + D | 315 | 13¢ | 26¢ | $7.80 | Citrate | 50 | — |
| GNC Calcium Citrate | 250 | 7¢ | 14¢ | $4.20 | Citrate | — | "No preservatives" claim superfluous |
| K-Mart/American Fare Vita-Smart Natural Oyster Shell Calcium | 500 | 6¢ | 6¢ | $1.80 | Carbonate | — | Best to avoid oyster shell |
| Nature Made Calcium | 500 | 8¢ | 8¢ | $2.40 | Carbonate | — | "Recommended by pharmacists" claim superfluous |
| Nature Made Calcium and Magnesium with Zinc | 333 | 5¢ | 10¢ | $3.00 | Carbonate | — | Magnesium and zinc not proven necessary in calcium pills |
| One A Day Calcium Plus | 500 | 10¢ | 10¢ | $3.00 | Carbonate | 25 | "High potency" claim superfluous |
| Os-Cal 500 + D | 500 | 11 ¢ | 11¢ | $3.30 | Carbonate | 31 | Best to avoid oyster shell |

**Table 46.1.** A Bare-Bones Look at Calcium Supplements, from previous page, continued on next page.

| Product | Calcium per Tablet in mg | Cost per Tablet | Cost per 500 mg* | Cost per 30 Days† | Form of Calcium | % DV Vit. D** | Comments |
|---|---|---|---|---|---|---|---|
| Osco Calcium Lactate | 83 | 3¢ | 18¢ | $5.40 | Lactate | — | 6 tablets necessary for 500 mg of calcium |
| Posture-D | 600 | 17¢ | 17¢ | $5.10 | Phosphate | 63 | Calcium from phosphate not well absorbed |
| Rolaids | 220 | 4¢ | 12¢ | $3.60 | Carbonate | — | Sold as antacid |
| Safeway Select Calcium | 600 | 9¢ | 9¢ | $2.70 | Carbonate | — | "Premium quality" claim superfluous |
| Schiff Calcium Lactate | 100 | 3¢ | 15¢ | $4.50 | Lactate | — | "Free of milk" claim superfluous |
| Schiff Super Calcium '1200' | 600 | 12¢ | 12¢ | $3.60 | Carbonate | 100 | Did not dissolve when tested |
| Solgar Calci-Chews | 500 | 10¢ | 10¢ | $3.00 | Carbonate | — | "Free of yeast" claim superfluous |
| Sundown Calcium 600 | 600 | 6¢ | 6¢ | $1.80 | Carbonate | — | — |
| Tums 500 | 500 | 9¢ | 9¢ | $2.70 | Carbonate | — | "Physician recommended" claim superfluous |

**Table 46.1.** A Bare-Bones Look at Calcium Supplements, from previous page.

| Product | Calcium per Tablet in mg | Cost per Tablet | Cost per 500 mg* | Cost per 30 Days† | Form of Calcium | % DV Vit. D** | Comments |
|---|---|---|---|---|---|---|---|
| **Twinlab Calcium Citrate Caps** | 300 | 8¢ | 16¢ | $4.80 | Citrate | — | Did not dissolve when tested |
| **Walgreens Calcium Lactate** | 84 | 3¢ | 18¢ | $5.40 | Lactate | — | 6 tablets needed for 500 mg of calcium |
| **Walgreens Finest Natural Chewable Calcium Plus Vitamin D** | 300 | 5¢ | 10¢ | $3.00 | Carbonate | 25 | "Natural" claim superfluous |
| **Your Life Calcium + D** | 600 | 12¢ | 12¢ | $3.60 | Carbonate | 31 | "Proven release" claim superfluous |

*Rounded to the nearest whole pill.
†Cost of 500 milligrams (mg) a day over 30 days.
**The DV (Daily Value) for vitamin D is 400 International Units.

# Chapter 47

# *Magnesium:*
# *Good for Your Bones*

To head off osteoporosis, a potentially crippling loss and embrittling of bone, doctors have been advocating that adults down plenty of bone-building calcium as a lifelong habit. Magnesium, however, may also prove pivotal in preserving bone, a new study hints.

Bone stores about 60 percent of the body's magnesium. Though certain bone cells use the mineral, uncertainties abound as to how it affects bone growth and breakdown. In the past decade, however, supplements have been found to build up bone in people with a deficiency, notes K.H. William Lau of the J.L. Pettis Memorial Veterans Administration Medical Center in Loma Linda, Calif.

For instance, in postmenopausal women, magnesium supplements are more important than calcium in reversing bone loss, according to a May 1990 report in the *Journal of Reproductive Medicine*. Indeed, its authors argued, late-onset osteoporosis in women may largely represent "a skeletal manifestation of chronic magnesium deficiency."

In the new study, Lam says, "we wanted to see whether magnesium supplementation in nondeficient individuals—especially young and healthy people—also benefits bone." So, together with researchers at the University of Graz Medical School in Austria, he launched a pilot study of 24 healthy young men who had already been eating the recommended daily allowance (RDA) of magnesium, about 350 milligrams. For 30 days, half of the men doubled their magnesium consumption by taking a supplement.

Because the body excretes any magnesium it doesn't need, the researchers could compare amounts of the metal in blood and urine throughout the trial to evaluate whether and how the body used the supplements. The team also monitored blood concentrations of several biomarkers of bone turnover—its continual breakdown and reformation. Young people usually rebuild at least as much bone as they break down, but in people with osteoporosis, each cycle of bone breakdown can lead to a net loss of bone.

In the August *Journal of Clinical Endocrinology and Metabolism*, Lau's team reports that while bone turnover continued unchanged throughout the trial in the unsupplemented men, it appeared to slow dramatically in all who received the extra magnesium.

One possibility is that the supplements may be suppressing all phases of bone turnover, Lau says. "But we believe that most action is on the osteoclast," cells important to bone breakdown. Therefore, he says, the supplements are preserving bone—and possibly fostering a net buildup.

These data are "suggestive" that magnesium cuts bone loss, agrees Connie M. Weaver of Purdue University in West Lafayette, Ind. "What is needed now to prove this hypothesis is a large clinical trial measuring the effect of supplementation on bone density or [osteoporotic] fracture."

Burton M. Altura of the State University of New York Health Science Center at Brooklyn remains perplexed, however, by the Graz study's blood data on magnesium ions, the biologically active form. His data have invariably shown that supplementation raises blood levels of these ions—the opposite of what Lau's team found.

Lau also was initially surprised by this finding, but he says a follow-up study has confirmed it. For him, however, the main issue is whether magnesium supplementation increases bone. If future studies show it does, he says, "that would mean the current RDA is too low."

Altura doesn't challenge that. Work by his group and others over the years has shown numerous benefits of magnesium in reducing risks of heart disease, stroke, and even migraine headaches. The mineral is especially prevalent in nuts, legumes, unmilled grains, bananas, and green vegetables. If everyone made an effort to consume 500 to 600 milligrams of magnesium daily, Altura maintains, "maybe we could prevent much cardiac disease, hypertension, and stroke, saving the nation a lot of money and visits to the doctor."

He says the data from a host of studies are already bearing out that suspicion.

*—by Janet Raloff*

# Chapter 48

# *Exercise and Osteoporosis*

## Staying Active—Safely

Osteoporosis can steal the strength from your bones, leaving you stoop-shouldered and prone to fractures. But there's something you can do with your muscles to help lower your risk for a break—exercise.

Research indicates that exercise may not only help prevent osteoporosis, but treat it as well. The key is knowing which exercises you should (and shouldn't) do and how to do them properly.

## Porous Bones

Osteoporosis means "porous bones." With the disease, bone strength decreases because your bones slowly lose mineral content and their internal supporting structure. Eventually, bones can become so weak they easily fracture.

The bones in your spine can actually compress (compression fractures), much like a stack of cardboard boxes in a damp basement. The result can be a severely stooped posture and perhaps an even greater risk for fractures.

Hip fractures are another common type of osteoporotic fracture. They often result from falls.

You can help prevent osteoporosis by keeping your bones strong. That means, among other things, exercising, consuming adequate calcium and vitamin D, not smoking and, for women during and after menopause, considering supplemental estrogen through hormone replacement therapy.

If you've already been diagnosed with osteoporosis, you're probably taking a medication to treat it. Exercise may also help.

## A Strong Combination

Exercise can slow mineral loss, help maintain posture and improve overall fitness to reduce risk of falls. Often, a combination of activities is recommended to help prevent or treat osteoporosis. All are designed to provide benefits while minimizing the risk of osteoporotic fractures during exercise. Exercises typically include:

- **Weight-bearing activities.** These include activities you do on your feet with your bones supporting your weight. Walking, jogging and stair climbing are examples. They work directly on bones in your legs, hips and lower spine to slow mineral loss. If you have osteoporosis, walking—preferably at least a mile a day—is generally the best weight-bearing exercise because it minimizes jarring to your bones.

- **Weightlifting.** Weightlifting, also called strength training and resistance training, can strengthen muscles and bones in your arms and upper spine. It can also work directly on bone to slow mineral loss. If you have osteoporosis, you'll need the assistance of your doctor or physical therapist in designing a strength-training program that includes proper lifting techniques and is appropriate for your degree of bone loss.

- **Back-strengthening exercises.** These exercises primarily work on muscles rather than bone. Research indicates that strengthening your back muscles may help treat osteoporosis by maintaining or improving posture. That's because the stooped posture caused by osteoporotic compression fractures may cause increased pressure along the spine, leading to even more compression fractures. Exercises that gently arch your back (see illustrations) can strengthen back muscles while minimizing stress on bones.

382

## *Exercises to Improve or Maintain Posture*

These exercises help strengthen back and abdominal muscles to maintain or improve posture, which is important in avoiding fractures due to osteoporosis. If you don't have osteoporosis and you're otherwise healthy, these exercises are generally safe to do. If you have osteoporosis, your doctor can advise you on the appropriateness of each of these exercises, based on your individual condition:

1. For the upper back exercise shown in 1, lie flat on a firm surface with a large pillow under your hips and the lower part of your abdomen. Place your hands at your sides. With chin tucked in, pull your shoulder blades together and raise your head and chest.

2. For the neck flexion, 2, rest your arms comfortably at your sides. Tighten your abdominal muscles as you raise your head.

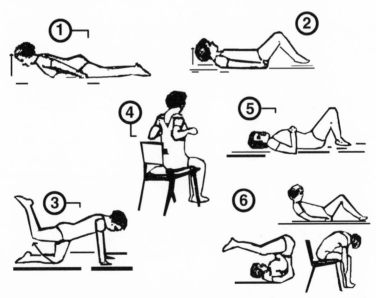

*Figure 48.1. Exercises. Exercises courtesy M. Sinaki, Mayo Clinic*

3.  For the lower back exercise, 3, from a hands-and-knees posi-
    tion, raise one leg at the hip, keeping your knee bent. Repeat
    with other leg.

4.  For the upper back exercise, 4, tuck in your chin and relax
    your shoulders. Bend elbows and pull shoulder blades to-
    gether as you straighten your upper back.

5.  For the pelvic tilt, 5, lie as shown. Tighten your abdominal
    muscles as you roll your pelvis up and back while flattening
    the small of your back against the surface. Avoid using leg
    and buttock muscles.

6.  Avoid these exercises if you have osteoporosis. If you have os-
    teoporosis, avoid exercises that round your back (see illustra-
    tions). They can cause increased pressure on your spine.

## Playing it Safe

Before starting any exercise program, check with your doctor if
you're a man over age 40 or a woman over 50, you have a family history of early onset cardiovascular disease, or you have health problems. Also check with your doctor if you're unsure of your health.

If you have osteoporosis, it's particularly important to get help from
your doctor in designing an exercise program that's safe for you.

# Chapter 49

# *Keeping Old Bones Whole*

## *Injury Prevention*

**Abstract:** Osteoporosis affects around 25 million Americans, 80 percent of whom are women. The main risk factors are a family history of the disease, an early hysterectomy and a diet low in calcium and vitamin D. The type of fall and a person's body weight can also affect the severity of a fracture. Methods to prevent or minimize fractures include averting falls by removing potential hazards, increasing flexibility and bone density through exercise, and wearing padded undergarments that cushion the fall. Estrogen replacement therapy also seems to offer benefits.

Although ice skaters and gymnasts practice falling safely so that they won't be hurt if they slip, rehearsing falls is not an option for most seniors. Instead, scientists are studying exercises that they may prevent falls and developing special kinds of gear to protect older people when they do take a spill.

The stakes are high: among people who lived independently before a hip fracture, 15-25 percent are still in long-term care institutions a year after the injury.

Bone is a remarkable material: although it is one of the hardest of human tissues, it is flexible and light enough to enable people to run, jump, bend, and twist. But when osteoporosis sets in, bones may become

Excerpted from the September 1996 issue of the *Harvard Health Letter*, © 1996, President and Fellows of Harvard College. Reprinted with permission.

so weak that they can barely support the body's weight. Low bone density, structural deterioration of the tissue, and increased susceptibility to fractures characterize this disease, which affects 25 million Americans, 80 percent of them women.

Women usually have smaller, thinner bones than men and lose mass more rapidly after menopause. Nevertheless, five million American men are affected by osteoporosis and one out of eight over age 50 will develop fractures. Factors that increase the risk for developing osteoporosis include a family history of the disease, an early hysterectomy, a diet low in calcium and vitamin D, thin build, Caucasian or Asian race, an inactive lifestyle, cigarette smoking, and having more than two alcoholic drinks a day.

People are often unaware that they have osteoporosis until their bones become so weak that a sudden bump or fall causes a hip fracture or the collapse of a vertebra. The good news is that specialized x-rays can detect osteoporosis before a break occurs, determine the rate of bone loss, and track the effects of treatment.

In the past, physicians thought osteoporosis was the overriding factor in late-life fractures. But recent research has shown that several other predictors are equally as important. Both a person's body weight and the characteristics of the fall—the location, direction, and force exerted on the bone—influence the chance of fracture.

A high-risk incident, for example, is one in which a standing person falls sideways so that her hip lands on a hard surface. When this occurs, a plump person is less likely to be seriously injured than a thin one, possibly because soft tissue overlying the hip acts as a shock absorber.

## Don't Fall Prey

There are three basic approaches to preventing fractures: averting the fall, decreasing the severity when one occurs, and keeping bones strong.

Ways to avoid falls include:

- getting rid of throw rugs,
- making sure electric cords are kept away from traveled areas,
- avoiding high-heeled shoes, and
- staying away from poorly lit stairs.

People whose eyeglass prescriptions are up-to-date are more likely to see household hazards. It may also be a good idea to review current medications with a physician and eliminate those that can cause hypotension, confusion, or impaired balance. If the doctor recommends a cane or a walker, by all means use one.

Another promising way to prevent falls is exercise to improve balance, flexibility, muscle strength, and reaction time. A study in the May 1996 issue of the *Journal of the American Geriatrics Society* showed that Tai Chi—an ancient Chinese martial art that employs slow, precise movements—helped improve balance and strength among seniors. Those who underwent Tai Chi training for 15 weeks reduced their risk of falling by 47.5 percent compared with those who didn't take classes. Another major benefit was a decreased fear of falling—a worry that often prevents older people from being as active as they'd like.

## Extra Padding

At least 90 percent of hip fractures are associated with a fall, so the next best thing to remaining upright is to reduce a fall's severity. Here scientists have taken some tips about protective gear from sports. In 1993, Danish researchers showed that wearing hip pads provided a 53 percent reduction in hip fracture incidence among older people.

There are several padding systems under development; only a few are available to the general public. The pads are built into a tight-fitting undergarment that looks like a girdle or a pair of bicycle shorts. Although most reduce the impact of a fall by absorbing energy, a newer system designed at Beth Israel Hospital in Boston transfers energy away from the bone and into surrounding tissues. One recent study found that this approach reduced the amount of force absorbed by the hip by 65 percent, providing twice the cushioning of conventional protective garments.

The energy-shunting model is filled with a gel-like substance that comfortably conforms to the body during normal activities but stiffens rapidly on impact, deflecting force away from the hip bone. It is also more comfortable than energy-absorbing pads that ride directly on the thigh bone. Further testing is needed before it becomes available commercially.

## Back to Basics

In the end, increasing or maintaining bone density is the staple of fracture prevention. Regular weight-bearing exercise increases bone mass, and proper nutrition—especially calcium and vitamin D in-take—is essential for protecting bone.

For women, estrogen replacement therapy effectively prevents postmenopausal bone loss. Medications such as calcitonin and fluo-ride and the bisphosphonates—alendronate sodium (Fosamax) and etidronate (Didronel)—can help both women and men preserve bone.

Though the statistics are sobering-over 300,000 hip fractures, 500,000 vertebral fractures, and 200,000 wrist fractures a year—bro-ken bones do not have to be an inevitable consequence of aging. The bottom line is that taking preventive steps can help seniors stay on their feet.

*—by Elizabeth R. Myers; Gabrielle I. Weiner.*

# Part Six

# Diagnosis, Treatment, and Coping Strategies

# Chapter 50

# *How to Find a Doctor*

Isabel Johnson, 64 years old, picked up a brochure on osteoporosis at her local pharmacy. What she read about the "silent disease" concerned her. She learned that she had several of the risk factors: she had gone through menopause at an early age, and her mother had suffered several fractures in her seventies and eighties.

Isabel called her neighbor, a registered nurse, who suggested that she call the National Osteoporosis Foundation for information on how to find an appropriate physician.

Our experience reveals that, for many individuals, finding a doctor who is knowledgeable about osteoporosis can be problematic. There is no physician specialty dedicated to osteoporosis, nor is there a certification program for health professionals who treat the disease. Therefore, a variety of medical specialists are treating people with osteoporosis, including internists, gynecologists, family physicians, endocrinologists, rheumatologists, physiatrists, and orthopedists.

There are a number of ways to find a doctor who treats osteoporosis patients. If you have a primary care physician or a family doctor, discuss your concerns with him or her. Your doctor may be able to refer you to an osteoporosis specialist.

If you are enrolled in an HMO or managed care health plan, consult your assigned physician about osteoporosis. This doctor should be able to give you an appropriate referral.

---

If you do not have a personal physician or your doctor cannot help you, you should contact your nearest university hospital or academic health center and ask for the department that cares for patients with osteoporosis. The department will vary from institution to institution. For example, in some facilities, the department of endocrinology or metabolic bone disease treats osteoporosis patients. In other medical centers, the appropriate department may be rheumatology, orthopedics, or gynecology. Some hospitals have a separate osteoporosis program or women's clinic that treats osteoporosis patients.

Once you have identified a doctor, you may wish to inquire about such things as whether the physician has specialized training in osteoporosis, how much of the practice is dedicated to osteoporosis, and whether he or she makes use of bone mass measurement.

Your own doctor, whether a gynecologist, orthopedist, or internist, is often the best person to treat you because she or he knows your medical history, your lifestyle, and your special needs.

## *Medical Specialists Who Treat Osteoporosis (in Alphabetical Order)*

**Endocrinologists** treat the endocrine system, which comprises the glands and hormones that help control the body's metabolic activity. In addition to osteoporosis, endocrinologists also treat diabetes and thyroid and pituitary diseases.

**Family physicians** have a broad range of training that includes surgery, internal medicine, gynecology, and pediatrics. They place special emphasis on caring for an individual or family on a long-term, continuing basis.

**Geriatricians** are family physicians or internists who have received additional training on the aging process and the conditions and diseases which often occur among the elderly, including incontinence, falls, and dementia. Geriatricians often care for patients in nursing homes, the patient's home, or in office or hospital settings.

**Gynecologists** diagnose and treat conditions of the female reproductive system and associated disorders. They often serve as primary care physicians for women, and follow their patients' reproductive health over time.

**Internists** are trained in the essentials of overall care of general internal medicine. Internists diagnose and treat non-surgically all diseases of the body. They provide long-term comprehensive care in the hospital and office, developing expertise in many areas, and often act as consultants to other specialists.

**Orthopedic surgeons** are physicians trained in the care of patients with musculoskeletal problems. Congenital skeletal deformities, skeletal trauma and infections, and metabolic disturbances are within the purview of orthopedists.

**Physiatrists** are physicians who specialize in physical medicine and rehabilitation. Physiatrists evaluate and treat patients with impairments, disabilities, or pain arising from musculoskeletal, neurologic, or other system problems. Physiatrists focus on restoring the physical, psychological, social and vocational functioning of the individual.

**Rheumatologists** diagnose and treat diseases of the joints, muscles, bones, and tendons, including arthritis and collagen diseases. The rheumatologist may work closely with other specialists such as orthopedists, physiatrists, and physical therapists.

This information has been brought to you by:

Osteoporosis and Related Bone Diseases—National Resource Center
1150 17th Street, N.W., Suite 500,
Washington, DC 20036-4603
Tel (202) 223-0344
Fax (202) 223-2237
TTY (202) 466-4315

# Chapter 51

# *The Diagnosis*

Osteoporosis is a disease that progresses silently over a long period of time. If diagnosed early, the fractures associated with the disease can be prevented. Unfortunately, osteoporosis often remains undiagnosed until a fracture occurs.

An examination to diagnose osteoporosis can involve several steps: an initial physical examination, including checking your height for changes and your posture to note any curvature of the spine (kyphosis); various x-rays, which detect skeletal abnormalities; laboratory tests, which reveal important information about the metabolic processes of bone breakdown and formation; and a bone densitometry test, which can confirm the diagnosis of osteoporosis.

Before performing any tests, your doctor will record information about your medical history and lifestyle, and will ask questions related to factors that increase the likelihood of your developing osteoporosis. These are called "risk factors" and include the following:

- Being female
- Thin and/or small frame
- Advanced age
- A family history of osteoporosis
- A personal history of previous fracture

From *The Osteoporosis Report,* Winter 1992, updated Spring 1999, © NOF, 1999. Reprinted with permission from the National Osteoporosis Foundation, Washington, D.C. 20037.

- Post-menopause, including early or surgically induced menopause
- Abnormal absence of menstrual periods (amenorrhea)
- Anorexia nervosa or bulimia
- A diet low in calcium and/or vitamin D
- Use of certain medications, such as corticosteroids and anti-convulsants
- Low testosterone levels in men
- An inactive lifestyle
- Cigarette smoking
- Excessive use of alcohol
- Being Caucasian or Asian, although African Americans and Hispanic Americans are at significant risk as well.

## X-ray Tests

If you have back pain, your doctor may order an x-ray of your spine to determine if you have had a fracture. An x-ray also may be appropriate if you have experienced a loss of height or a change in posture. However, since an x-ray can only detect bone loss after 25-40 percent of the skeleton has been depleted, the presence of osteoporosis may be missed.

## Bone Mineral Density Tests

A bone mineral density test (BMD) that measures bone mass can confirm a diagnosis of osteoporosis and determine your risk for fractures. The BMD test is non-invasive and painless. During a BMD test, either an extremely low energy source is passed over part, or all, of the body, or high frequency sound waves are used. The information is evaluated by a computer program that allows the physician to see how much bone mass you have and, since bone mass serves as an approximate measure of bone strength, helps the physician accurately detect low bone mass, make a definitive diagnosis of osteoporosis, and determine your risk of future fractures.

In addition to diagnosing osteoporosis, results from a BMD test can help the physician decide whether to begin a prevention or treatment program. Also, physicians may repeat a BMD test to monitor the effectiveness of a treatment regimen.

According to the World Health Organization, a person's BMD test measures current bone mass and compares it to a specific standard or number value that reflects optimal or peak bone density. For women, this number value reflects the bone density of a 30 year old woman. A computer program then compares the person's bone mass to the optimal bone mass and prints out the findings in terms of "standard deviations," or how far above or below the norm a person falls.

For BMD tests, individuals who are within one standard deviation of the "norm" are considered to have normal bone density. A score from 1 to 2.5 standard deviations below the norm indicates low bone mass or osteopenia, and a score of more than 2.5 standard deviations below the norm is considered a diagnosis of osteoporosis.

## Bone Scans

In some patients, a bone scan may be ordered. A bone scan is different from the bone mass measurement (BMD) test just described, although the term "bone scan" often is used incorrectly to describe a bone density test. A bone scan can tell the physician whether there are changes that may indicate cancer, bone lesions, inflammation, or new fractures. To perform a bone scan, the patient is injected with a dye that allows a scanner to identify differences in the condition of different areas of bone tissue.

## Laboratory Tests

A number of laboratory tests may be performed on blood and urine samples. The results of these tests may help your doctor identify conditions that may be contributing to your bone loss. The most common blood tests are:

- Blood calcium levels
- Thyroid function tests
- Parathyroid hormone levels
- Estradiol levels to measure estrogen (in women)
- Follicle Stimulating Hormone (FSH) test to establish menopause status (in women)
- Testosterone levels (in men)
- Osteocalcin levels to measure bone formation
- 25-hydroxyvitamin D test to measure vitamin D

The most common urine tests are:

- Twenty-four hour urine collection to measure calcium metabolism

- Biochemical marker tests to measure the rate at which a person is breaking down or resorbing bone

## *Treatment*

Once you and your physician have definitive information based on your history, physical examination, and diagnostic tests results, a specific treatment program can be developed for you. Recommendations for optimizing bone health include a comprehensive program that consists of adequate calcium and vitamin D intake, appropriate exercise, and a healthy lifestyle (including not smoking, avoiding excessive alcohol, sodium, fast foods and colas, and recognizing that some prescription medications and chronic diseases can cause bone loss).

In addition, your doctor may prescribe specific medical treatment to help you preserve and build bone mass and prevent fractures. If you already have experienced a fracture, your doctor may refer you to a specialist in physical therapy or rehabilitation medicine to help you with daily activities, safe movement, and exercises to improve strength and balance.

**Editor's Note:** We would like to thank Theresa Galsworthy, R.N., Director of The Osteoporosis Center, Hospital for Special Surgery, New York City, for her assistance in writing this article.

# Chapter 52

# *Changing Perceptions in Osteoporosis*

**Abstract:** One of the primary concerns about the potential for and progression of osteoporosis is vulnerability to fracture, but bone density cannot identify who will sustain osteoporotic fracture or who will not. This is because antiresorptive treatments prevent fracture, whether they are given at the menopause or decades later, and bone density does not change much with antiresorptive treatment such as hormone replacement therapy, but bone turnover falls dramatically. Bone turnover may be the responsive element in treatments to prevent osteoporotic fracture. Since impact and repetition of impact are the main risk factors for fracture, and these rise dramatically with age, treatment should be focused on infirm older people, without regard for measurement of bone density.

## *Summary Points*

- Bone densitometry cannot identify people who will sustain osteoporotic fracture.

- Bone density changes little with antiresorptive treatment (hormone replacement therapy and bisphosphonate drugs), whereas bone turnover falls dramatically

- Bone turnover may be the responsive element in treatments to prevent osteoporotic fracture

- Antiresorptive treatments prevent fracture, regardless of whether they are given at the menopause or decades later

- Since frequency of impact, which rises exponentially with age, is the main risk factor for fracture, treatment should be focused on infirm older people, irrespective of their bone density

- A recent meta-analysis of 11 separate study populations and over 2000 fractures concluded that bone mineral density "cannot identify individuals who will have a fracture."[1] So why do we measure it? The question is worth asking when the number of dual energy x ray absorptiometry machines installed in the United Kingdom exceeds 130 (National Osteoporosis Society, personal communication), and the number of Medline citations incorporating the term dual energy x-ray absorptiometry has grown from 26 in 1988 to 464 in 1997. The concept of "fracture threshold" has led to the recommendation that preventive treatment be given to women once their bone density lies (arbitrarily) more than 1 SD below the mean for premenopausal women—a state of osteopenia, according to the WHO definition. But should we be managing osteoporosis by numbers?

## Osteoporosis and Osteomalacia

Bone comprises a matrix framework on which mineral is deposited. Osteoporosis is caused by the disintegration of the matrix, and osteomalacia by a failure to mineralize it. When mineralized matrix disintegrates, calcium is inevitably lost. The negative calcium balance observed with matrix loss gave rise to erroneous beliefs that the calcium requirements of postmenopausal women were higher than those of premenopausal women and that osteoporosis could be prevented by calcium supplementation.[2] Calcium is crucial during the development of bone, but it cannot replace disintegrating matrix or prevent its loss.[3] As Heaney has pointed out, calcium is a nutrient and not a drug, and the only disorder it can be expected to alleviate is calcium deficiency.[4] What is more, excess calcium supplementation will suppress the secretion of parathyroid hormone and slow the natural turnover of bone. "Fossilized" bone is at risk from microfractures. Calcium intakes of between 1 g and 1.5 g daily, commonly recommended in postmenopausal women, are associated with an increased rather than decreased risk of fracture.[5] Preventing osteoporosis does not depend on calcium, but rather on preserving bone matrix, a living tissue whose structure, strength, and integrity depend, in turn, on fine control of its turnover.

Bone turnover is maintained by two groups of cells—osteoclasts, which dig pits in mineralized matrix, and osteoblasts, which refill the pits. Osteoclastic activity is constrained by the action of sex steroids, and coordination with the osteoblasts is normally maintained such that there is no net change in bone mass during early adult life. After the menopause, circulating oestrogen concentrations fall rapidly and osteoclastic activity accelerates, outstripping the attempts of osteoblasts to keep pace. The net result is bone loss which, over a period of years, may amount to 20 percent or more of the skeleton.

## Effect of Antiresorptive Drugs

The widespread view that treatment with antiresorptive drugs restores lost bone, and that the increase in bone density observed is responsible for the subsequent reduction in the fracture rate, needs careful rethinking.[6] There is no evidence that treatment for osteoporosis restores bone, although (unlike calcium supplements) antiresorptive drugs undoubtedly prevent its further loss. The small increases in bone mineral density gained during the early years of treatment with hormone replacement therapy or bisphosphonate drugs soon level off,[7] and probably reflect no more than the filling by osteoblasts of the myriad pits dug before treatment by uncontrolled osteoclasts.[7 8] The challenge to the view that there is a causal relation between bone mineral density and risk of fracture lies in the results of large, placebo controlled, double blind, multicenter trials of bisphosphonate drugs (even those conducted in ageing women with established osteoporosis). These show a reduction in the risk of fracture at the hip and spine of more than 50 percent, but an increase in bone mineral density at these sites of only 5-8 percent,[9] and even less in earlier studies of spinal fracture.[7] It is difficult to attribute such a spectacular clinical result to such a small increase in bone mass.

## Factors in Fracture Risk

Hui et al constructed a family of curves relating fracture risk to bone density in different age groups. For the same bone density, the risk of fracture rose 8-fold to 10-fold from age [is less than] 45 years to [is greater than or equal to] 80 years?[10] In a sample of 5800 Dutch men and women over 55 years of age, the risk of hip fracture rose

13-fold with age, to which the decrease in bone density contributed only 1.9 in women and 1.6 in men.[11] These are important observations, because they suggest that something very important in the ageing process influences fracture risk independently of bone density.

Apart from further undermining the validity of bone density as a surrogate for individual fracture risk and its clinical use in identifying those to whom treatment should be given, the observation calls for an explanation. One obvious mechanism is that ageing people fall more frequently and, for a given bone density, sustain fracture more often as a result. Fractures seldom occur without some impact, however fragile the bone, but there may be an additional and more subtle explanation to account for the differences in risk, one which can reconcile the data from clinical trials on fracture risk, bone density, and bone resorption.

It is intuitively likely that bone depends for strength more on its architecture than on its mass. Bone in a younger person is structurally normal, whereas in ageing people its architecture is compromised in two ways. Firstly, the progressive erosion of trabeculas will leave them weakened and, in some cases, disconnected.[7] Microscopy shows that trabecular erosions and disconnectivity cannot be reversed by treatment,[12] Secondly, and possibly more importantly, the rate of bone turnover in women who are deficient in oestrogen will inevitably be higher, mass for mass, than in women who are oestrogen replete. If a bolt or two at a time were removed from a cantilever bridge for replacement, architectural strength might not be affected—but if a thousand were removed at one time (a high turnover state), architectural strength could be compromised critically, with little loss in mass. Fractures occur in situations in which high bone turnover is combined with frequent impact. Bone density does not contribute greatly to the individual's risk.

While measurements of bone density emphasize how little bone is regained during antiresorptive treatment, measures of matrix loss show a dramatic and immediate slowing of bone turnover. In postmenopausal women, N-telopeptide type I collagen (a marker for osteoclast activity) fell from 3 SD above the mean to the premenopausal mean within one month of starting treatment, an effect which remained throughout the 15 month study.[13] The bone specific alkaline phosphatase value (a marker for osteoblastic activity) showed a similar pattern within six months (the delay probably contributed to the 5 percent increase in spinal bone mass observed over the study period). The fossa intervention trial (FOSIT) observed over 1000 postmenopausal women with low bone density in a placebo controlled trial of alendronate that lasted more than 12 months. It showed an 80 percent reduction in the bone resorption rate in relation to increases in bone density of 5 percent at the lumbar spine and just 2 percent at the neck of the femur.[14]

Critics have pointed out that markers of bone turnover are "poorly predictive of bone mineral density... and cannot be used to diagnose osteoporosis or to select patients for subsequent densitometry" but this is to miss the point.[15] If the modest gain in bone density seen with treatment is insufficient to account for the substantial reduction in fracture risk, a state of high bone turnover, rather than its prevailing mass, may be the responsive element in fracture prevention, no matter at what age it is encountered. The clinical implications are important, as there is no evidence that bone density identifies those people who will sustain a fracture, but abundant evidence that restoring bone turnover to normal values universally reduces the risk. A switch in emphasis from bone density, which declines irreversibly, to bone turnover, which rises, but is fully reversible, makes reducing the risk of fracture a viable consideration at any age after the menopause.

A fall in bone mass, erosion of trabeculas, and ultimately their loss of connectivity must, in themselves, render bone progressively more fragile. However, the evidence cited suggests that fracture risk can be reduced appreciably, even in older women who are already osteoporotic, and without a noticeable restoration of bone mass. The widely held notion that it is too late to treat women with established osteoporosis because bone cannot be restored once it is lost is flawed because bone density and fracture risk are poorly correlated and a high turnover of bone can be normalized at any age or bone density. Bone densitometry might arguably have only a limited role in strategies to prevent osteoporotic fracture.

If high bone turnover rather than low bone density is the major component of fracture risk, antiresorptive drugs should reduce the risk of fracture to the same extent at any age after the menopause, independently of bone density, and when they are stopped their protective effect should be lost before bone density decreases. A recent report by Michaelsson et al provides the first evidence that bears out both these predictions.[16] In a large, population based, case-control study, hormone replacement therapy reduced the risk of hip fracture to the same extent, whether treatment began at the menopause or decades later. After hormone replacement therapy was stopped, protection against fracture fell rapidly in relation to the interval since it was last used, and became statistically insignificant after five years.

In 1995, it was claimed that "it is now possible to accurately determine individuals' risk of osteoporosis, and to monitor their response to treatment, by means of bone densitometry."[7] In the light of current understanding, this is probably not the case. People who will sustain a fracture cannot be identified by bone densitometry, and if bone turnover is the key responsive element in treatment, measures of bone resorption rather than of its density should be the focus of technical developments in monitoring response to treatment.

## Programs for Preventing Osteoporotic Fracture

How much, then, can we be certain of in formulating programs for the prevention of osteoporotic fracture? We know that antiresorptive drugs taken at the time of the menopause will maintain bone density for as long as they are continued. However, we also know that without them few women sustain fractures before the age of 65 years, probably because they tend not to fall. So has anything been gained in prescribing treatment during 15 years of low fracture risk? Certainly, the NHS can afford neither to screen the perimenopausal population nor to treat blindly. We also know that antiresorptive drugs reduce the risk of fracture equally at any age after the menopause, and that this protection is lost rapidly when they are stopped. Finally, bone density benefits little from antiresorptive agents, while bone turnover returns to its premenopausal state.

If bone density determination cannot distinguish between those who will and will not sustain osteoporotic fractures, it has no place in selecting people for prophylaxis—notwithstanding recent Department of Health guidelines.[17] Current knowledge indicates that prophylaxis should be targeted not at maintaining bone density throughout menopausal life but at restoring normal bone turnover in those who, for whatever reason, become infirm and at greatest risk of impact. Such an approach to the prevention of osteoporotic fracture would be evidence based, could be budgeted for, and would rationalize management of the individual patient—something that treatment by numbers does not.

*—by Terence J Wilkin.*

Terence J Wilkin, professor
Plymouth Postgraduate Medical School,
University of Plymouth, Plymouth PL4 8AA
twilkin@plymouth. ac.uk
BMJ 1000;318:862-5

## References

1. Marshall D, Johnell O, Wedel H. Meta-analysis of how well measures of bone mineral density predict occurrence of osteoporotic fractures. *BMJ* 996;312:1254-9.

2. Nordin BE, Horsman A, Marshall DH, Simpson H, Waterhouse GH. Calcium requirement and calcium therapy. *Clin Orthop* 1979;140:216-39.

3. Kreiger N, Gross A, Hunter G. Dietary factors and fracture in post-menopausal women: a case-controlled study, *Int J Epidemiol* 1992;21:953-8.

4. Heaney RP. Calcium in the prevention and treatment of osteoporosis. *J Intern Med* 1992;231:169-80.

5. Cumming RG, Cummings SR, Nevitt MG, Scott J, Ensrud KE, Vogt TM, et al. Calcium intake and fracture risk; results from the Study of Osteoporotic Fractures. *Am J Epidemiol* 1997;145:926-34.

6. Liberman UA, Weiss SR, Broll J, Minne HW, Quan H, Bell NH, et al. Effect of oral alendronate on bone mineral density and the incidence of fractures in postmenopausal osteoporosis. *N Engl J Med* 1995;333: 1437-43.

7. Peel N, Eastell R. Osteoporosis. *BMJ* 1995;310:989-92.

8. Christiansen C. Skeletal osteoporosis. *J Bone Mincr Res* 1993;8(suppl 2):S475-80.

9. Black DM, Cummings SR, Karpf DB, Cauley JA, Thompson DE, Nevitt MC, et al. Randomised trial of effect of alendronate on risk of fracture in women with existing vertebral fractures. *N Engl J Med* 1996;348:1535-41.

10. Hui SL, Slemenda CW, Johston CC Jr. Age and bone mass as predictors of fracture in a prospective study. *J Clin Invest* 1988;81:1804-9.

11. DeLaet CEDH, Van Hoar BA, Banger H, Hotman A, Pols HA. Bone density and risk of hip fracture in men and women: cross sectional analysis. *BMJ* 1997;315:221-5.

12. Kanis J. Treatment of osteoporotic fracture. *Lancet* 1984;i:27-33.

13. Garnero P, Shih WJ, Gineyts E, Karpf DB, Delmas PD. Comparison of new biochemical markers of bone turnover in late post-menopausal osteoporotic women in response to alendronate treatment. *J Clin Invest* 1994;79:1693-700.

14. Wilkin TJ. Multi-national, placebo-controlled study of alendronate in post-menopausal osteoporosis—results of 1000 patients from the FOSIT study. *Acta Obstet Gynecol Scand* 1997;76 (suppl 167):61.

15. Eastell R, Blumsohn A. The value of biochemical markers of bone turnover in osteoporosis. *J Rheueuttol* 1997;24:1215-7.

16. Michaelsson K, Baron JA, Farahmand BY, Johnell O, Magnusson C, Persson P-G, et al. Hormone replacement therapy and risk of hip fracture: population based case-control study. *BMJ* 1998;316:1858-63.

17. Department of Health. Clinical guidelines for strategies to prevent and treat osteoporosis. London: Department of Health, 1998. (http://www.open.gov.uk/doh/pub/docs/doh/osteoq.pdf)

# Chapter 53

# *A Step-by-Step Approach to Osteoporosis Treatment*

## *Screening Women at Risk*

**Abstract:** Primary care physicians are encouraged to follow this seven-step protocol in order to screen the predisposition to osteoporosis in postmenopausal women. The steps include measuring bone density and trying estrogen before considering alternatives.

Now that baby boomer women are arriving at menopause in large numbers, you need an effective plan for preventing and treating osteoporosis. This seven-step protocol gives you a practical approach to screening and treating women at risk.

Osteoporosis is a systemic skeletal disease characterized by decreased bone mass and microarchitectural deterioration of bone tissue, which consequently increases bone fragility and susceptibility to fracture. In women, most cases of osteoporosis are caused by two major factors: estrogen deficiency and aging. While the mechanisms by which these factors cause osteoporosis are not fully known, excess osteoclast-mediated bone resorption appears to override osteoblast-mediated bone formation. The keys to preventing and treating osteoporosis, therefore, are to inhibit osteoclast activity and, to a lesser degree, to stimulate osteoblast activity.

*Patient Care*, April 30, 1998, Vol. 32, No. 8, p. 138(9). ©1998 Medical Economics Publishing and the author, Robert L. Barbieri. Reprinted with permission of *Patient Care*.

Osteoporosis is an important health problem for postmenopausal women. Approximately 1.5 million osteoporotic fractures occur in the United States each year, with a direct cost exceeding $10 billion. Of the total, about 300,000 are hip fractures, the most serious complication of osteoporosis, two thirds of them in women. In the year following a hip fracture, 20 percent of victims will die, 25 percent of survivors will be confined to long-term care facilities, and 50 percent will experience long-term loss of mobility.[1] Primary care physicians can make a significant dent in morbidity and mortality figures by following the seven steps outlined in this article.

### Step 1: Measure Bone Density

In the past, osteoporosis was diagnosed only after a woman suffered a "low-trauma" fracture. The development of accurate, noninvasive bone mineral density (BMD) measurement, however, now allows physicians to identify women at risk before a fracture occurs. The World Health Organization defines osteoporosis as a BMD that is more than 2.5 standard deviations below the young adult mean.[2,3] Osteopenia, a condition characterized by low bone density, is a BMD between 1 and 2.5 standard deviations below the young adult mean. For each 1 standard deviation decrease in bone density from the young adult mean, there is a twofold to three fold increased risk of fracture.[4]

Osteoporosis and osteopenia can be identified through BMD measurement. The benefit of determining a woman's bone density is that you can predict her risk of fracture and take steps to prevent one before it occurs.

With a precision of measurement of 1 percent and a radiation dose of less than 5 mrem, dual-energy x-ray absorptiometry (DEXA) is currently the best test for measuring BMD. Advantages of DEXA include a 5-minute (or less) scanning time and the ability either to measure total-body bone mass or to assess bone density at selected sites such as the spine and hip. Many researchers also believe DEXA measurements at one site are strongly predictive of the likelihood of fracture throughout the entire body. Just as cholesterol screening can predict vascular disease and blood pressure readings can predict stroke, DEXA is useful for determining risk of hip, spine, and wrist fracture. While qualitative CT also can be used to measure bone mass, it delivers a large radiation dose and tends to be more expensive than DEXA.

My current recommendation, which is also shared by The American College of Obstetricians and Gynecologists and the American College of Physicians, is that menopausal women at risk for osteoporosis should undergo a bone-density measurement if they are not taking estrogen (see Table 53.1). BMD testing also may be warranted in premenopausal women who have significant risk factors such as prolonged amenorrhea, eating disorders, glucocorticoid treatment, or renal disease.

**Table 53.1** Clinical Risk Factors for Osteoporosis

- Alcohol intake greater than 3 standardized glasses per week
- Caucasian or Asian race
- Certain medications such as glucocorticoid treatment at dosages greater than the equivalent of prednisone 10 mg daily
- Cigarette smoking
- Family history of osteoporosis
- Long interval of hypoestrogenism: many years of menopause, early menopause and oophorectomy, long intervals of amenorrhea in premenopausal women
- Sedentary lifestyle
- Small skeletal frame

### *Step 2: Focus on the T-score*

The standard BMD report is rich with information--in fact, many of the numbers may be irrelevant. Most bone density measurement reports include the following:

- An absolute value for the bone mass expressed as grams per square centimeter
- A value for bone mass relative to a sex- and age-matched reference population, usually called a Z-score
- A value for bone mass relative to the young adult mean bone density, usually called a T-score or a young adult Z-score.[6]

The key to interpreting a bone density test is the T-score. A T-score of 22.5 indicates that the bone mass is 2.5 standard deviations below the mean peak bone mass and is associated with a marked increased risk of osteoporotic fracture.

## *Step 3: Review the Differential Diagnosis*

For most osteoporotic women, estrogen deficiency and the aging process are the two major contributors to their low BMD. However, a few women have bone metabolism diseases such as hyperparathyroidism that contribute to the osteoporosis. Table 53.2 lists some of the major diseases that affect bone metabolism. The best screening test for hyperparathyroidism is a measurement of the circulating total calcium level.

**Table 53.2** Clinical Laboratory Data Associated with Common Metabolic Bone Diseases

| Bone disorder | Serum calcium |
|---|---|
| Osteoporosis | Normal |
| Osteomalacia | Decreased |
| Hyperparathyroidism | Increased |
| Renal failure/renal osteodystrophy | Decreased |
| Paget's disease | Normal |

| Bone disorder | Serum phosphorus |
|---|---|
| Osteoporosis | Normal |
| Osteomalacia | Decreased |
| Hyperparathyroidism | Decreased |
| Renal failure/renal osteodystrophy | Increased |
| Paget's disease | Normal |

| Bone disorder | Alkaline phosphatase |
|---|---|
| Osteoporosis | Normal |
| Osteomalacia | Increased |
| Hyperparathyroidism | Increased |
| Renal failure/renal osteodystrophy | Increased |
| Paget's disease | Markedly increased |

## *Step 4: Try Estrogen First*

Estrogen is the principle treatment for all hypoestrogenic women. You do not necessarily need to take another BMD measurement if a patient has started estrogen therapy and continues treatment. Screening should be done, however, in women who do not take estrogen or do not continue with estrogen treatment. Also recommend BMD measurement to menopausal women with risk factors for osteoporosis who decline estrogen therapy. Women with a T-score of 22.5 or more below the peak adult mean bone density should be offered estrogen, alendronate, or calcitonin-salmon.

Estrogen therapy is the key to preventing and treating osteoporosis because it reduces osteoclast activity, decreases bone loss, reduces spine and hip fractures, and prevents loss of height.[7-10] When estrogen treatment is initiated early in menopause, the rapid bone loss associated with menopause decreases and the risk of fracture is cut in half. Estrogen also achieves similar effects even when it is started years after menopause begins.[11]

Estrogen inhibits osteoclast bone resorption, which is an important goal in the prevention and treatment of osteoporosis. This effect can be well documented by demonstrating the effect of estrogen treatment on markers of bone resorption such as urinary N-telopeptide collagen cross-links (NTx). In one study, urinary NTx was significantly suppressed by estrogen within 1 month of the initiation of therapy.[8] Measuring urinary NTx may help determine whether estrogen treatment is effective in reducing osteoclast bone resorption.

Estrogen therapy is the best approach to the prevention and treatment of osteoporosis because it reduces osteoclast-mediated bone resorption and has other beneficial effects, such as reducing risk of myocardial infarction, improving vasomotor symptoms, and helping to maintain the function of secondary sexual tissues such as the vaginal epithelium.[12] For other approaches to strengthening bone, see "Supplements: Calcium and vitamin D."

### *Step 5: Be Flexible about Dosage*

In menopausal women, estrogen treatment clearly improves bone density. However, the ideal minimum dosage for preventing and reducing bone loss has yet to be established. Since side effects associated with standard estrogen dosages often deter women from continuing treatment, a minimal ideal dosage is necessary.

Recent studies suggest that there is a dose-response curve between estrogen treatment and bone mass. Lower dosages of estrogen preserved bone density more effectively than a placebo in some studies. For example, one group demonstrated a 32 percent increase (95 percent Cl, 0.06-5.84 percent) in lumbar spine bone density in menopausal women who had taken a daily regimen of 0.3 mg of conjugated equine estrogen combined with 2.5 mg of medroxyprogesterone for 2 years.[13] This is a major contrast to the decrease in bone density at the lumbar spine (22 percent) that resulted in menopausal women who had taken a placebo. Interestingly, treatment with 0.3 mg of conjugated equine estrogen daily was associated with less uterine bleeding than a regimen containing 0.625 mg.

This study and others suggest that lower-dose estrogen treatment is better than no estrogen treatment to preserve bone mass. [14] Clinicians should be flexible in the dosage of estrogen treatment prescribed to hypoestrogenic women. Use of "low" dosages of estrogen may help minimize symptoms that might otherwise cause a woman to discontinue this therapy.

### Step 6: Consider Alternatives When Needed

Many menopausal women decline estrogen treatment or discontinue it within their first year of treatment because they experience side effects or have fears about long-term adverse effects, such as the small increased risk of breast cancer. Offer BMD testing if a menopausal woman at risk for osteoporosis declines or discontinues estrogen treatment. If the measurement indicates osteoporosis or osteopenia, consider prescribing alendronate or calcitonin.

**Alendronate.** This bisphosphonate inhibits osteoclast activity and increases bone density, reducing the risk of fracture by approximately 50 percent and the risk of multiple vertebral fractures by approximately 90 percent.[15] A benefit of these risk reductions is that they help preserve a woman's height. To treat osteoporosis, the recommended alendronate dosage is 10 mg/d for 3 years. For osteopenia and prevention of osteoporosis, the daily dosage is 5 mg.

The main problems with alendronate are that only 1 percent is absorbed from the GI tract and the drug can cause GI symptoms such as abdominal pain. Contraindications to alendronate include abnormalities of esophageal emptying, such as stricture or achalasia, which might increase the risk of GI side effects. When using alendronate, make sure you reinforce the prescribing instructions: Alendronate should be swallowed upon arising for the day with a full glass of water (6-8 oz), and patients should not lie down for at least 30 minutes and until after their first food of the day.

A potential advantage of alendronate is that it remains tightly bound to the bone surface for many years, probably providing some protection against osteoclast resorption of bone for a period after discontinuation of therapy.

No published clinical trials provide data to evaluate the clinical utility of combining alendronate with estrogen in the treatment of osteoporosis. It is likely that some women who fail to achieve an increase in bone density with a single agent will benefit with combined therapy. Future trials will likely evaluate the clinical utility of combining low dosages of estrogen (conjugated equine estrogen, 0.3 mg/d) and alendronate (5 mg/d) in the hope of minimizing side effects and maximizing improvement in bone density.

**Calcitonin.** This hormone is produced endogenously by the perifollicular C cells of the thyroid gland and inhibits osteoclast-mediated bone resorption. Given intranasally, calcitonin provides 200 IU per spray, increases bone mass, and may reduce fracture risk.[16,17] The most common side effect of nasal calcitonin is rhinitis. While this hormone may be slightly less potent than estrogen and alendronate in inhibiting osteoclast bone resorption, it has few side effects and a very good safety profile.

### *Step 7: Prepare to Use New Agents*

During the next few years many new agents are likely to be released for treatment of osteoporosis and osteopenia. One recently approved agent, raloxifene, is a selective estrogen receptor modulator (SERM) that holds promise as an agent to prevent osteoporosis. Another is tibolene, a synthetic progestin with androgenic and some estrogenic effects.

**Raloxifene.** This nonsteroidal compound works as an estrogen agonist in the bone, increasing bone density, and in the liver, decreasing low-density lipoprotein (LDL) cholesterol secretion. It works as an estrogen antagonist in the breast, endometrium (treatment is associated with endometrial atrophy and amenorrhea), and CNS (treatment is associated with an increase in vasomotor symptoms).

In a preliminary report at the 1997 National Osteoporosis Foundation, one group observed that treatment with raloxifene, 30-150 mg/d, plus calcium supplementation, 500 mg/d, resulted in a 2-4 percent bone-mass increase compared with placebo. Raloxifene also produced a 10 percent decrease in LDL cholesterol levels and a 6 percent decrease in total cholesterol levels. Treatment was associated with almost no uterine bleeding.

**Tibolone.** At dosages of 1.25 mg/d and 2.5 mg/d, tibolone increases lumbar spine and distal forearm bone density.[18] Vasomotor symptoms of menopause are also reduced. There is a 15 percent rate of vaginal bleeding and an 18 percent rate of breast tenderness in women taking this agent. The major adverse effect that is associated with tibolone therapy is a significant decrease in high-density lipoprotein cholesterol levels. Tibolone is currently approved for the treatment of menopause in many European countries.

## References

1. Cummings SR, Kelsey JL, Nevitt MC, et al: Epidemiology of osteoporosis and osteoporotic fractures. *Epdemiol Rev* 1985;7:178-208.

2. World Health Organization 1994. Assessment of fracture risks and its application to screening for post-menopausal osteoporosis. Technical Report Series. WHO Geneva.

3. Kanis JA, Melton LJ, Christiansen C, at al: The diagnosis of osteoporosis. *J Bone Miner Res* 1994;9: 1137-1141.

4. Melton LJ, Atkinson EJ, O'Fallon WM, et al: Long-term fracture prediction by bone mineral assessed at different skeletal sites. *J Bone Mineral Res* 1993; 8:1227-1234.

5. Jergas M, Genant HK: Current methods and recent advances in the diagnosis of osteoporosis. *Arthritis Rheum* 1993;36:1649-1662.

6. Compston JE, Cooper C, Kanis JA: Bone density in clinical practice. *BMJ* 1995;310:1507-1015.

7. Breslau NA: Calcium, estrogen, and progestin in the treatment of osteoporosis. *Rheum Dis Clin North Amer* 1994;20:691-716.

8. Rosen CJ, Chestnut CH, Mallinak NJS: The predictive value of biochemical markers of bone turnover for bone mineral density in early postmenopausal women treated with hormone replacement or calcium supplementation. *J Clin Endocrinol Metab* 1997;82:1904-1910.

9. Lindsay R, Tohme JF: Estrogen treatment of patients with established postmenopausal osteoporosis. *Obstet Gynecol* 1990;76:290-295.

10. Ettinger B, Genant HK, Cann CE: Long-term estrogen replacement therapy prevents bone loss and fractures. *Ann Intern Med* 1985;102:319-324.

11. Lufkin EG, Wenner HW, O'Fallon WM, et al: Treatment of postmenopausal osteoporosis with transdermal estrogen. *Ann Intern Med* 1992;117:1-9.

12. Barrett-Connor E, Bush TL: Estrogen and coronary heart disease in women. *JAMA* 1995;273:199-208.

13. Mizunuma H, Okano H, Soda M, at al: Prevention of postmenopausal bone loss with minimal uterine bleeding using low dose continuous estrogen/ progestin therapy: A 2-year prospective study. *Maturitas* 1997;27:69-76.

14. Naessen T, Berglund L, Ulmsten U: Bone loss in elderly women prevented by ultra low doses of parenteral 17 beta-estradiol. *Am J Obstet Gynecol* 1997; 177:115-119.

15. Liberman UA, Weiss SR, Broll J, et al: Effect of oral alendronate on bone mineral density and the incidence of fractures in postmenopausal osteoporosis: The Alendronate phase II osteoporosis treatment study group. *N Engl J Med* 1995;333:1437-1443.

16. Overgaard K, Hansen MA, Jensen SB, et al: Effect of salcaltonin given intranasally on bone mass and fracture rates in established osteoporosis: A dose-response study. *BMJ* 1992;305:556-561.

17. Rico H, Hernandez ER, Revma M, et al: Salmon calcitonin reduces vertebral fracture rate in postmenopausal crush fracture syndrome. *Bone Miner* 1992; 16:131-138.

18. Bjamason NH, Bjamason K, Haarbo J, at al: Tilbolone: Prevention of bone loss in late postmenopausal women. *J Clin Endocrinol Metab* 1996;81:2419-2422.

## Supplements: Calcium and Vitamin D

While estrogen remains the most effective treatment for reversing osteoporosis, women should also be encouraged to supplement their diets with calcium and vitamin D. It should be noted that clinical trials evaluating the impact of calcium and vitamin D on osteoporosis

**Table 53.3.** Calcium Recommendations

| Age | Minimum daily intake |
|---|---|
| <6 mo | 210 mg |
| 6-12 mo | 270 mg |
| 1-3 yr | 500 mg |
| 4-8 yr | 800 mg |
| 9-18 yr | 1,300 mg |
| 19-50 yr | 1,000 mg |
| ≥ 51 yr | 1,200 mg |

SPECIAL CONSIDERATIONS

| | |
|---|---|
| Pregnant/lactating women <19 yr | 1,300 mg |
| Pregnant/lactating women >19 yr | 1,000 mg |

**Note:** National Institute of Medicine, National Research Council, recommended dietary allowance for calcium should exceed these minimum intakes. Maximum calcium intake should exceed 2,500 mg/d.

**Table 53.4.** Selected Sources of Calcium

| Agent | Calcium per tablet (mg) |
|---|---|
| *Calcium carbonate* | |
| Biocal | 500 |
| Caltrate | 600 |
| Generic USP | 500 |
| Os-Cal 5W Chewable | 500 |
| Tums | 200 |
| Tums E-X | 300 |
| | |
| *Calcium citrate* | |
| Citracal | 200 |
| Generic calcium gluconate | 45, 87.7 |
| Generic calcium lactate | 84.5 |

**Source:** *Heaney RP: Calcium supplements: Practical considerations. Osteoporos Int 1991;1:65-71.*

*Vitamin D is recommended in dosages ranging from 400 IU/d (the recommended dietary allowance) to 800 IU/d if absorption is impaired.*

are inconsistent, with some demonstrating benefit and others not clearly indicating clinical utility. However, calcium and vitamin D treatment may be effective in women with low calcium intake, the elderly, and women confined to long-term-care facilities.(1)

The following are the national recommended intake guidelines for calcium and vitamin D.

According to the Institute of Medicine's recently revised recommendations, women older than 50 should take at least 1,200 mg/d of calcium (see Table 53.3). Dietary sources rich in calcium include dairy products, vegetables such as broccoli and collard greens, and sardines. Calcium supplements, which can be taken to achieve this recommended dietary goal, are described in Table 53.4.(2)

## *References*

1. Chapuy MC, Arlot MR, Delmas PD, et al: Effect of calcium and cholecalciferol treatment for three years on hip fractures in elderly women. *BMJ* 1994;309:1081-1082.

2. Heaney RP: Calcium supplements: Practical considerations. *Osteoporosis Int* 1991;1:65-71.

*— by Robert L. Barbieri*

ROBERT L. BARBIERI, MD, is Kate Macy Ladd Professor, Department of Obstetrics, Gynecology, and Reproductive Biology, Harvard Medical School, Boston, Mass.

Edited by Tanya Gregory, Managing Editor

# Chapter 54

# *New Ways to Heal Broken Bones*

The body's 206 dynamic, living bones renew themselves lifelong through a continual breakdown, buildup process known as remodeling.

Jacqueline Wallace, of Phoenix, sat enjoying the December 1993 holidays at her son's home in Gaithersburg, Md. But when she stood up and took a step, her holiday took a turn for the worse. Wallace fell and fractured her hip.

"My foot dragged a little, not exactly a stumble," Wallace says. "I don't know whether the bone broke because I fell, or I fell because the bone broke."

Despite her 84 years and weak heart, Wallace had a lot going for her after her fall: modern medical practice and determination to walk again. Surgery to implant an artificial hip joint took under 45 minutes. Spinal anesthesia and sedation were administered instead of general anesthesia because they are thought to pose less risk. And her physical therapy began the day after the operation.

"I fussed," she says. "I was afraid it was going to hurt or I'd fall. But they said if you want to go home, you have to do this. And I did. It was more scary than painful."

Wallace's fracture was one of 1.5 million—including 336,000 hip fractures—reported in 1993, the latest year for which the National Center for Health Statistics has figures.

Besides surgical repair, treatments for broken bones include bone manipulation to reduce the fracture, use of a cast, and bone stimulation.

U.S. Food and Drug Administration (FDA), *FDA Consumer* magazine, April 1996.

Central to fracture healing is bone biology. Many treatments, some on the horizon, are designed to improve the natural course of healing.

## Bones at Work

For skeletal growth and maintenance, the body's 206 dynamic, living bones renew themselves lifelong through a continual breakdown, build-up process known as remodeling. This process is also involved in the remodeling of fractures, says Martin Yahiro, M.D., a Baltimore orthopedist in private practice and a consultant on fracture treatment devices to the Food and Drug Administration's Center for Devices and Radiological Health.

In remodeling, complex chemical signals prompt cells called osteoclasts to break down and remove (resorb) old bone, and others called osteoblasts to deposit new bone. Many elements influence remodeling. Among them: weight-bearing, vitamin D, growth factors, prostaglandins, and various hormones, including estrogen, thyroid, parathyroid, and calcitonin.

As 80 percent of the mature skeleton, compact *cortical bone* supports the body, providing extra thickness mid-shaft in long bones to prevent their bending. *Cancellous bone,* whose porous structure with small cavities resembles a sponge, predominates in the pelvis and the 33 vertebrae from the neck to the tailbone. A fibrous membrane called the *periosteum* covers bone.

For healing and health, living bone must have a steady supply of nutrients. Blood vessels permeate bone to provide this lifeline. Blood-forming elements fill the long bone inner canals.

## When a Bone Breaks

Fracture breaks continuity of bone and of important attached soft tissue—including blood vessels, which spill their contents into surrounding tissue.

Even before treatment, the body automatically seeks to repair the injury. Inflammatory cells rush to destroy, dilute or isolate invaders and injured tissue. Tiny new blood vessels called capillaries begin growing into the site. Cells proliferate. The injured person usually must endure pain, swelling, and increased heat at the breakage site for one to three days.

New tissue bonds the fractured bone ends with a soft callus, a mass of connective tissue and exudate (matter escaped through blood vessel walls). Remodeling begins. Within a few months, hard callus replaces the soft one. Remodeling restores the inner canal.

Once restoration is complete, which may take years, the healed area is brand new, without a scar. Usually thicker, the new bone may even be stronger than the old, Yahiro says, adding that if the bone should break again, it's unlikely to be at the same place.

And children's bones have a healing boost: They're growing.

"The growing skeleton is just geared to make bone," Yahiro says. "A very young child's wrist bones grow a millimeter a month, to rapidly correct misalignment or length defects. An adult may take six to eight weeks to heal a wrist fracture, a 5-year-old only three."

When the ends of a fractured bone, such as an arm bone, form an abnormal angle, the doctor must decide whether to push the ends together (manipulation) to reduce the fracture, possibly under anesthesia. Simple x-rays aid evaluation.

"If it's a large angle, we'd want to reduce that fracture," Yahiro says. "But if it's a small angle, especially in a young child whose growth will correct it, we'd probably just put the limb in a cast."

## Surgery for Joint Fractures

Joint fractures usually require surgery, Yahiro says. "We try to restore the joint to perfect, like putting a jigsaw puzzle back together."

An artificial joint can be used to replace a fractured head of the long bone in the hip, like Wallace had, or in the shoulder.

Total hip joint replacements are mainly made of titanium or cobalt-chrome alloys or other metals. Each replacement has a stem that goes into the thigh bone inner canal, a ball for the head, and a plastic cup socket—the latter usually only used if the joint is badly arthritic. Yahiro often uses bipolar joints—a big ball atop a smaller one. All these joint replacements are approved by FDA.

Approved replacements for fractures in shoulder joints also consist of a ball and stem.

Andrew Bender, M.D., the orthopedist who implanted Wallace's partial replacement, says this simple model has been in use 30 to 40 years. "It has different size balls, one size stem, so it's not an exact fit. But it gives what we call a three-point fixation for some immediate tightness. The stem has holes for bone to grow through and across for more permanence."

Bender pressed in Wallace's device without cement, a snug fit. He cements only if the fit is very, very loose. "Modern day hip replacement without cement is relatively quick, both sides. She had only one side done and good bone, so it didn't take long."

If a replacement fails, it usually does so within 5 to 10 years. Simple models tend not to fail in the very old, Yahiro says. "A person in a chair or bed most of the time won't put demands on the joint that, say, Bo Jackson does." (Jackson had a hip replacement in 1992 due to a football injury.)

For higher demand, there are more precisely fitted models.

A robot that drills a more precise hole for the stem, to possibly keep the joint intact longer, is under investigation for use in cementless hip joint replacements.

An external fixator—a pin-and-rod frame—can keep the joint from being compressed by other bones, to heal before a load, or stress, is put on it again. Pins are inserted on one side of the limb through the skin, muscle and bone, out the other side, and attached to the external rod, forming the frame.

About 30 percent of patients get infected at the pin site, so meticulous hygiene is crucial. "It's a race," says Kenneth McDermott, who reviews the devices for the Center for Devices and Radiological Health. "The pin goes through the skin, and infection can go right down the pin."

Internal fixation devices pose less risk of infection. These metal plates, rods, wires, screws, nails, pins, staples, and anchors may sometimes be left in. A tiny pin may not be felt, but plates or screws may cause irritation or pain. The decision whether to remove the device in a second surgery is made on a case-by-case basis.

Surgery to remove a screw in the very old may be too risky. For a 20-year-old, benefits of a second surgery may outweigh risks. In the ankle, plates and screws are customarily removed. Yahiro says, "The bones are so superficial, the device often rubs on the shoe." McDermott gives another reason for removing a plate or screw: "It can take the load off the bone, causing the bone to resorb and weaken."

Fixators and internal fixation devices are used also for some midbone fractures.

## Grafts

The surgeon may graft bone to replace a missing segment that had to be surgically removed due to infection.

For a small segment, tissue can be taken from the patient's own bone (autologous graft).

Cadaver bone (allograft) may be used, especially for a large segment. Though dead tissue, cadaver bone provides a scaffold for living bone to grow into and remodel the graft. For healing to occur—and sometimes it doesn't—the body must put blood vessels into the graft to nurture the new living bone as it replaces the dead tissue. Healing takes longer than with an autologous graft.

Another option is a substitute bone graft, fashioned with help from nonhuman substances. FDA recently approved two such grafts:

- **Pro Osteon Implant 500 Coralline Hydroxyapatite Bone Void Filler** (1992)—Fills holes near the ends of long bones in adults. It derives from marine coral, whose spongy calcium structure resembles human cancellous bone.

- **Collagraft Bone Graft Matrix** (1993)—Treats long-bone fractures and other injury-caused areas of missing bone of 30 milliliters (1.8 cubic inches) or less. The product—consisting of purified cow collagen and a chemical, hydroxyapatite-tricalcium phosphate—is mixed with the patient's marrow into a paste and put into the area of missing bone to encourage new bone growth. It's not for use in certain patients, such as those with osteomyelitis (bone inflammation) at the fracture site, severe allergies, or allergy to cow collagen, and those being desensitized to meat products, as the treatment injections may contain cow collagen.

When these substitute grafts are placed next to healthy bone, the body remodels them in the same way it remodels human grafts. But according to Center for Devices and Radiological Health reviewer Nadine Rosile, "The substitute grafts aren't strong enough for use without a fixation device to stabilize the fracture."

A bone filler paste now under investigation, however, is as strong as bone within 12 hours, according to a report of a study of patients whose wrist fractures were injected with the paste. The report, in the March 24, 1995, issue of *Science*, stated that the paste stabilized the bone during healing and was eventually remodeled. The patients had greater grip strength at six months than historical controls (other patients in the past who had not been treated with the paste) had at two years, the report stated.

Also under investigation are injections of growth factor proteins, such as morphogenic protein and transforming growth factor-beta, found naturally in the body in very small amounts.

"The proteins turn on cells to produce bone," Yahiro says. "Animal studies show growth with injections similar to that with autologous grafts." The hope, he says, is that injected fractures, even with large areas of missing bone, will heal faster and be stronger, without grafts.

## Healing Helpers

FDA has approved seven electrical bone growth stimulators, mainly for fractures at the middle of long bones, such as the shinbone (tibia), that have not healed over at least nine months. Although exactly how the stimulators heal is unknown, manufacturers'studies showed the devices did in fact affect cellular processes.

Yahiro explains that loading (stressing) a bone produces in it a small electrical field called piezo electric force, believed to stimulate new bone formation. "It's believed that electrical stimulation does something like that on a large scale," he says.

For direct stimulation, an electrode is implanted at the fracture, linked through the skin to a generator. For indirect stimulation, electric coils outside the limb on the non-fracture side induce an electrical field at the fracture side.

In 1994, FDA approved the first ultrasound bone growth stimulator. The Sonic Accelerated Fracture Healing System (SAFHS) is for adults with small fractures in the lower leg or lower forearm. A cast or splint is used. It is the first stimulator for the treatment of fractures occurring within seven days before treatment. Studies suggest that mechanical forces of the ultrasound waves transform into electrical impulses as they travel through the tissues.

The SAFHS consists of a portable generator cabled to a small, square treatment module that emits ultrasound pulses at about the same low intensity as sonogram fetal monitors. In some instances, the patient may use the unit at home. Recommended treatment is 20 minutes once a day until the fracture heals.

The SAFHS is not for patients who need additional fixation or surgery, are pregnant or breast-feeding, have bone disease or circulatory problems, or take medicines that may adversely affect remodeling.

In studies, all treated patients—and especially older people— healed faster than those using a placebo. In those age 50 and older, arms healed 40 days faster, and legs 85 days faster. Six years' follow-up did not suggest long-term adverse effects.

Stimulation, grafts, manipulation, joint replacements, casts. Whatever the treatment, fracture healing is monitored by x-rays and physical examination to answer such questions as: Does it hurt or move when pushed on? On x-ray, does the fracture look healed? On x-ray, are the bones aligned?

For Wallace, healing is now complete. She is indeed walking again, using a cane as she did before the replacement surgery.

"If I don't use the cane, my leg aches," she says. "I'm still careful to use my good leg stepping up a curb, and my bad leg stepping down, like I learned in therapy."

## Boning up

The most important influences on fracture healing are nutrition and overall health, including bone health, before the injury, says orthopedist Martin Yahiro, M.D., a consultant to FDA. "That's why it's so important all your life to do weight-bearing exercise such as walking and get enough calcium and vitamin D, so you lay down as much bone as possible during growth and keep as much as you can later on."

The Recommended Dietary Allowance (RDA) for calcium is 1,200 milligrams a day for people ages 11 to 24 and for pregnant or breast-feeding women. For men and women older than 25 who no longer have to meet the greater demands of growth, the calcium RDA is 800 milligrams a day.

In general, genes decide bone shape and size. But mechanical stress by muscle, body weight, and physical activity influence bone shape and density—and health—throughout life.

Simply put, loaded (stressed) bone strengthens, and unloaded bone weakens. As examples, astronauts' bones weaken in outer space with no gravity pull on them, and the shaft of the humerus (long upper arm bone) in a professional tennis player's dominant arm gets denser and thicker from the extra load.

The body increases its bone mass until, usually, the mid-30s, after which a gradual loss begins.

Age-related bone loss can lead to osteoporosis, a condition of thin, weakened bone that fractures easily. The condition affects many postmenopausal women, because bone loss increases with menopause due to lower estrogen levels.

In announcing its recent approval of Fosamax and Miacalcin Nasal Spray for osteoporosis, FDA advised that patients also exercise and get adequate calcium and vitamin D. Drugs approved by FDA to prevent or treat osteoporosis are:

- estrogen—Premarin, Ogen, and Estrace tablets; Estraderm patch

- estrogen packaged with progestin hormone tablets—Prempro; Premphase

- alendronate—Fosamax
- calcitonin—Miacalcin Nasal Spray, Calcimar Injection, Miacalcin Injection, and Cibacalcin for injection.

*—by Dixie Farley*

Dixie Farley is a staff writer for FDA Consumer.

# Chapter 55

# *What's New in Prevention and Treatment*

**Abstract:** Osteoporosis affects mainly women, and is characterized by low bone density caused by poor metabolism of osteoblasts and
osteoclasts. The risks of developing the condition can be reduced with
newly-developed medicines and supplements of vitamin D and calcium. Screening techniques are described.

For women with osteoporosis, independence is as fragile as the
bones that may suddenly fail to support them. Fortunately, new methods of diagnosis and management are available to help prevent fractures in those at risk.

Conservation of bone mass relies on a delicate partnership between
two types of cells. Osteoblasts, the cells that manufacture the protein
matrix of new bone, ordinarily keep pace with osteoclasts, the cells
that clear away old bone. But this tidy process can be jostled by a
number of factors, causing resorption to outstrip formation. The dis-
ruption, technically known as uncoupling, can be generated by an
event as mundane as a few days of bed rest. Bone loss continues until equilibrium is restored between osteoblasts and osteoclasts.

Persistent bone loss threatens the skeletal integrity of an estimated
25 million people in the United States, most of them women (see "Primarily a female problem"). Some 8 million have osteoporosis, a metabolic disease marked by bones so fragile they can shatter with

*Patient Care*, August 15, 1996, p. 24. ©1996 Medical Economics Publishing
and the author, Robert Lindsay. Reprinted with permission of *Patient Care*.

apparent spontaneity. The remaining 17 million have diminished bone mass, putting them at increased risk for osteoporosis.

Reductions in bone mass are more easily prevented than treated. Although dissipation can be stalled once it begins, none of the available treatments can replace bone equal in quantity or quality to what has already been lost. All female patients are candidates for some measure of prophylaxis. The earlier you intervene with bone-conserving tactics, the better the outcome is likely to be. Still, women are never too old for treatment.

It's also clear that fracture and its attendant disability can be prevented in those who already have diminished bone density. A simple approach, consisting of supplementation with calcium and vitamin D, has been shown to reduce the risk of fracture in one study of women with an average age of 84 years.(1) Study participants taking the active regimen had 32 percent fewer nonvertebral fractures and 43 percent fewer hip fractures over a period of 18 months than those taking placebo.

## Gauging Risk

The primary risk factor for osteoporosis is advancing age. Postmenopausal osteoporosis is spurred by a decline in circulating estrogen levels, thus explaining another critical risk factor—female gender. Associated with accelerated bone loss, postmenopausal osteoporosis mainly affects cancellous trabecular bone and is assumed to be a consequence of increased bone resorption. Another age-related form of the disease, also known as senile osteoporosis, generally affects men and women older than 75 and is blamed on decreased bone formation. It's characterized by gradual erosion of both cancellous and cortical bone.

While aging is the most prominent culprit in bone loss, it's hardly the only one in osteoporosis. Bone mass at any point in life is a function of what's already been formed and what has been lost. Patients who don't form adequate peak bone mass in their younger years can be at severe risk of fracture even if they manage not to lose more later on. Diseases, drug therapies, and personal habits all can influence bone metabolism (see Table 55.1). For example, high levels of circulating corticosteroids speed bone loss, whether they're endogenously produced as a result of Cushing's syndrome or administered therapeutically for a chronic condition.

Definitive diagnosis of low bone mass or osteoporosis can't be made without a measurement of bone density, currently the most dependable predictor of fracture risk. However, a careful history can help you determine which patients are more likely to be near the so-called fracture threshold, the point where bones are so brittle they can snap with a cough or the hoisting of a grocery bag. It's particularly important to ask patients about medical problems that occurred during the adolescent growth spurt, since more than half of a woman's final bone mass is gained during that period. Disorders that delay or disrupt menstrual function, severe dietary deficits, or physical immobilization can reduce peak bone acquisition. So a bout with anorexia nervosa during the teenage years can have repercussions on the middle-aged skeleton.

**Table 55.1.** Osteoporosis Risk Factors

Advanced age

Alcohol, excessive use

Asian or Caucasian race

Caffeine, excessive use

Chronic drug therapy
Anticonvulsants
Corticosteroids
Cyclosporine (Sandimmune)
Heparin
Methotrexate

Cigarette smoking

Dietary deficiencies
Calcium
Vitamin C
Vitamin D

Disease
Anorexia nervosa
Cystic fibrosis
Hepatic insufficiency
Homocystinuria
Inflammatory bowel disease
Mastocytosis
Multiple myeloma

Disease, continued
Osteogenesis imperfecta
Rheumatoid arthritis
Sarcoidosis
Waldenstrom's macroglobulinemia

Early menopause

Endocrine disorders
Cushing's syndrome
Diabetes mellitus, type 1
Hypogonadism
Hyperparathyroidism
Hyperthyroidism

Family history of osteoporosis

Female gender

Idiopathy

Immobilization
Extended bed rest
Lengthy casting or splinting
Paralysis,
Routine inactivity

Low body weight

Small frame

Be alert to a history of bone-thinning ailments. Ask the patient about her use of alcohol, cigarettes, or chronic medication. Find out whether the patient's mother or grandmothers ever endured fractures or had evidence of vertebral deformity. Family history carries considerable weight.

One recent study identified a set of elements that independently increase the risk for hip fracture, regardless of bone density.(2) Data from more than 9,500 women indicated that those whose mother had experienced a hip fracture had twice the hip-fracture risk of women without such a maternal history, particularly if the maternal fracture occurred before age 80. Other traits that boosted the likelihood of hip fracture included a history of any type of fracture since age 50 and a tendency to spend four hours or less per day on the feet.

Inexplicably, tall stature at age 25 appeared to increase the risk of hip fracture. Researchers have suggested that tall women fall farther than their shorter counterparts or that a longer distance between the greater trochanter and inner pelvic brim is an inherent hazard. Risk also rose with increased caffeine intake and with benzodiazepine use. Clearly, some factors reflect an influence on the risk of falling and the consequences of a fall rather than a direct effect on bone.

## Primarily a Female Problem

Of the 25 million people with low bone mass in the United States, 80 percent are women. In fact, an estimated 1 of every 2 women 50 and older will have an osteoporosis-related fracture, compared with 1 in 8 men in that age-group. Here are some other numbers worth noting:

- Some 1.5 million fractures per year, including more than 300,000 hip fractures, 500,000 vertebral fractures and 200,000 wrist fractures, are attributed to osteoporosis.

- The national tab for osteoporosis-related hospital and nursing home stays has been placed at $10 billion a year and is expected to rise as the population ages.

- Women can lose up to 20 percent of their bone mass in the 5-7 years following menopause.

- White women 60 or older have at least twice the incidence of fractures as black women. Nonetheless, 1 in 5 black women are at risk of developing osteoporosis.

- Spinal osteoporosis is eight times more likely to afflict women than men.

- The rate of hip fracture is 2-3 times higher in women than men, though the death rate for men within one year after a hip fracture is 26 percent higher than in women.

- Patients with hip fracture have a 5-20 percent greater risk of dying within the first year following that injury than others in their age-group.

- Among those who were living independently before a hip fracture, 15-25 percent remain in long-term care a year after the injury.

- *Source:* Osteoporosis and Related Bone Diseases—National Resource Center.

## Bone Densitometry

The possibility of low bone mass increases with the number of patient risk factors—and the length of time those risk factors have existed. For example, a tall, thin Caucasian smoker who'd entered menopause at 43 would be at high risk, even more so if her mother had sustained a hip fracture. A technical definition of low bone mass, devised by the World Health Organization, is a bone density value that's within 1-2.5 standard deviations below the normal premenopausal mean value. Lower values signify osteoporosis.

Several radiographic methods are available for measuring bone mass. The technique currently considered most useful is dual energy X-ray absorptiometry (DXA), which provides fast, precise measurements with minimal doses of radiation (see Table 55.2). DXA can be used to measure any part of the body, though the forearm, hip, or spine—common fracture sites—are most commonly scanned. What's not yet clear is whether measurements at more than one site allow more reliable assessments of bone mass. At present, the spine is considered the site of choice when testing patients in early menopause, and a hip measurement is thought to be more useful in older women.

Generally, bone densitometry isn't considered until menopause. One excellent candidate for testing is the patient who is contemplating either starting or discontinuing estrogen replacement therapy and who might be swayed by an evaluation of her skeletal strength. A bone measurement may help decide whether the patient with primary hyperparathyroidism should undergo surgery or long-term follow-up.

431

**Table 55.2.** Techniques for Measuring Bone Mass

| Technique | Scan Charges ($) | Site | Scan Time (minutes) | Precision Error (percent)[1] | Accuracy Error (percent)[2] | Radiation Exposure (millirem) |
|---|---|---|---|---|---|---|
| Dual energy X-ray Absorptiometry | 150-300 | Spine, hip | 5-10 | 0.5-3 | 3-9 | <5 |

Comment: An X-ray energy source releases photons of two distinct energies, permitting imaging of thicker body parts. Advantages include scanning speed, low radiation dose, and precision. A total body scan can be accomplished in 20 minutes, minimizing errors from patient motion.

| | | | | | | |
|---|---|---|---|---|---|---|
| Dual Photon Absoptometry | 150-300 | Spine, hip | 20-40 | 2-5 | 3-10 | 5-10 |

Comment: Can quantify total body mass. Uses an isotopic ($^{153}$Gd) energy source that emits photons of two distinct energies.

| | | | | | | |
|---|---|---|---|---|---|---|
| Quantitative Computed Tomography (QCT) | 150-400 | Spine | 10-30 | 2-6 | 5-15 | 100-1,000 (100-300 for newer scanners) |

Comment: Uses conventional CT and commercially available software to measure bone in three-dimensional sections. Can separate cortical from trabecular bone with great anatomic detail. Exposes patients to more radiation than other methods—about the dose received with a chest film. A version known as peripheral OCT measures bone density at the wrist.

**Table 55.2.** Techniques for Measuring Bone Mass

| Technique | Scan Charges ($) | Site | Scan Time (minutes) | Precision Error (percent)[1] | Accuracy Error (percent)[2] | Radiation Exposure (millirem) |
|---|---|---|---|---|---|---|
| Radiographic Absorptiometry | 90-160 | Hands | 5-10 | 2-4 | 5-10 | 10-100 |
| Comment: Used mainly to measure the phalanges, which are a mixture of cortical and trabecular bone with minimal overlying soft tissue. A computer-assisted densitometric measurement is made from the resulting x-ray image. | | | | | | |
| Single Photon Absorptiometry (SPA) | 50-150 | Heel, forearm | 5-15 | 2-5 | 3-8 | 2-5 |
| Comment: The iodine ([125]) radiation source must be replaced several times a year, possibly reducing instrument reliability. SPA is being supplanted by a similar x-ray-based method called single energy x-ray absorptiometry, which offers improved precision and speed. | | | | | | |

[1]Variability in measurements occurring with repeated measurements of the same object. Particularly important when serial measurements are used to document bone loss over time.
[2]Degree to which the measurement varies from the accepted standard value.

Source: Agency for Health Care Policy and Research: Bone Densitometry: Patients with Asymptomatic Primary Hyperparathyroidism, Rockville, Md., US Dept of Health and Human Services, 1995.

433

Testing should be considered for patients coping with bone-wasting medical conditions or drug regimens. It's also advisable when another event trips your suspicions. For example, consider densitometry for the patient who sustains a fracture after relatively minor injury or for the one whose X-ray film suggests osteopenia.

You do not need to measure bone density in the patient with multiple fractures and the two body changes typical of osteoporosis: kyphosis—commonly known as dowager's hump—and height loss. The evidence is clear in such a case. Similarly, densitometry may not be necessary for the patient who wants to take hormone replacement therapy since the test results will not alter the course of her treatment.

Densitometry can be used to follow patients' progress after they've begun treatment for osteoporosis. An interval of 1-2 years between tests is usually sufficient. The longer you wait, the more apt you are to see a perceivable difference. Measurements should be made on a more frequent basis, perhaps every six months, when patients are likely to be losing bone rapidly, as in those taking long-term corticosteroid therapy.

Undoubtedly, new diagnostic techniques will be developed in the next 5-10 years, making widespread screening a more feasible option. Ultrasound techniques are under scrutiny, though their usefulness in determining fracture risk has yet to be defined. Evidence suggests that ultrasound may be able to estimate bone mass and also provide information about bone architecture, biomechanical properties, and geometry, all elements that contribute to bone quality.

## Metabolic Milestones

Another strategy measures serum or urine markers of bone remodeling. Urinary tests quantify breakdown products of collagen, specifically deoxypyridinoline, pyridinoline, pyridinium collagen cross-links, and other substances. This provides an indication of how fast bone is being resorbed. Levels of these elements should decrease as bone destruction slows. Serum markers of bone formation include bone-specific alkaline phosphatase, osteocalcin, and procollagen-1 extension peptides.

Two such tests—Osteomark and Pyrilinks—are approved for monitoring the effect of osteoporosis treatments, but whether they can help predict fracture risk is still to be established. While levels of these substances are a manifestation of bone turnover, they don't disclose absolute information about bone status. Densitometry remains the only way to estimate bone mass. A high remodeling rate in a patient with very high bone density would suggest rapid bone loss even in the patient who is not at serious risk of fracture. Then again, a moderate metabolic rate would be falsely reassuring in a patient who has very low bone mass. Some experts believe that markers of bone metabolism have more prognostic value in patients 65 and older since bone density has, presumably, already been compromised to some degree.

Nonetheless, metabolic benchmarks have potential applications. Mainly they can be used to monitor patient compliance and drug efficacy. These tests produce evidence of progress faster than densitometry. Some change in marker levels should be apparent within six months of beginning treatment. That can help motivate patients who have yet to develop symptoms of disease. Measures of biochemical markers may also provide information about the effect of menopause on bone remodeling. Or they may ultimately help physicians choose the best therapy for individual patients.

## Estrogen Replacement Therapy

Like bone densitometry, prescription drug therapy for prevention and treatment of osteoporosis generally isn't considered until the patient approaches menopause. An exception might be the younger woman with risk factors for osteoporosis who has experienced fractures following minor trauma, a strong suggestion of bone fragility. Alendronate sodium, calcitonin-salmon, and estrogen replacement therapy (ERT) are approved for treatment of women with post-menopausal osteoporosis. All inhibit bone resorption. ERT remains the treatment of choice. Its ability to preserve bone mass and prevent fractures is firmly established, and the long-term risks of therapy have been well-documented.

ERT can reduce the risk of osteoporotic fracture by as much as 50 percent. Unlike the other therapies prescribed for patients with low bone mass, it also provides significant protection against cardiovascular disease and alleviates the symptoms of menopause. And ERT is not particularly expensive (see Table 55.3).

Then again, ERT's effect on multiple body systems poses potential dilemmas. The recurrence of menstrual-like bleeding and premenstrual symptoms is a nuisance many women would prefer to avoid. More worrisome is the possible connection between ERT and cancers of the breast and uterus. In addition, ERT's protective effects on bone endure only as long as therapy continues. It appears that durable skeletal preservation requires indefinite administration of estrogen. Cessation of treatment precipitates a period of accelerated bone lose.

**Table 55.3.** Drugs Used in Prevention and Treatment of Osteoporosis

| Drug | Dosage | Cost ($) |
| --- | --- | --- |
| Alendronate sodium (Fosamax) | 10 mg/d | 1.67 per 1 0-mg tablet |
| Calcitonin-salmon, injection(Calcimar, Miacalcin) | 100 IU/d SC or IM | 27.48-42.45 per 2-mL vial (200 IU/mL) |
| Calcitonin-salmon, nasal spray (Miacalcin) | 200 IU/d intranasally (alternating nostrils daily) | 25.03 per 2-mL bottle (2,200 IU/mL) |
| Conjugated estrogens (Premarin) | 0.625 mg/d cyclically, 3 wk on followed by 1 wk off | 0.39 per 0.625-mg tablet |
| Conjugated estrogens and medroxyprogesterone acetate (Premphase) | 0.625 mg/d conjugated estrogens, d 1-14; 0.625 mg conjugated estrogens/5 mg medroxyprogesterone, d 15-28 | 16.39 per 28-d cycle |
| Conjugated estrogens and medroxyprogesterone acetate (Prempro) | 0.625 mg conjugated estrogens/2-5 mg medroxyprogesterone daily | 17.88 per 28-d cycle |
| Estradiol, micronized (Estrace) | 0.5 mg/d cyclically, 23 d on followed by 5 d off | 0.26 per 0.5-mg tablet |
| Estradid transdermal system (Climara, Estraderm, Vivelle) | 0.05 mg/24 h (Estraderm and Vivelle are applied twice aweek; Climara, once every 7 d) | 2.23 per Estraderrn patch, 2.45 per Vivelle patch, 4.94 per Climara patch |
| Estropipate (Ogen) | 0.625 mg/d for 25 d of a 31-d cycle | 0.33-0.53 per 0.625-mg tablet |
| Etidronate disodium (Didronel—unlabeled use) | 400 mg/d for 2 wk every 3 mo. Daily calcium supplementation is givenfor remainder of cycle. | 3.63 per 400-mg tablet |

**Note:** *Cost shown is average wholesale price, based on information in* PDP Generics *1996 and* Red Book Update, *May 1996. Both are publications of Medical Economics, Montvale, N.J.*

The threat of endometrial malignancy is reduced by prescribing combined estrogen-progestin therapy for any patient with an intact uterus. Conjugated estrogens are generally paired with medroxyprogesterone acetate. (Unlabeled use for medroxyprogesterone.) Higher dosages of the progestin-5-10 mg—administered on a cyclical basis provide predictable periods of withdrawal bleeding. Cycles need not occur monthly. For example, you can prescribe a daily 0.625-mg dose of estrogen for a two-month cycle with medroxyprogesterone taken in combination during the first or last 12 days of that interval.

Continuous daily administration of medroxyprogesterone, 2.5 mg, may circumvent vaginal bleeding altogether in most women. An uninterrupted regimen of estrogen and progestin usually causes some spotting and irregular bleeding for several months, then bleeding stops completely. Occasionally, women have erratic bleeding episodes that show no sign of abating after six months or more. This situation is more likely to develop when patients are in early menopause. A cyclical regimen may prove more convenient in such cases.

But there's no evidence that concomitant use of progestin protects breast tissue. Fear of breast cancer discourages many prospective ERT users. While the issue has yet to be settled, the risk of breast cancer from ERT—if it indeed confers a risk—is believed to be less powerful than age, family history, and other risk factors for the disease.

In fact, considerations other than bone density usually prompt the decision to initiate therapy. Generally, any woman who has no contraindications—the primary one being a history of breast cancer—and is willing to try ERT can do so, whether she's interested in preventing bone loss, cardiovascular disease, or menopausal symptoms. Those taking ERT should be especially conscientious about obtaining an annual clinical breast exam and mammogram. An endometrial biopsy is advisable for the woman who has persistent abnormal postmenopausal vaginal bleeding before beginning ERT or off-cycle bleeding during therapy.

More bone is conserved when ERT begins shortly after menopause begins. Perhaps as much as 20 percent of the skeleton is maintained under the influence of estrogen, and that component slips away without the hormone. One recent study found that current use of estrogen diminished the risk for hip, wrist, and nonspinal fractures but was more effective if started within five years of menopause and used for longer than 10 years? The risk of hip, fracture was reduced by 80 percent in women older than 75 who were using estrogen at the time of the study.

Although estrogen doesn't build new bone, there is an initial rise in bone mass early in treatment, followed by stabilization. The increase is modest—an estimated 1-3 percent in cortical bone and possibly 8-10 percent in the more metabolic cancellous bone.(4) A daily dosage of conjugated estrogens, 0.625 mg, is protective for most women whether or not they've endured previous fractures. Higher dosages are frequently required for the patient who's seeking relief from menopausal symptoms. Transdermal estrogen therapy has been credited with a 5.3 percent increase in lumbar spine bone mineral density and a more than 50 percent reduction in the vertebral fracture rate.(5) Both oral and transdermal estrogen work well, although vaginally applied estrogen preparations don't provide reliable systemic effects.

## Other Treatment Options

In the second half of 1995, the FDA approved two new therapeutic alternatives to estrogen for the treatment of postmenopausal osteoporosis, alendronate sodium and calcitonin-salmon nasal spray. Both inhibit bone resorption. Alendronate, a member of the bisphosphonate class of compounds, is adsorbed onto bone, apparently fortifying it against osteoclasts. Calcitonin, a hormone secreted by the mammalian thyroid gland, helps moderate calcium and bone metabolism. Neither has an effect on any body system other than the skeleton. That fact clarifies safety issues to some degree but creates questions about cost-effectiveness since the newer therapies, unlike estrogen, offer no additional benefits. Before prescribing either drug, make sure the patient has low bone density or a history of osteoporotic fracture.

### *The Bisphosphonates*

Data from a study of nearly 900 women show that 10 mg of alendronate administered daily for three years provided significant increases in bone mineral density of the spine, hip, and total body.(6) Patients taking the drug had an overall increase of about 8 percent in spine bone mineral density, compared with a loss of bone mass in those taking placebo. A 50 percent decrease in the proportion of women with new vertebral fractures was also noted. The results suggest an effect comparable to that of estrogen therapy.

Alendronate does not seem to be metabolized, and it has a lengthy terminal half-life—more than 10 years. That means that the drug remains in the body long after therapy stops. It's not yet clear if this has any harmful consequences since alendronate hasn't been administered to anybody for longer than six years. Postmarketing studies

438

have yet to disclose signs of skeletal toxicity. Until information about extended use is available, alendronate is probably most appropriate for women who can't or won't take estrogen and who have low bone mass and a history of fracture.

Women with disorders of the upper GI tract, such as esophageal strictures, gastroesophageal reflux disease, or hiatal hernia, may be more vulnerable to drug-related GI disturbances. The bisphosphonates are irritating as well as poorly absorbed. Patients must be instructed to take alendronate upon awakening with 6-8 oz of water. At least 30 minutes must elapse before food, other liquids, or additional medications are ingested. During this interval, patients must remain upright. Lying down within one half hour of administration can provoke esophageal irritation.

Another bisphosphonate, etidronate disodium, has regularly been used to prevent bone loss in postmenopausal women, although it has not been approved for that purpose. Etidronate has been shown to increase bone mass, but study data did not convince the FDA that the drug reduced the incidence of vertebral fractures. In contrast to alendronate, etidronate is administered cyclically, for two weeks every three months. Also poorly absorbed, it should be taken with a full glass of water two hours before or two hours after eating. Patients must be instructed not to ingest calcium-rich foods or metal-containing vitamins and antacids within two hours of a dose of etidronate.

An IV bisphosphonate has also been used on an unlabeled basis. Pamidronate disodium sidesteps GI adverse reactions, but patients have to be willing to endure a monthly four-hour IV infusion. Doses range from 60-90 mg.

## *Calcitonin-salmon*

Even though injectable calcitonin-salmon carries a general indication for the treatment of postmenopausal osteoporosis, the nasal formulation is specifically labeled for women who have low bone mass, are five years past menopause, and can't or won't take estrogen. Calcitonin does not have as large an effect on bone mass as alendronate or estrogen. And definitive evidence that calcitonin reduces fracture risk is not yet available, though fracture studies are under way.

Nonetheless, calcitonin might be an appropriate choice when estrogen replacement is not an option for the older patient with a GI disorder or an already complicated medication regimen. The nasal spray is easy to administer, and patients don't have to juggle each dose with dietary intake. They do however, have to take in at least 1,000 mg of elemental calcium and 400 IU of vitamin D per day, and that means faithful adherence to supplementation. As with estrogen, the benefits of therapy last only as long as treatment.

Calcitonin has its advantages. It's very safe and has a low incidence of adverse reactions. Nausea, which occurs in perhaps 10 percent of patients treated with the injectable form, tends to decrease with continued use. The nasal version is associated with a 1-3 percent incidence of nausea. Rhinitis is more common, occurring in some 12 percent of patients. The drug also provides an analgesic effect, an asset for patients with pain from osteoporotic fractures.

### Unestablished Strategies

There's currently no information suggesting that a patient who's taking estrogen can't take alendronate too, but scientific evidence supporting the value of such a composite is still being accrued. A trial comparing alendronate to estrogen to a combination of the two is scheduled to continue into next year. Some experts may begin treating a patient who has fractures with calcitonin, later moving on to alendronate once pain is controlled and a stronger bone-sparing effect is desired, even though no formal protocol for doing so exists.

The FDA's Endocrinologic and Metabolic Drugs Advisory Committee recently endorsed the use of slow-release sodium fluoride in the treatment of patients with bone loss, but the agency has yet to confer final approval. Fluoride directly stimulates bone formation, an observation backed by studies demonstrating an increase in bone density for treated patients. Concerns about its narrow therapeutic window and its effect on fracture rate have existed for more than a decade, since studies of immediate-release agents suggested that fluoride propels formation of abnormal bone with reduced elasticity and tensile strength—bone that is actually more breakable. In addition, fluoride is irritating to the GI tract and can cause ulcers. The sustained-release agent circumvents that problem by gradually discharging small doses.

Tamoxifen citrate, (Unlabeled use.) which is primarily but not purely an antiestrogen, has a bone-sparing effect at the usual dosage of 20 mg/d. For that reason, it can be useful in the treatment of menopausal women who have had breast cancer. Tamoxifen does stimulate endometrial tissue, and therapy should be limited to five years. After that, the risk of adverse reactions outweighs any benefits.

Thiazide diuretics reduce calcium excretion and, for that reason, have been considered possibly useful in preservation of bone. While studies have suggested that the thiazides might be beneficial in women with osteoporosis, data have not been explicit enough to spur ardent recommendations. One recent study indicated that use of thiazide or non-thiazide diuretics was associated with a positive effect on bone mass density? But weight proved most highly predictive of bone-mass density—greater weight was tied to greater bone mass. Another trial found thinner women to be at considerably more risk of hip fracture than heavier women but discovered no significant protective effect of thiazide diuretics once researchers made adjustments for body-mass index. The resulting interpretation was that heavy women were simply more likely to be using thiazide diuretics.

A number of new compounds are under investigation for their ability to build or retain bone. These include a recombinant human parathyroid hormone, a bisphosphonate, and estrogen analogs (see "Drugs in development"). The last, also known as designer estrogens, are constructed to deliver beneficial hormonal effects without detrimental ones. In essence, these agents would be good for the bones, the heart, and the urogenital system without stimulating breast or endometrial tissue.

## Lifestyle Tactics

All women should be advised to eliminate the risk factors for osteoporosis that are within their control. Nicotine poisons bone as well as other tissues. Smokers should be encouraged to quit (see "The growing problem of smoking in women"). Advise patients to limit their use of alcohol.

Good nutrition is also important. To maximize peak bone mass or reduce bone loss, women need to ingest adequate amounts of calcium—approximately 1,000 mg/d for adults, 1,200 mg/d for adolescents, and 1,500 mg/d for postmenopausal women. It is estimated that the average American diet furnishes about 500 mg daily. An 8-oz glass of skim milk will provide approximately 300 mg of calcium, as will 8 oz of calcium-fortified orange juice, 1 1/2 cups of boiled broccoli, or about 6 oz of canned salmon. Dietary sources of calcium are preferable, but supplementation is a useful alternative for those who won't increase their calcium intake from food sources.

Of the available calcium salts, calcium carbonate supplies the greatest percentage of elemental calcium at 40 percent; calcium glubionate the least at 6.5 percent. Preparations of calcium acetate (25 percent), calcium citrate (21 percent), calcium gluconate (9 percent), calcium lactate (13 percent), and tricalcium phosphate (39 percent) are also available. Most patients should be able to take calcium carbonate with no problem. One increasingly popular source is the chewable antacid Tums. Calcium citrate may be preferable for the patient with GI problems, including constipation, or those who are prone to calcium-based kidney stones. Whatever the form chosen, recommend administration with meals to maximize absorption.

Adequate vitamin D intake, necessary as well, is most likely to be a problem for those wintering in the northern United States. Daily use of a multivitamin containing 400 IU of vitamin D should overcome deprivation due to a lack of sunshine. Patients should also be advised to take in adequate amounts of vitamin C and protein, as deficiencies in these nutrients can affect bone metabolism.

Urge patients to undertake some sort of weight-bearing exercise, particularly walking, for a minimum of 30 minutes 3-4 times per week. The skeleton is designed to accommodate the burden that it habitually receives.

Regular stress does more than conserve bone. It also helps maintain flexibility and muscle strength, assets in preventing falls and subsequent injury. Patients who make exercise a social activity are more likely to stick with it. Suggest ways of incorporating exercise into the daily routine. For instance, advise patients to take steps instead of elevators or park the car farther from their destination than they ordinarily might.

Patients should also do what they can to minimize the chance of injury. Remind women that certain medications can affect attentiveness or balance. Any condition that reduces visual acuity can also be troublesome. Recommend that grab bars be installed in the bathtub and in any other locations where a fall is likely. Tell them that clutter may also prove hazardous to health. Scatter rugs, extension cords, or other objects that increase the chance of a stumble should be kept to a minimum.

## References

1. Chapuy MC, Arlot ME, Duboeuf F: Vitamin D3 and calcium to prevent hip fractures in elderly women. *N Engl J Med* 1992;327:1637-1642.

2. Cummings SR, Nevitt MC, Browner WS: Risk factors for hip fracture in white women. *N Engl J Med* 1995;332:767-773.

3. Cauley JA, Seeley DG, Ensrud K, et al: Estrogen replacement therapy and fractures in older women. *Ann Intern Med* 1995;122:9-16.

4. Lindsay R: Criteria for successful estrogen therapy in osteoporosis. *Osteoporos Int* 1993(suppl 2):9-13.

5. Lufkin EG, Wahner HW, O'Fallon WM, et al: Treatment of postmenopausal osteoporosis with transdermal estrogen. *Ann Intern Med* 1992;117:1-9.

6. Liberman UA, Weiss SR, Broil J, et al: Effect of oral alendronate on bone mineral density end the incidence of fractures in postmenopausal osteoporosis. *N Engl J Med* 1995;333:1437-1443.

7. Orwoll ES, Bauer DC, Vogt TM, et al: Axial bone mass in older women. *Ann Intern Med* 1996;124:187-196.

8. Grisso JA, Kelsey JL, Strom BL: Risk factors for hip fracture in black women. *N Engl J Med* 1994;330:1555-1559.

### Suggested Reading

Black DM: Why elderly women should be screened and treated to prevent osteoporosis. *Am J Med* 1995;98(suppl 2A):67S-75S.

Christiansen C: What should be done at the time of menopause? *Am J Med* 1995;98(suppl 2A):56S-59S.

Dargent-Molina P, Favier F, Grandjean H, et al: Fall-related factors and risk of hip fracture: The EPIDOS prospective study. *Lancet* 1996;348:145-149.

Delmas PD: Biochemical markers of bone turnover I: Theoretical considerations and clinical use in osteoporosis. *Am J Med* 1993(suppl 5A);95:11S-16S.

Gambert SR, Schultz BM, Hemdy RC: Osteoporosis: Clinical features, prevention, and treatment, *Endccrinol Metab Clin North Am* 1995;24:317-371.

Kanis JA: Treatment of osteoporosis in elderly women. *Am J Med* 1995;98(suppl 2A):60S-66S.

Kaplan FS: Prevention and management of osteoporosis. *Clin Syrup* 1995;47:2-32.

Khosla S, Riggs BL: Concise review for primary-care physicians: Treatment options for osteoporosis. *Mayo Clin Proc* 1995;70:978-982.

Lindsey R: Hormone replacement therapy for prevention and treatment of osteoporosis. *Am J Med* 1993;95(suppl 5A):37S-39S.

Marshall D, Johnell O, Wedel H: Meta-analysis of how well measures of bone mineral density predict occurrence of osteoporotic fractures. *BMJ* 1996;312:1254-1259.

Odell WD, Heath H: Osteoporosis: Pathophysiology, prevention, diagnosis, and treatment. *Dis Mon* 1993;39:791-667.

Riggs BL, Melton L.J III: The worldwide problem of osteoporosis: Insights afforded by epidemiology. *Bone* 1995(suppl 5);17:505S-511S.

Riis BJ: The role of bone loss. *Am J Med* 1995;98(suppl 2A):29S-32S.

Riis BJ: Biochemical markers of bone turnover II: Diagnosis, prophylaxis, and treatment of osteoporosis. *Am J Med* 1993(suppl 5A);95:17S-21S.

# Chapter 56

# *Treating Fractures: Wrist, Vertebral, and Hip*

## *Wrist Fracture*

Mrs. M., 61 years old, slipped on the ice this winter. When she tried to break her fall, she landed on her outstretched hand and broke her wrist.

### *Definition*

Wrist fracture is the most common type of fracture before the age of 75. In women, the number of wrist fractures increases at menopause and plateaus after age 65. This increased incidence is most likely related to the rapid loss of bone in the years following, menopause. Since men do not experience menopause, the incidence of wrist fracture in men remains fairly constant. Wrist fracture occurs most often in women who are relatively healthy and active and have good reflexes. In fact, the majority of wrist fractures occur outdoors during the winter months when snow and ice make walking treacherous, and falls are common.

The wrist is made up of two bones in the lower arm, the radius and ulna, plus the small bones of the hand. The most common wrist

This chapter contains text from three documents in the National Osteoporosis Foundation's "Strategies for People with Osteoporosis" series: "Wrist Fracture," "Recovering from Hip Fracture," and "After the Vertebral Fracture,"© NOF, 1997. Reprinted with permission from the National Osteoporosis Foundation, Washington, DC 20037.

445

fracture occurs when a person extends an arm to break a fall. The hand and forearm take all the weight and force from the fall, and one of the wrist bones breaks. When the radius breaks within one or two inches of the wrist (the distal radius), the fracture is called a Colles fracture, named after the doctor who first described it. Colles fractures occur most frequently in postmenopausal women. The risk for Colles fracture appears to be related to the bone density of the distal radius. A wrist fracture can be a sign of underlying problems such as low bone density, balance problems, vision problems, or hearing loss.

### Diagnosis

Following a fall, you may be bruised and sore. Sometimes, a fracture may be misdiagnosed as a bad sprain, and the pain, limited movement, and weak hand grasp in the affected arm is ignored. If you have persistent pain, swelling near the wrist, changes in finger movement, or numbness, your wrist is probably fractured rather than sprained. Usually, an x-ray can confirm the diagnosis. Once the fracture is diagnosed, appropriate treatment begins.

### Treatment and Rehabilitation

The primary goal of treatment and rehabilitation is to return normal movement to the affected hand and wrist. Throughout the healing process there will be exercises that you must do to preserve movement and flexibility, and build strength.

The appropriate treatment depends on the location and severity of the fracture. A simple fracture means that the bone has broken, but the broken edges remain close enough together that simple manipulation realigns the involved bone (known as reduction of the fracture). A more complex fracture means that multiple pieces of bone are broken or that the joint is involved. In this case, a cast alone may be inadequate and surgery may be required.

The first cast or splint will extend above the elbow to restrict movement of both the elbow and wrist. Your health care provider will teach you exercises for your fingers and shoulder on the affected side. It is important that you perform these exercises for short periods of time several times a day, even while in the cast. This will prevent finger stiffness later on, one of the side effects of the Colles fracture.

Over the first two to three weeks, your wrist will be x-rayed weekly. If the bones have slipped out of position, an operation may be needed to reposition the bones and pin them in place. In any case, the cast or splint is removed after six or eight weeks. Both active and passive exercises for the hand, wrist, forearm, elbow and shoulder will help you regain your strength and maintain mobility. After the cast or splint is removed, you may occasionally use a wrist splint or elastic wrap to support and protect the joint. Sometimes, the wrist may not look exactly the same as it did before the fracture, but with proper physical therapy, little function will be lost.

Initially, you will need assistance with your daily routine. If the break is in your dominant arm, you may need help with the easiest tasks: getting dressed, combing your hair, even brushing your teeth. Very independent people will find this a frustrating experience, but it helps to focus on the fact that wrist fractures heal and exercises strengthen the arm quickly. Before you know it, you will be back to normal.

The secondary goal of treatment is to determine whether osteoporosis is present. Since wrist fractures occurring in women ages 40-60 can be the result of osteoporosis, or may be an early warning sign of it, a bone density test would be appropriate at this time. A bone density test measures your current bone health and is the only way to predict your risk for future fractures.

### Prevention of Future Fractures

If osteoporosis is present, or the risk of your developing it is high, appropriate steps must be taken to maintain existing bone density. If your bone density is in the normal range, you should focus on preserving your bone health. Studies have shown that an adequate calcium and vitamin D intake and weight-bearing exercises preserve bone density. If the test shows that your bone density is low, calcium, vitamin D, and exercise may not be enough to protect against osteoporosis. Your doctor may prescribe a medication to prevent or slow further bone loss.

If you have not had a vision and hearing test in some time, this would be a good time to do so. Corrected vision and the best hearing possible can help prevent falls.

## After the Vertebral Fracture

Osteoporosis is a disease that causes bone to become weak and easily broken. Osteoporotic fractures can result from a fall, the lifting of a heavy object, or a sudden twisting motion. Sometimes an activity that is not considered stressful or dangerous, such as bending over to pick up a newspaper, sneezing, turning a key in a lock, or receiving an affectionate hug, can result in a fractured vertebra, a broken wrist, or a cracked rib.

When Mr. Johnson, 72, broke two vertebrae, he had many questions about what to expect. Would there be a cast or a brace put on his back? How long would it be before he could resume gardening and his other hobbies? Mr. Johnson's doctor scheduled a special appointment with Mr. and Mrs. Johnson to answer their questions about what they could expect in the next several months. This is what he and his wife learned:

### Q. Mr. Johnson: How long will it take for me to recover from these broken bones?

**A. Dr. Smith:** A fractured vertebra can take anywhere from 6 to 8 weeks for the bone to set and up to 12 weeks to heal completely. But recovery from a vertebral fracture goes beyond healing the bone. Recovery becomes an ongoing process to enable you to regain strength and mobility and to resume your daily activities.

Everyone experiences a slightly different recuperation. You may find your posture changing and have some nagging pain. This is because a vertebral fracture results in a deformity of the vertebra itself, which affects the muscles, tendons, ligaments, and nerves near the fractured bone. Fortunately, there are steps you can take to minimize these consequences of vertebral fracture.

### Q. Will I need surgery to correct the fracture?

**A.** No, surgery is not required with a vertebral fracture.

### Q. Will I have to stay in bed the whole time?

**A.** Bed rest for the first 2-3 days following a fracture is important. The body has suffered a trauma—a broken bone—and needs time and rest in order to heal. How long you stay in bed depends on how much pain you feel and how long you can be up before your back starts hurting again. In general, we encourage people to be active as soon as pain permits.

During the healing period, you may find that you need help doing things you ordinarily do for yourself, like dressing, bathing, getting in and out of bed or chairs. It's okay to ask for help during this time. Just remember, you won't remain in this dependent condition if you give yourself time to heal and take the proper steps toward recovery.

While it's important to rest after you've had a vertebral fracture, it is also important to get up and around as soon as you can. Bones and muscles respond well to movement and activity and, in the long run, you'll improve more quickly if you are able to slowly ease back into your usual routine. If you have access to a pool, walking in the water is a great way to maintain and use your muscles without putting stress on the bone that is healing.

## Q. What medications will I be taking now?

**A.** You will be given pain medication and a different medication to prevent further bone loss so you'll be less likely to fracture again. For pain control, we'll start you on simple, over-the-counter analgesics. We'll also use heating pads, ice packs, and gentle massage to alleviate the pain. If the pain does not subside with these methods, you may be given prescription pain-killers. The duration and intensity of pain is different for every person and often depends on how many vertebral fractures one has had.

To prevent further bone loss and reduce the risk of future fractures, your physician may prescribe estrogen (for women), alendronate, or calcitonin. Research currently is underway for additional medications to prevent and treat osteoporosis.

I will also want you to be sure to get 1,000 mg per day of calcium and at least 400 IU of vitamin D each day.

## Q. Will osteoporosis cause my back to curve over? I would like to avoid developing stooped posture if I can.

**A.** The back curvature you refer to is called Kyphosis. Kyphosis is the result of physical changes in the spine and adjacent muscles, tendons, and ligaments that occur after vertebral fractures. The degree of kyphosis varies with the number of fractures and muscle strength. To minimize the curvature, you will need to learn flexibility and strengthening exercises for your back and torso. I know a rehabilitation clinic with specialties in physical medicine and rehabilitation who can work with you on these exercises. You probably won't start the therapeutic exercise for about two to four weeks after the fracture, depending on how you're feeling. You'll start out slowly at first; the therapy can be painful, but in the long run you will have the benefits of a stronger back, increased flexibility, and straighter posture.

## Q. Should I wear a back brace?

**A.** A back brace or support may be beneficial during the healing period for several reasons: 1) it helps the patient avoid strenuous bending; 2) it provides some pain relief by supporting the spine; and 3) it helps reduce the degree of kyphosis. If a brace is used too much or for too long a time, the back muscles will weaken, which is actually worse for spinal osteoporosis because strong, muscles help support the spine. Physical therapy, in the form of exercises to strengthen the back and torso, can be performed even while the individual is wearing the brace.

There are several different types of braces to choose from. If you find that your pain persists or if your posture starts to stoop drastically, we can fit you with the appropriate brace.

Another type of support you might find useful is a cane or walker. While you are recovering from the fracture, you may be a little unsteady on your feet and a cane or walker will give you better balance. Also, these devices take weight off of your spine, which can ease some of the pain you feel in the first few weeks.

**Q. Will I have to buy a special mattress to protect my back?**

**A.** A very firm mattress is best for people with spinal osteoporosis. For comfort, you can cover it with synthetic sheepskin or an egg crate mattress pad. If you have a very soft mattress, you may have to buy a new one. But before you do that, try putting a piece of plywood on top of the box spring beneath the mattress. This may provide the support your spine needs.

**Q. What kinds of changes will I have to make in my life? My wife and I have plans to do some traveling.**

**A.** You will be able to resume nearly all of your normal activities with minimal change to your routine. You can still travel and garden. In fact, being active is beneficial to your health.

The chances you do have to make involve the way you move and the safety of your environment. For example, no more bending from the waist to pick something up. You'll have to learn to bend your knees. Activities that require a twisting motion of the torso, such as golf, put a heavy strain on the spine and should be avoided. And no lifting of anything heavier than a light bag of groceries, depending on the severity of the osteoporosis.

You should fall-proof your home to minimize the chances of tripping and falling. Be careful when taking medications that might make you dizzy, and be aware of the effects of alcohol on your balance.

**Q. I'm usually not the kind of person to talk about my troubles, but this osteoporosis is pretty serious and I'm worried about it. Is there a group of people I could get together with to discuss some of these changes?**

**A.** Attending a support group is great way to share information and discuss feelings as you learn to cope with these changes. The purse can give you the name and phone number of the osteoporosis support group leader in the area. Many of my patients and their family members attend meetings regularly. Quite often a speaker comes to the meetings to present information on different aspects of osteoporosis prevention and treatment. I have spoken at a couple of the meetings myself.

## Recovery from Hip Fracture

Fran Smith, 78, fractured her hip last night. Her hospital admission physical exam revealed osteoporosis. Fran asked her doctor what to expect in terms of recovery. The doctor assured Fran that, in time, she would be able to get back on her feet and return to independent living. The doctor did stress that treatment, participation in rehabilitation activities, and a positive attitude are important for a successful recovery.

### Definition

A hip fracture is a broken bone near the top of the femur or thigh bone. The femur is the long, straight bone that runs from the knee to the hip joint. The top of the femur angles in towards the body where its rounded ball-shaped end fits into a C-shaped cavity in the pelvic bone. This kind of joint is called a ball and socket joint. The hip most commonly fractures near the top of the femur or at the angle where the bone connects to the body.

An operation is usually necessary to repair a fractured hip. The surgeon repairs some fractures by inserting a pin to hold the bones together while they heal. Other fractures require a hip replacement which is done with a prosthesis or artificial ball and/or joint socket.

### Recovery and Rehabilitation

After surgery, rehabilitation begins so that weight bearing, standing, and attempting to walk are possible in the first week. At this time, your doctor may prescribe medications to prevent further bone loss as well as appropriate amounts of calcium and vitamin D.

When you are sent home after surgery, you may have frequent, scheduled appointments with specialists such as physiatrists, doctors who specialize in physical medicine and rehabilitation, visiting nurses, physical therapists, and occupational therapists. If you are being discharged to your home, you may remain in the hospital from one to three weeks before discharge. If you are discharged to a rehabilitation facility, your hospital stay may be shorter.

If there is no one to help you at home, you may be sent to a rehabilitation facility or nursing home. Here, people will help you learn to care for yourself again. As you become stronger and more mobile, you may continue physical therapy as an outpatient, coming into the hospital or rehabilitation facility daily or several times a week to ensure continued progress.

You will begin physical therapy immediately after surgery. Physical therapists focus on getting you back on your feet even though you feel unsteady and initially it hurts to move. You will do exercises to increase the strength, flexibility, and stamina of your hip muscles. In the beginning, you may need to use a wheelchair to get around. As you get stronger and the pain decreases, you will graduate to a walker, crutches, or a cane. Physical therapists will instruct you on walking with the aid of crutches, a walker, or a cane, getting up and down stairs, maneuvering around obstacles in your home, and getting, into and out of a car. By the end of three months, you may need assistive devices only occasionally.

Occupational therapists teach you how to dress, bathe, and care for your personal needs and can assess your home environment and identify appliances and aids to help you function independently. They can also make recommendations that make your home environment safer for you. Some changes may include a chair or grasp rails in the tub, removal of scatter rugs, and the substitution of a tall, high-backed chair instead of a low, soft easy chair.

Recovery from a hip fracture can take four to eight months. In the early weeks of rehabilitation, your activities will be limited, and you will need to rely on others for shopping, cooking, cleaning, bathing, and even dressing yourself. For some people, acknowledging how dependent they are on others is very hard. No one else does things the way you do, and this may cause frustration and friction in the best of families. Hopefully, the people helping you will be sensitive to how you feel about being so dependent, but you need to remind yourself that this is only temporary.

According to rehabilitation studies, recovery is positively affected by a strong social support system, living with others, and being, able to go shopping or visiting outside the home even once a month. Although pain, fear, and depression are common following a hip fracture, your ability to fight these negative feelings and maintain a positive attitude can help move your recovery forward. You may have periods of feeling very tired or weak. At these times it's important to look back over all the progress you have made.

One important mental exercise to do every day is to repeat positive steps to yourself. Unfortunately, we are more comfortable telling ourselves negative things like "I'll never be able to walk like I did before," or "It hurts too much." Instead, try telling yourself, "I walked 10 steps further today than yesterday." "I was able to make breakfast today." "I will go to the hairdresser next week. " Remember that all the small steps add up when you're recovering from a broken hip. Write down at least one positive change every day. It may deal with exercising, walking, doing an errand, going to a movie, or even putting away the breakfast dishes

If you continue to feel depressed, ask your doctor, hospital discharge planner, or rehabilitation facility for a referral to a knowledgeable counselor. A few counseling sessions may help you to feel more positive about your recovery.

### *Safety*

Since many hip fractures result from tripping, slipping, or loss of balance, fallproofing the home, balance training, and exercises to increase muscle strength should be part of the rehabilitation process. As people age, they move more slowly, their reflexes are slower, and they are less able to catch themselves once they start to fall. Also, medications for existing medical conditions may affect balance, vision, or sensations in the feet.

You can reduce your risk for falling by having regular physical exams, including vision and hearing tests, and by reviewing with your doctor the medications you are taking. Avoid alcohol, and wear sturdy, low-heeled shoes. Also, balance training can help you improve your posture, control your body position and coordination, and increase muscle strength and joint flexibility.

This information has been brought to you by:

Osteoporosis and Related Bone Diseases—National Resource Center
1150 17th Street, N.W., Suite 500
Washington, D.C. 20036-4603
Tel (800) 624- BONE or (202) 223-0344
Fax (202) 223-2237; TTY (202) 266-4315

Text used with permission of the National Osteoporosis Foundation. ORBD—NRC is supported by the National Institute of Arthritis and Musculoskeletal and Skin Diseases, National Institutes of Health.

Chapter 57

# Bone Scans

## A High-Tech Debate over Women's Bones

**Abstract:** Women now have available to them a number of new choices, in the form of bone scans and drugs, when faced with the onset of osteoporosis. Doctors, however, are still divided over the value of bone-density measurements, of which there are no formal guidelines.

Jessica Finnegan, 61, walks a mile a day, rain or shine. She also drinks milk. That means she has taken two important steps—getting regular exercise and including calcium in her diet—toward building and keeping strong bones. What's more, she spent her young adulthood chasing after her five children in a big old Victorian house in Ho-Ho-Kus, N.J., hauling laundry up and down two flights of stairs and, in her spare time, playing tennis. Finnegan menstruated until her late 50s, another protector of strong bones.

But last winter, Finnegan took advantage of a free bone scan offered by her employer. The test showed that she was heading straight toward osteoporosis, a disease that makes bones porous, which means that hips can easily shatter and spines slowly collapse. After the test, she learned of a risk factor she could do nothing about—Irish ancestry.

She began taking Fosamax, a drug from Merck & Co. that slows bone loss—and may even rebuild lost bone—in women who have had a fracture. Her doctor suggested Fosamax after Finnegan decided against estrogen supplements. Estrogen slows the rapid bone loss that occurs right after menopause, and it protects against heart disease. But estrogen taken with progestin—a combination recommended because it protects against cancer of the uterus—renews monthly bleeding. "I menstruated for a long time—long enough," says Finnegan.

More women are having bone scans because new testing technology is becoming available. And new osteoporosis drugs are giving women wider choices. But whether to take advantage of these options is not as obvious as it might seem.

Fosamax received Food and Drug Administration approval in 1995 for treating osteoporosis, not for preventing it. But Finnegan's doctor, like many physicians, believes that if Fosamax works for women who have already broken a bone, it's a good bet it will also help women before they break a bone. Research presented at a meeting of the American Society for Bone and Mineral Research earlier this month backs up that belief. Two-year results of a study of 1,609 women showed that Fosamax slowed bone loss and restored up to 3.5 percent of lost bone in postmenopausal women ages 45 to 59 who were not diagnosed with osteoporosis. (Fosamax costs about $1.55 a day, compared with about 40 cents for Premarin, a popular estrogen supplement.)

**Fracture logic.** Bone scans like the one Finnegan had are relatively new. Not too long ago, osteoporosis was diagnosed if a minor fall or bump resulted in a broken bone. Tests of bone density were almost irrelevant, since all patients got the same advice: Take up weight-bearing exercise; make sure the daily diet includes 1,000 milligrams of calcium (1,500 for postmenopausal women not on estrogen); and, for women entering menopause, begin taking estrogen.

More sophisticated scanning devices have permitted a new and precise diagnosis. Since 1994, the World Health Organization has determined that osteoporosis is a level of bone mass below a specific numerical threshold, based on age and computed from X-ray readings.

But many doctors argue that bone density measurements still have limited value. Formal guidelines—setting out which women should have their bone density tested and why—don't yet exist, and experts generally believe healthy women don't need to be tested until menopause. If they then decide to take estrogen, they don't need to be tested because estrogen is the recommended preventive therapy. But if they are reluctant to take estrogen, a bone density test could help them decide; or they might consider Fosamax or Miacalcin, another bone-saving drug approved in 1995 in the form of a nasal spray.

Most experts agree that postmenopausal women who have specific risk factors for osteoporosis should either take estrogen or be tested. Risk factors include a family history of the disease, Northern European or Asian descent, a thin frame, early menopause or smoking. Certain drugs, such as corticosteroids and thyroid hormones, can deplete bone mass, putting both men and women at increased risk for the disease.

Checking all postmenopausal women simply isn't practical. With relatively few state-of-the-art machines available, mass testing would take 6 to 12 years and cost a fortune. The current gold standard is a technology called DEXA (dual energy X-ray absorptiometry), which checks bone density at the hip, spine or forearm. Measurements in the spine and hip are the most significant, since a break can mean immobility and loss of independence.

**Cost and geography.** But a DEXA test costs $125 to $150, and only about half of insurers pay for it. Most Medicare carriers currently reimburse $110 to $120 of the cost. And with only about 2,000 DEXA machines in use in the United States, the device is not available everywhere. (The National Osteoporosis Foundation, 800-464-6700, can send a list of DEXA locations.) Another device, quantitative computed tomography, is a mini-CT scanner that produces sharp, three-dimensional images, but the test costs up to $300 and gives patients a higher dose of radiation than DEXA does. A lot of physicians prefer DEXA for the lower radiation dose.

A third device, the pDEXA forearm densitometer, has the virtue of portability and the defect of selectivity. Some studies suggest that forearm tests don't precisely predict the fate of the hip or spine — though many experts believe such a test is an acceptable first step. "If the only option is to look at only the forearm, I'd take it," says Susan Greenspan, director of the Osteoporosis Prevention and Treatment Center at Beth Israel Hospital in Boston. The pDEXA test is available in clinics and private doctors' offices.

Last summer, Walgreens, with educational materials provided by Merck, peppered central Florida with pDEXA machines in 150 drugstores for two months. Some 6,000 women paid $27 for the test. The response shows the need for more devices, says Michael Kleerekoper, professor of medicine at Wayne State University in Michigan. A menopausal woman who has risk factors but who is reluctant to take estrogen, he says, should be tested with "whatever is available," since limited information is better than none.

*— by Susan Brink.*

Chapter 58

# Screening for
# Osteoporosis Gets Easier

While the consequences of osteoporosis—bone fractures and loss of mobility—can be severe, the disease develops silently and painlessly. Thus, people don't usually know they have it until they break one or more bones.

Measuring bone density is the only way to detect osteoporosis before it causes out—and–out damage so that steps can be taken to stall its advance. But for many, access to high—tech bone-scanning devices has been limited. Bone scans using DEXA (dual energy x-ray absorptiometry)imaging, the current "gold standard" method, are expensive–and aren't available in rural areas far from major medical centers.

But that will start to change, now that the Food and Drug Administration has approved a new bone-scanning device called the Sahara. Unlike the large, bulky DEXA scanners, the portable Sahara machine fits easily in a primary-care physician's office.

The device uses high-frequency sound waves to measure bone density at the heel, which is rich in the same type of bone found in the spine and hips. To get a measurement, the patient simply rests her foot in the device for 10 seconds. A DEXA scan, by contrast, involves 6 to 8 minutes of lying on a table while the scanner slowly passes over the hips or spine. The Sahara test is expected to cost around $40, as opposed to $130 or more for a DEXA scan.

"Screening for Osteoporosis Gets Easier," from *Tufts University Health and Nutrition Letter*, June 1998, Vol. 16, No. 4, p. 1, © 1998. Reprinted with permission, Tufts University Health and Nutrition Letter, telephone: 1-800-274-7581.

The new scanner is not without drawbacks. "If you think of DEXA as the Cadillac of bone scanners, the Sahara is a Ford," says Bess Dawson-Hughes, MI, chief of the Calcium and Bone Metabolism laboratory at Tufts. "It isn't as precise—and it's not quite as good at predicting fractures of the spine and hips because it doesn't measure bone density at those sites."

But the fact remains that some 10 million Americans have osteoporosis and 18 million more are at risk for the disease—and many of them have never been checked for bone loss at all. That's where the Sahara comes in. "It should be very useful as a screening tool to see who has low bone mineral density and identify who needs to be treated," explains Dr. Dawson-Hughes. "Then, if osteoporosis is present, DEXA scanning can track changes in bone density over time."

Because the rate of bone loss jumps dramatically after menopause, the Sahara scanner should be a special boon to post-menopausal women, who are at increased risk for the disease.

# Chapter 59

# *Strong Recommendation for Bone Density Testing*

All postmenopausal women are at risk of osteoporosis (weak bones that break easily), and about one—half eventually develop the condition. Osteoporosis also occurs among older men, though the condition is much less common. Sufferers are prone to hip fractures, a leading cause of disability and death, and spinal fractures, which can he extremely painful and lead to a stooped posture. Until recently, osteoporosis could he diagnosed only by standard x-rays, which can detect the condition only after significant bone loss has occurred. Often, it wasn't detected until after a fracture—and few treatments were available.

Today, the situation is dramatically different. There are now three effective drug options: hormone replacement therapy (HRT), alendronate (Fosamax), and calcitonin (Calcimar and Miacalcin)—and more are on the way, including the "designer" estrogen raloxifene. All three of the currently approved medications preserve bone strength, and studies show that HRT and alendronate also reduce fracture risk. Furthermore, a relatively new non-invasive imaging technique can help identify osteoporosis at an early stage, before any bones break. And several recently approved laboratory tests can help guide treatment.

---

"Our Strong Recommendation for Bone Density Testing," from *The Johns Hopkins Medical Letter Health After 50*, October 1997. Reprinted with permission from *The Johns Hopkins Medical Letter Health After 50*, © Medletter Associates, 1997. To order a one year subscription, call 800-829-9170.

461

Unfortunately, many women are unaware that they should have an evaluation, and diagnostic techniques and treatment options are so new that many doctors have not yet incorporated them into routine practice.

## How Bones Change

Although adult bones may seem to be unchanging structures, they are constantly built up and broken down in a dynamic process known as bone remodeling. Two types of bone cells are involved: osteoblasts (which form new bone) and osteoclasts (which remove, or resorb, old bone). During the first half of life, more bone is formed than resorbed. As a result, bone density increases, peaking at around age 30. After that, the rate of bone resorption gradually begins to surpass the rate of bone formation, Thus, bone mass begins a slow hut steady decline, which rapidly accelerates in women after menopause.

Osteoporosis typically occurs among those who never accumulated enough bone mass, and those who lose bone too rapidly. Eventually, these patients may lose so much bone that their skeletal mass declines beneath the "fracture threshold," the point at which bones are likely to break under minimal stress. Once osteoporosis occurs, ordinary activities (such as sneezing, picking up a light bundle, or stepping off a curb) can lead to a fracture. Remodeling rates differ widely from one person to another and are greatly affected by sex hormones (estrogen in women and testosterone in men), which help keep calcium bound to bone.

Older women are vulnerable to osteoporosis because estrogen levels decline markedly after menopause. Other risk factors include:

- Being white or Asian;

- A family history of osteoporosis;

- Continued use or high doses of certain medications, including corticosteroids, thyroid hormone, anticonvulsants, heparin, and chemotherapy drugs;

- Moderate to heavy alcohol consumption;

- Hyperthyroidism;

- Smoking;

- Being very thin;

- Immobilization and lack of exercise;

- A diet that lacks calcium (the main component of bone) and vitamin D (which is necessary for the proper use of calcium);

- Possibly heavy caffeine consumption.

### *Who Should Be Tested?*

Any postmenopausal woman who is not already on HRT, which is beneficial because estrogen is its principal component, should consider undergoing bone densitometry. This noninvasive imaging study measures bone density. The current gold standard is dual energy x-ray absorptiometry (DEXA), which provides hip, spine, and sometimes wrist measurements. DEXA findings are compared to the normal peak bone density of someone of the same sex (see Figure 59.1). By DEXA machine standards, 1.0 to 2.0 standard deviations (SDs) below normal peak indicates osteopenia (reduced bone mass); more than 2.0 SDs below normal peak indicates osteoporosis. Each SD below peak represents a 10 to 12 percent loss of total bone mass.

# Sample DEXA Findings for the Hip
## (Femoral Neck)

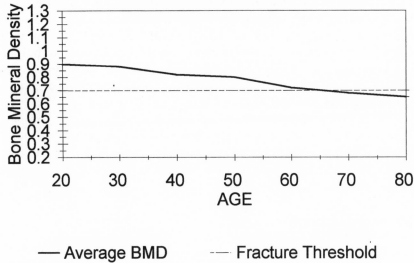

*Figure 59.1. Sample DEXA Findings for the Hip (Femoral Neck)*

DEXA takes about 15 minutes and delivers less radiation than a standard chest x-ray. However, DEXA machines are not available in all parts of the country, and testing may not be covered by insurance. The cost ranges from $125 to $250. Portable DEXAs are sometimes used at malls and in other non-health care settings. Although much less expensive, they do not provide enough data for a thorough assessment. Other imaging techniques that may be useful include single-photon absorptiometry (SPA), dual-photon absorptiometry (DPA), and quantitative computed tomography (QCT).

If osteoporosis has developed, treatment with HRT, calcitonin (usually in nasal spray form), or alendronate (a pill), is necessary. Unlike HRT, which has many other health benefits, calcitonin and alendronate act only on bone. If osteopenia is diagnosed, osteoporosis may be prevented with HRT or alendronate.

The main side effect of alendronate is esophagitis (inflammation of the esophagus), which can cause heartburn and lead to ulcers of the esophagus if neglected. However, taking alendronate properly—on an empty stomach, at least 30 minutes before breakfast, with an 8-ounce glass of water—can nearly always circumvent the problem. It's also important not to lie down again for at least 30 minutes (preferably an hour) after taking the medication. Calcitonin seems to be particularly helpful for patients who suffer from the chronic pain of spinal fractures. Side effects of calcitonin include nausea, flushing, and nasal irritation.

In women treated for bone thinning, a second bone density study should be performed in about a year to evaluate treatment. At the very least, bone density should have stabilized, and may even have increased. In the interim, new laboratory tests can be used to help assess response to therapy. These tests measure the biochemical markers of bone remodeling (substances that are released into the blood and urine as byproducts of bone formation and resorption). At least four have recently been approved: Pyrilinks, Pyrilinks D, Osteomark (all of which measure the rate of bone resorption), and Ostase (which measures the rate of bone formation). But because biochemical markers are highly variable, laboratory testing should not be used as a substitute for densitometry.

## Measuring Bones

A woman reaches peak bone density (BMD) in her hip between the ages of 20 and 30 (the normal peak averages about 0.895 g/cm$^2$). Two standard deviations (SDs) below this peak indicate osteoporosis, or the fracture threshold (dotted line), the point below which bones are more likely to break. At least one-half of all postmenopausal women eventually reach this point. The 67-year-old sample patient who provided the data for chart 59.1 is an example. Her BMD score is 0.535, which is 3.6 SDs below normal peak, indicating osteoporosis and the need for aggressive treatment.

### *For More Information*

Call 800-464-6700
The National Osteoporosis Foundation
www.nof.org

Chapter 60

# Selective Estrogen Receptor Modulators (SERMs)

### Encouraging News from the SERM Frontier. (Selective Estrogen Receptor Modulators)

**Abstract:** The drug raloxifene is an example of a drug that mimics the action of estrogen in some parts of the body, but blocks the action of estrogen in other parts of the body. Drugs that do this are called selective estrogen receptor modulators, or SERMs. Estrogen has beneficial effects such as keeping bones strong and lowering the risk of heart disease but it also increases the risk of breast and endometrial cancer. SERMs may mimic the positive aspects of estrogen while minimizing its negative aspects. A 1999 study found that raloxifene significantly reduced the risk of breast cancer among postmenopausal women with osteoporosis.

The discovery that pharmacologic agents can be estrogenic in some tissues while antiestrogenic in others has led to intense interest in better understanding the mechanism by which molecular structure interacts with cellular receptors to selectively affect DNA transcription in different organs. Appreciation for these selective estrogen receptor modulators (SERMs) has inevitably given way to the hope of developing one that could confer all of the benefits of estrogen without any

Franks, Adele L., and Karen K. Steinberg, "Encouraging News from the SERM Frontier," from *JAMA, The Journal of the American Medical Association*, June 16, 1999, Vol. 281, Issue 23, p.2243, © 1999 American Medical Association. Reprinted with permission.

of its risks. The first widely used SERM, tamoxifen citrate, has been found to have the antiestrogenic effect of reducing risk for breast cancer as well as beneficial estrogenic effects on serum lipids and bone density in women. [1] However, tamoxifen also has the undesirable antiestrogenic effect of causing hot flashes and the undesirable estrogenic effects of increasing risk for endometrial cancer and venous thromboembolism in women. [1] Because raloxifene hydrochloride, a second-generation SERM, has been shown to increase women's bone density without increasing risk for endometrial cancer, [2,3] results of clinical trials designed to study its protective effects against breast cancer have been eagerly awaited.

In this issue of the journal, Cummings and colleagues [4] report results from a large, well-designed, randomized controlled trial (RCT), the Multiple Outcomes of Raloxifene Evaluation (MORE), which show that raloxifene significantly reduced the risk for estrogen receptor-positive breast cancer among postmenopausal women with osteoporosis. These findings, as well as the finding that raloxifene does not cause endometrial hyperplasia, provide a welcome confirmation of what was anticipated on the basis of prior human and animal studies. [2,5] Although clinicians need to be cautious in generalizing from the findings of the MORE study, which lasted only 3 years and included only women with low bone density, the results do suggest that raloxifene may be a welcome alternative for women who are considering estrogen therapy for treatment or prevention of osteoporosis but who fear the increased risk for breast or endometrial cancer associated with estrogen.

In addition to interest in SERMs as a way to treat osteoporosis and prevent breast cancer, there is avid interest in determining whether SERMs may someday prove superior to exogenous estrogen after menopause for the multitude of reasons for which estrogen is now prescribed. One of the greatest expected benefits of estrogen is the primary prevention of ischemic heart disease (IHD), the leading cause of death among women in the United States. [6] Because the data suggesting a substantial reduction in risk for IHD among women who use estrogen emerged from observational studies rather than from RCTs, these effects have not been universally accepted. [7] Although one RCT has clearly shown estrogen to have a beneficial effect on serum lipid levels, women in that study were not followed up long enough to measure the effects of estrogen on IHD risk. [8] Of greater concern is a recent large and well-designed RCT of postmenopausal women with preexisting IHD that failed to show a protective effect of estrogen against subsequent ischemic events, despite affecting lipid levels in the same positive manner as shown in the previous trial. [9] These disappointing findings have increased suspicion that some of the previously reported cardioprotective effects of estrogen may have been due to uncontrolled bias (e.g., that women who chose to take estrogen were at lower risk for heart disease for other reasons or that women who became ill discontinued taking estrogen). Fortunately, several large RCTs designed to help clarify the role of estrogen in preventing IHD (including the Women's Health Initiative in the United States) are currently under way.

Evidence suggests that raloxifene, like tamoxifen, lowers women's total and low-density lipoprotein cholesterol levels in a manner similar to estrogen but does not increase high-density lipoprotein cholesterol levels as estrogen does. [10] Since the extent of cardioprotective effects of estrogen is currently in question, physicians should not assume that SERMs have cardioprotective effects solely because they have estrogen-like effects on lipid levels. Furthermore, the nonlipid-related cardioprotective effects of estrogen [11] have not been demonstrated for the SERMs. In fact, results of a study of raloxifene in menopausal monkeys showed no cardioprotective effect. [12]

The effect of estrogen and SERMs on cognitive function is yet another area of major interest. Although there is evidence suggesting that estrogen use may improve cognitive function, this effect is unconfirmed. [13,14] Results of recent animal studies that showed the newly isolated estrogen receptor-[beta] to be concentrated in regions of the brain associated with learning and memory support the biological plausibility of the role of estrogen in cognitive function, [15] as do those of a small RCT among women which showed that estrogen use was associated with the activation of certain regions of the brain during cognitive tasks. [16] Although raloxifene appears to have antiestrogenic effects on some central nervous system functions,[5] one small study showed that raloxifene use had no detrimental effect on selected cognitive tasks. [17] Thus, the comparative effects of estrogen and raloxifene on cognitive function is far from well understood at this time.

Moreover, women who initiate menopausal estrogen therapy commonly give as their reason a desire for relief of menopausal symptoms such as hot flashes and night sweats. [18] Thus; relief of menopausal symptoms may be of more immediate concern for decision making than weighing the long term risks and benefits. That currently available SERMs do not alleviate such symptoms and may even exacerbate some of them [19] suggests that much work remains before a widely acceptable alternative to estrogen will be available.

In the context of bone density and cancer chemoprevention, the study reported by Cummings et al [4] in this issue of *JAMA* confirms one anticipated improvement of raloxifene over tamoxifen: raloxifene not only preserves bone and protects against breast cancer, it also eliminates the excess risk of endometrial cancer previously associated with both estrogen and tamoxifen. Whether raloxifene provides similar degrees of breast cancer protection as tamoxifen will be determined by RCTs that directly compare the two SERMs; the National Surgical Adjuvant Breast and Bowel Project has announced plans for such a trial. [20]

In the larger context of our hopeful exploration of the molecular frontier, seeking to create the perfect SERM that will duplicate or improve on the beneficial effects of estrogen while protecting against its risks, the raloxifene findings provide solid encouragement. Raloxifene should not be considered suitable for use by most women at this time, but its contributions to knowledge intensify the anticipation of finding something even better on this new frontier.

*— by Adele L. Franks; Karen K. Steinberg.*

**Author Affiliations:** The Prudential Center for Health Care Research (Dr Franks) and Molecular Biology Branch, Centers for Disease Control and Prevention (Dr Steinberg), Atlanta, Ga.

**Corresponding Author and Reprints:** Adele L. Franks, MD, The Prudential Center for Health Care Research, 2859 Paces Ferry Rd, Suite 820, Atlanta, GA 30339 (e-mail: adele.franks@prudential.com).

### References

1.  Fisher B, Costantino JP, Wickerham DL, et al. Tamoxifen for prevention of breast cancer: report of the National Surgical Adjuvant Breast and Bowel Project P-i Study. *J Natl Cancer Inst*. 1998:90:1371-1388.

2.  Delmas PD, Bjarnason NH, Mitlak BH, et al. Effects of raloxifene on bone mineral density, serum cholesterol concentrations, and uterine endometrium in post-menopausal women. *N Engl J Med*. 1997:337:1641-1647.

3.  Lufkin EG, Whitaker MD, Nickelsen T, et al. Treatment of established post- menopausal osteoporosis with raloxifene: a randomized trial. *J Bone Miner Res*. 1998;13:1747- 1754.

4.  Cummings SR, Eckert 5, Krueger KA, et al. The effect of raloxifene on risk of breast cancer in postmenopausal women: results from the MORE randomized trial. *JAMA*. 1999:281:2189-2197.

5.  Khovidhunkit W, Shoback DM. clinical effects of raloxifene hydrocholoride in women. *Ann Intern Med*. 1999:130:431-439.

6.  Wenger NK, Speroff L, Packard B. cardiovascular health and disease in women. *N Engl J Med*. 1993:329:247-256.

7.  Petitti DB. Coronary heart disease and estrogen replacement therapy: can compliance bias explain the results of observational studies? *Ann Epidemiol*. 1994:4: 115-118.

8.  The Writing Group for the PEPI Trial. Effects of estrogen or estrogen/progestinregimens on heart disease risk factors in postmenopausal women: the Postmenopausal Estrogen/Progestin Interventions (PEPI) Trial. *JAMA*. 1995:273:199-208.

9.  Hulley, Grady D, Bush T, et al. Randomized trial of estrogen plus progestin for secondary prevention of coronary heart disease in postmenopausal women. *JAMA*. 1998:280:605-613.

10. Walsh W, Kuller LH, Wild RA, et al. Effects of raloxifene on serum lipids and coagulation factors in healthy postmenopausal women. *JAMA*. 1998:279:1445- 1451.

11. Stevenson JC, crook D, Godsland IF, Collins P, Whitehead Ml. Hormone replacement therapy and the cardiovascular system: nonlipid effects. *Drugs*. 1994: 47(suppl 2):35-41.

12. Clarkson TB, Anthony MS, Jerome CP. Lack of effect of raloxifene on coronary artery atherosclerosis of postmenopausal monkeys. *J Clin Endocrinol Metab*. 1998:83:721-726.

13. Haskell SG, Richardson ED, Horwitz RI. The effect of estrogen replacement therapy on cognitive function in women: a critical review of the literature. *J Clin Epidemiol*. 1997;50:149-164.

14. Yaffe K, Sawaya G, Lieberburg I, Grady D. Estrogen therapy in postmenopausal women: effects on cognitive function and dementia. *JAMA*. 1998:279: 688-695.

15. Shughrue PJ, Lane MV, Merchenthaler I. Comparative distribution of estrogen receptor-[gamma] and -[beta] mRNA in the rat central nervous system. *J Comp Neural*. 1997:388:507-525.

16. Shaywitz SE, Shaywitz BA, Pugh KR, et al. Effect of estrogen on brain activation patterns in postmenopausal women during working memory tasks. *JAMA*. 1999:281:1197-1202.

17. Nickelsen T, Lufkin EG, Riggs BL, Cox DA, Crook TH. Raloxifene hydrochloride, a selective estrogen receptor modulator: safety assessment of effects on cognitive function and mood in postmenopausal women. *Psychoneuroendocrinology*. 1999:24:115-128.

18. Newton KM. LaCroix AZ, Leveille SG, et al. Women's beliefs and decisions about hormone replacement therapy. *J Womens Health*. 1997:6:459-465.

19. Davies GC, Huster WJ, Lu Y, Plouffe L, Lakshmanan M. Adverse events reported by postmenopausal women in controlled trials with raloxifene. *Obstet Gynecol*. 1999:93:558-565.

20. Goldhirsh A, Coates AS, Castiglione-Gertsch M, Geiber RD. New treatments for breast cancer or just steps in the right direction? *Ann Oncol*. 1998:9: 973-976.

# Chapter 61

# *Raloxifene:*
# *A New Alternative to Estrogen*

### *A New Class of Anti-Estrogens for the Prevention of Osteoporosis*

**Abstract:** Selective estrogen receptor modulators (SERMs), such as raloxifene, can provide female patients the benefits of estrogen therapies while avoiding some of their risks. Benefits include cardio-vascular performance and improved bone mass, making them useful in preventing osteoporosis. Estrogen therapy risks that SERMs circumvent include harmful impacts on uterine and breast tissue.

As the number of elderly women continues to rise, the incidence of postmenopausal osteoporosis will continue to increase. Historically, hormone replacement therapy (HRT) has been a mainstay of pharmacologic treatment for this large group of women. However, many women have been unable or unwilling to comply with the therapeutic regimen.

In recent years, several new therapies have been developed and successfully used as alternatives to estrogen therapy for postmenopausal osteoporosis. In fall 1995, both alendronate (Fosamax, Merck) and intranasal calcitonin (Miacalcin, Novartis) were approved by the FDA for the management of postmenopausal osteoporosis.[1] While these therapies have demonstrated safety and efficacy in a variety of clinical trials, there is still room for additional weapons in the fight

Used with permission from Kessenich, C.R.: "Raloxifene: A New Class of Anti-Estrogens for the Prevention of Osteoporosis," in *The Nurse Practitioner*, 23(9):91-93, © 1998 Springhouse Corporation/www.springnet.com.

against the low bone mass and increased susceptibility to fracture that characterize postmenopausal osteoporosis.

### Pharmacology

Raloxifene (Evista, Eli Lilly) is the first of a new classification of drugs developed as an alternative therapy for postmenopausal osteoporosis. Approved by the FDA early this year, this benzothiophene derivative belongs to a new class of drugs called selective estrogen receptor modulators (SERMs) or anti-estrogens. These drugs mimic estrogen in some parts of the body and block estrogen's cancer-promoting effects in others. The drug's selection to act as either an agonist or antagonist is based on the molecular structures of the various receptor sites in the body.[2]

The goal of raloxifene therapy is to reduce the rate of bone resorption and decrease the rate of overall bone turnover. At the cellular level, raloxifene binds to estrogen receptors and stimulates estrogen receptor-specific genes that are present in a variety of tissues. Ultimately, raloxifene therapy should result in an increase in bone mineral density and a concomitant decrease in total and LDL cholesterol levels.

Following oral administration, about 60 percent of a raloxifene dose is rapidly absorbed via the gastrointestinal tract. Raloxifene exhibits a significant first-pass effect and as a result has an elimination half-life of about 27 hours. The liver metabolizes it almost exclusively. Primary excretion occurs in the feces and 0.2 percent appears unchanged via the urine.[3] Efficacy has not been established for persons with hepatic insufficiency.

### Clinical Trials

The search for an effective SERM for the prevention of osteoporosis began as a serendipitous finding in tamoxifen trials. In these trials, SERMs were found to have a beneficial effect on bone density. Tamoxifen is a SERM that has been widely used as an adjuvant therapy in women with breast cancer. Tamoxifen has been shown to reduce the risk of breast cancer relapse by 30 percent, while lowering serum cholesterol and producing a small positive effect on bone density.[4,5,6] Long-term therapy with tamoxifen has been shown to produce endometrial hypertrophy,[4] which makes it a poor choice for the long-term prevention of osteoporosis.

Raloxifene's approval by the FDA was based on preclinical animal trials and on Phase 3 trials with treatment of approximately 1,764 women. In vitro studies with mice show that raloxifene inhibits cancer development in breast tissue in a fashion similar to tamoxifen.[7] In two Phase 3 trials, women were randomly assigned to raloxifene or placebo.[8,9] In the third study,[10] women took raloxifene, placebo, or HRT. All women took calcium supplements in addition to their assigned treatment. In these studies, women given both raloxifene and calcium had a higher increase in bone mineral density than those taking calcium supplements alone. Raloxifene decreased serum lipids but was less effective than estrogen in increasing bone mineral density and decreasing serum lipids. Raloxifene did not affect endometrial tissue or breast tissue, and may have even caused a reduction in new breast cancers.[10]

In spring 1998, Eli Lilly and Company announced the initiation of a prospective clinical trial entitled Raloxifene Use for the Heart (RUTH). RUTH will be conducted by an independent group of nonindustry scientists. The trial will take place over 7 years in 25 countries and aims to enroll 10,000 postmenopausal women at risk of cardiac disease. The trial's primary objective is to evaluate chronic treatment with raloxifene and its effect on the incidence of coronary death, myocardial infarction, strokes, and breast cancer.

## Clinical Indications

Raloxifene is indicated for the prevention of postmenopausal osteoporosis. Women at risk for the development of postmenopausal osteoporosis due to family history, small bone structure, early onset of estrogen deficiency, low calcium diets, or sedentary lifestyles may consider this drug an attractive alternative to HRT. Treatment with raloxifene is acceptable for women at risk for endometrial and breast cancers who may be reluctant to use HRT. Additionally, it may be a good choice for protection against elevated total and LDL cholesterol.[10]

Raloxifene is contraindicated in women who have past or present histories of deep vein thrombosis, pulmonary emboli, or retinal vein thrombosis. The drug should not be taken by women with known sensitivity to the drug or those who are taking other forms of HRT. Raloxifene does not relieve hot flashes and may even increase their incidence, so it should not be prescribed for them.

## Dosage and Administration

Raloxifene is prescribed as one 60 mg tablet per day. It can be given without regard to time of day or meals. The drug should only be prescribed to postmenopausal women. While taking the drug, patients should be advised to take calcium and vitamin D supplements and to engage in weight bearing exercise to enhance osteoporosis prevention.

## Drug Interactions

Raloxifene is highly protein bound, but does not interact in vitro with the binding of warfarin, phenytoin or tamoxifen to plasma proteins. Despite this, the manufacturer recommends monitoring prothrombin times (PT) in patients receiving warfarin as raloxifene causes a 10 percent decrease in PT. Because raloxifene is more than 95 percent bound to plasma proteins, it should be used cautiously in conjunction with other highly protein-bound drugs such as indomethacin, ibuprofen, naproxen, and diazepam. Cholestryramine reduces the absorption of raloxifene by approximately 60 percent; thus co-administration is not recommended.[3]

## Adverse Effects

Raloxifene is generally well tolerated. In clinical trials, the adverse effects experienced most often by patients were venous thrombosis (especially during the first 4 months of therapy), hot flashes, leg cramps, headaches and sinusitis, with hot flashes the most commonly observed adverse effect. Women taking raloxifene reported a higher rate of hot flashes than women taking placebo (24.6 percent compared to 18.3 percent).[3]

Patients should avoid long periods of immobility and should discontinue the drug 3 days prior to a period of prolonged immobility. Patients should be educated to notify their provider immediately for any of the following symptoms: calf or leg pain, sudden chest pain, shortness of breath, hemoptysis, or any visual changes. If a woman becomes pregnant, the drug should be stopped immediately as it is a potential teratogen.

## Cost

At the recommended dosage of 60 mg per day, raloxifene will cost the pharmacist $59.40 per month.[11]

## Conclusion

SERMs are a class of drugs that may mimic the beneficial effects of estrogens on bone mass and cardiovascular risk factors, while avoiding estrogen's harmful effects on breast and uterine tissue. It is clear that this class of compounds is an exciting addition to current osteoporosis prevention options and will be of great interest in the future search for agents to prevent and treat osteoporosis.

Longitudinal data are needed to determine if the small increases in bone density due to raloxifene therapy will result in decreased fracture rates. Additional data are needed to evaluate the long-term effects on cardiovascular risk factors and protection against breast cancer. Time and additional research will help to clarify anti-estrogens' role in decreasing the incidence, morbidity, and mortality of osteoporosis.

*— by Cathy R. Kessenich*

Cathy R. Kessenich, ARNP, DSN, is an Associate Professor at Husson College, Bangor, Maine, and Research Associate for the Maine Center for Osteoporosis Research and Education.

## References

1. Kessenich CR: Update of pharmacologic therapies for osteoporosis. *Nurse Practitioner* 1996; 21(8):19-24.

2. Grasser WA, Pan LC, Thompson DD, et al: Common mechanisms for the estrogen agonist and antagonist activities of raloxifene. *Journal of Cell Biochemistry* 1997;65:159-71.

3. Evista (Raloxifene)—Product Package Insert, 1997.

4. Powles TJ: Efficacy of tamoxifen as treatment of breast cancer. *Seminars in Oncology* 1996; 24(Suppl 1):S1-48.

5. Rutqvist LE, Mattsson A: Cardiac and thromboembolic morbidity among postmenopausal women with early-stage breast cancer in a randomized trial of adjuvant tamoxifen. *Journal of the National Cancer Institute* 1993;85:1398-1406.

6. Grey AB, Stapleton JP, Evans MC, et al: The effect of the anti-estrogen tamoxifen on bone mineral density in normal late postmenopausal women. *American Journal of Medicine* 1995; 99:636-41.

7. Purdie, DW: Selective estrogen receptor modulation: HRT replacement therapy? *Br J Ob & Gyn* 1997;104:1103-05.

8. Balfour, JA, Goa, KL. Raloxifene. *Drugs & Aging* 1998;12:335-41.

9. Eli Lilly and Company. Raloxifene prescribing information. Indianapolis, IN.

10. Delmas PD, Bjarnason NH, Mitlak BH, et al: Effects of raloxifene on bone mineral density, serum cholesterol concentrations, and uterine endometrium in postmenopausal women. *N Engl J Med* 1997;337:1641-47.

11. Drug Topics: Redbook: Medical Economics Company. Montvale, NJ.

Chapter 62

# Minocycline:
# A Promising Treatment for
# Osteoporosis

Minocycline, an antibiotic related to tetracycline, has been shown to increase bone mineral density, improve bone strength and formation, and slow bone resorption in old laboratory animals with surgically-induced menopause. As a result of these promising effects, the National Institutes of Health (NIH) is funding a clinical trial of the drug in women to begin in January. The laboratory results underlying the clinical trial were obtained by Dr. C. Tony Liang, et al., of the National Institute on Aging (NIA) and are published in the December 1996 journal, *Bone*.

"Lack of estrogen in postmenopausal women leads to decreased bone formation and more bone resorption, resulting in a net loss of bone," says NIA scientist, Dr. Liang, who conducted the study. "Our results in animals suggest that an inexpensive antibiotic, minocycline, may not only prevent bone loss, but may increase bone mineral density beyond that of premenopausal bone mineral density. The next step would be to test the drug in humans."

Dr. Liang and his colleagues studied five groups of old female rats. They removed the ovaries to induce a postmenopausal state in four groups. The control group retained their ovaries and received no medication or hormone therapy. Of the 4 "menopausal" groups, 1 received 10 mg of minocycline daily, 1 group received 24 g of estrogen daily, 1 group received 10 mg of minocycline and 24 g of estrogen daily, and

National Institute on Aging, National Institutes of Health (NIH) New Release December 9, 1996. Available at http://www.nih.gov/news/pr/dec96/nia-09.htm.

479

the control group did not receive medication or hormone. The treatment phase of the study lasted for 8 weeks.

After the treatment was completed, researchers measured bone mineral density of the femur, or thigh bone, using dual energy X-ray absorptiometry, a sophisticated bone scan. The femur is made of a hard cortical bone on the outside, spongy trabecular bone inside, with an inner cavity of bone marrow. The trabecular bone (the name means "little beam") gives the bone its strength. There is more trabecular bone toward both ends of the femur, near the knee and hip joints. By measuring both total bone mineral density in the femur and specifically in the knee and hip joint regions, scientists can determine if the bone is weak or strong, thereby predicting fracture risk.

The control group of rats without ovaries lost 14 percent of their total femoral bone mineral density, 10 percent close to the hip joint, and 19 percent close to knee joint compared to the control group with ovaries. Rats treated with minocycline maintained bone mineral density levels similar to the group of rats with ovaries and significantly above levels observed in the control group without ovaries. Previous rat studies looking at the effects of estrogen also have shown an increase in bone mineral density.

Earlier studies have confirmed the benefits of taking estrogen to prevent bone loss in menopausal women. The studies also have linked estrogen to the development of endometrial cancer in some people. Minocycline has several potential advantages over estrogen in terms of its influence on bone. Not only does minocycline prevent bone resorption similar to estrogen, but also and unlike estrogen, minocycline increases bone formation and connectivity between bony trabeculae. Thus, minocycline has an additional mechanism of action and because it is not a hormone, it should not exert adverse effects on the uterine lining.

"The action of minocycline on bone formation and resorption is unique compared to estrogen and bisphosphonate, a commonly prescribed medication to treat osteoporosis,"Liang said. "Estrogen and bisphosphonate prevent the resorption of bone. Minocycline is very inexpensive, it accumulates in the bone, and it causes the synthesis of strong, hard bone." According to Liang, scientists do not understand fully how minocycline works, and he is beginning studies to find the answers.

Meanwhile, researchers at Johns Hopkins University and the NIA are launching a 1-year clinical trial at the General Clinical Research Center at the Johns Hopkins Bayview Medical Center in Baltimore to study the effects of minocycline in postmenopausal women with osteoporosis.

Osteoporosis is a major public health threat for 25 million Americans, 80 percent of whom are women. In the United States, 7 to 8 million individuals already have the disease and 17 million more have low bone mass, placing them at increased risk for osteoporosis.

Osteoporosis is responsible for 1.5 million fractures annually, including more than 300,000 hip fractures, 500,000 vertebral fractures, 200,000 wrist fractures, and more than 300,000 fractures at other sites. Moreover, individuals suffering hip fractures have a 5 to 20 percent greater risk of dying within the first year following that injury than others in their age group.

The estimated national direct costs for osteoporosis and associated fractures is $10 billion-$27 million each day—and the cost is rising. Prevention is the best hope for diminishing the personal and financial losses associated with osteoporosis.

A free fact sheet on osteoporosis, *"Osteoporosis: The Bone Thinner,"* is available by calling the NIA Information Center's toll-free number, (800) 222-2225.

The National Institute on Aging, a component of the National Institutes of Health, conducts and supports biomedical, social, and behavioral research related to the aging process, age-associated diseases, and other special needs of older people.

# Chapter 63

# *Miacalcin and Fosamax*

## *Two New Drugs Approved for Osteoporosis*

Government approval of two new drugs for osteoporosis has given clinicians new options for the treatment of this bone-weakening condition, which commonly affects postmenopausal women and leaves them susceptible to fracture of the spine and hip and at high risk for home placement.

One of the drugs is alendronate sodium, marketed under the brand name Fosamax. The other, marketed as Miacalcin, is a preparation of calcitonin that is administered as a nasal spray. Both act by preventing the loss of mineral from bone. The drugs may be used in combination.

According to Dr. Bruce M. Solitar of New York University School of Medicine, prevention of osteoporosis can also be accomplished with weight-bearing exercise such as walking, proper calcium intake by diet and calcium supplements; and limiting alcohol consumption. In addition, careful monitoring is needed for women with epidemiological characteristics known to be associated with osteoporosis. These include having a small frame and being Caucasian.

Further treatment options include estrogen and other female hormones, along with drugs such as Fosamax and Miacalcin.

The availability of new drugs does not, says Solitar, alter the recommendation that postmenopausal women should not smoke, should

*The Brown University Long-Term Care Quality Letter*, May 27, 1996, Vol. 8, No. 10, p. 5(1), © 1996. Reprinted with permission of Opus Communications.

drink in moderation and should exercise regularly to help preserve bone strength. With follow-up bone density measurements, treatment can be monitored and adjusted as needed.

# Chapter 64

# *Hip Replacement Surgery*

## *What Is a Hip Replacement?*

Hip replacement, or arthroplasty, is a surgical procedure in which the diseased parts of the hip joint are removed and replaced with new, artificial parts. These artificial parts are called the prosthesis. The goals of hip replacement surgery are to improve mobility by relieving pain and improve function of the hip joint.

## *Who Should Have Hip Replacement Surgery?*

The most common reason that people have hip replacement surgery is the wearing down of the hip joint that results from osteoarthritis. Other conditions, such as rheumatoid arthritis (a chronic inflammatory disease that causes joint pain, stiffness, and swelling), avascular necrosis (loss of bone caused by insufficient blood supply), injury, and bone tumors also may lead to breakdown of the hip joint and the need for hip replacement surgery.

Before suggesting hip replacement surgery, the doctor is likely to try walking aids such as a cane, or non-surgical therapies such as medication and physical therapy. These therapies are not always effective in relieving pain and improving the function of the hip joint. Hip replacement may be an option if persistent pain and disability

National Institute of Arthritis and Musculoskeletal and Skin Diseases (NIAMS), NIH Publication No. AR-149QA, May 1997. Available at http://www.nih.gov/niams/healthinfo/hiprepqa.htm

interfere with daily activities. Before a doctor recommends hip replacement, joint damage should be detectable on x rays.

In the past, hip replacement surgery was an option primarily for people over 60 years of age. Typically, older people are less active and put less strain on the artificial hip than do younger, more active people. In recent years, however, doctors have found that hip replacement surgery can be very successful in younger people as well. New technology has improved the artificial parts, allowing them to withstand more stress and strain. A more important factor than age in determining the success of hip replacement is the overall health and activity level of the patient.

For some people who would otherwise qualify, hip replacement may be problematic. For example, people who suffer from severe muscle weakness or Parkinson's disease are more likely than healthy people to damage or dislocate an artificial hip. Because people who are at high risk for infections or in poor health are less likely to recover successfully, doctors may not recommend hip replacement surgery for these patients.

## What Are Alternatives to Total Hip Replacement?

Before considering a total hip replacement, the doctor may try other methods of treatment, such as an exercise program and medication. An exercise program can strengthen the muscles in the hip joint and sometimes improve positioning of the hip and relieve pain.

The doctor also may treat inflammation in the hip with nonsteroidal anti-inflammatory drugs, or NSAIDs. Some common NSAIDs are aspirin and ibuprofen. Many of these medications are available without a prescription, although a doctor also can prescribe NSAIDs in stronger doses.

In a small number of cases, the doctor may prescribe corticosteroids, such as prednisone or cortisone, if NSAIDs do not relieve pain. Corticosteroids reduce joint inflammation and are frequently used to treat rheumatic diseases such as rheumatoid arthritis. Corticosteroids are not always a treatment option because they can cause further damage to the bones in the joint. Some people experience side effects from corticosteroids such as increased appetite, weight gain, and lower resistance to infections. A doctor must prescribe and monitor corticosteroid treatment. Because corticosteroids alter the body's natural hormone production, patients should not stop taking them suddenly and should follow the doctor's instructions for discontinuing treatment.

If physical therapy and medication do not relieve pain and improve joint function, the doctor may suggest corrective surgery that is less complex than a hip replacement, such as an osteotomy. Osteotomy is surgical repositioning of the joint. The surgeon cuts away damaged bone and tissue and restores the joint to its proper position. The goal of this surgery is to restore the joint to its correct position, which helps to distribute weight evenly in the joint. For some people, an osteotomy relieves pain. Recovery from an osteotomy takes 6 to 12 months. After an osteotomy, the function of the hip joint may continue to worsen and the patient may need additional treatment. The length of time before another surgery is needed varies greatly and depends on the condition of the joint before the procedure.

## What Does Hip Replacement Surgery Involve?

The hip joint is located where the upper end of the femur meets the acetabulum. The femur, or thigh bone, looks like a long stem with a ball on the end. The acetabulum is a socket or cup-like structure in the pelvis, or hip bone. This "ball and socket" arrangement allows a wide range of motion, including sitting, standing, walking, and other daily activities.

During hip replacement, the surgeon removes the diseased bone tissue and cartilage from the hip joint. The healthy parts of the hip are left intact. Then the surgeon replaces the head of the femur (the ball) and the acetabulum (the socket) with new, artificial parts. The new hip is made of materials that allow a natural, gliding motion of the joint. Hip replacement surgery usually lasts 2 to 3 hours.

Sometimes the surgeon will use a special glue, or cement, to bond the new parts of the hip joint to the existing, healthy bone. This is referred to as a "cemented" procedure. In an uncemented procedure, the artificial parts are made of porous material that allows the patient's own bone to grow into the pores and hold the new parts in place. Doctors sometimes use a "hybrid" replacement, which consists of a cemented femur part and an uncemented acetabular part.

## Is a Cemented or Uncemented Prosthesis Better?

Cemented prostheses were developed 40 years ago. Uncemented prostheses were developed about 20 years ago to try to avoid the possibility of loosening parts and the breaking off of cement particles, which sometimes happen in the cemented replacement. Because each person's condition is unique, the doctor and patient must weigh the advantages and disadvantages to decide which type of prosthesis is better.

For some people, an uncemented prosthesis may last longer than cemented replacements because there is no cement that can break away. And, if the patient needs an additional hip replacement (which is likely in younger people), also known as a revision, the surgery sometimes is easier if the person has an uncemented prosthesis.

The primary disadvantage of an uncemented prosthesis is the extended recovery period. Because it takes a long time for the natural bone to grow and attach to the prosthesis, people with uncemented replacements must limit activities for up to 3 months to protect the hip joint. The process of natural bone growth also can cause thigh pain for several months after the surgery.

Research has proven the effectiveness of cemented prostheses to reduce pain and increase joint mobility. These results usually are noticeable immediately after surgery. Cemented replacements are more frequently used than cementless ones for older, less active people and people with weak bones, such as those who have osteoporosis.

## What Can Be Expected Immediately after Surgery?

Patients are allowed only limited movement immediately after hip replacement surgery. When the patient is in bed, the hip usually is braced with pillows or a special device that holds the hip in the correct position. The patient may receive fluids through an intravenous tube to replace fluids lost during surgery. There also may be a tube located near the incision to drain fluid and a tube (catheter) may be used to drain urine until the patient is able to use the bathroom. The doctor will prescribe medicine for pain or discomfort.

## How Long Are Recovery and Rehabilitation?

On the day after surgery or sometimes on the day of surgery, therapists will teach the patient exercises that will improve recovery. A respiratory therapist may ask the patient to breathe deeply, cough, or blow into a simple device that measures lung capacity. These exercises reduce the collection of fluid in the lungs after surgery.

A physical therapist may teach the patient exercises, such as contracting and relaxing certain muscles, that can strengthen the hip. Because the new, artificial hip has a more limited range of movement than an undiseased hip, the physical therapist also will teach the patient proper techniques for simple activities of daily living, such as bending and sitting, to prevent injury to the new hip. As early as 1 to 2 days after surgery, a patient may be able to sit on the edge of the bed, stand, and even walk with assistance.

Usually, people do not spend more than 10 days in the hospital after hip replacement surgery. Full recovery from the surgery takes about 3 to 6 months, depending on the type of surgery, the overall health of the patient, and the success of rehabilitation.

## How to Prepare for Surgery and Recovery

People can do many things before and after they have surgery to make everyday tasks easier and help speed their recovery.

### Before Surgery

- Learn what to expect before, during, and after surgery. Request information written for patients from the doctor or contact one of the organizations listed near the end of this chapter.

- Arrange for someone to help you around the house for a week or two after coming home from the hospital.

- Arrange for transportation to and from the hospital.

- Set up a "recovery station" at home. Place the television remote control, radio, telephone, medicine, tissues, waste basket, and pitcher and glass next to the spot where you will spend the most time while you recover.

- Place items you use every day at arm level to avoid reaching up or bending down.

- Stock up on kitchen staples and prepare food in advance, such as frozen casseroles or soups that can be reheated and served easily.

### After Surgery

- Follow the doctor's instructions.

- Work with a physical therapist or other health care professional to rehabilitate your hip.

- Wear an apron for carrying things around the house. This leaves hands and arms free for balance or to use crutches.

- Use a long-handled "reacher" to turn on lights or grab things that are beyond arm's length. Hospital personnel may provide one of these or suggest where to buy one.

## What Are Possible Complications of Hip Replacement Surgery?

According the American Academy of Orthopaedic Surgeons, approximately 120,000 hip replacement operations are performed each year in the United States and less than 10 percent require further surgery. New technology and advances in surgical techniques have greatly reduced the risks involved with hip replacements.

The most common problem that may happen soon after hip replacement surgery is hip dislocation. Because the artificial ball and socket are smaller than the normal ones, the ball can become dislodged from the socket if the hip is placed in certain positions. The most dangerous position usually is pulling the knees up to the chest.

The most common later complication of hip replacement surgery is an inflammatory reaction to tiny particles that gradually wear off of the artificial joint surfaces and are absorbed by the surrounding tissues. The inflammation may trigger the action of special cells that eat away some of the bone, causing the implant to loosen. To treat this complication, the doctor may use anti-inflammatory medications or recommend revision surgery (replacement of an artificial joint). Medical scientists are experimenting with new materials that last longer and cause less inflammation.

Less common complications of hip replacement surgery include infection, blood clots, and heterotopic bone formation (bone growth beyond the normal edges of bone).

## When Is Revision Surgery Necessary?

Hip replacement is one of the most successful orthopaedic surgeries performed—more than 90 percent of people who have hip replacement surgery will never need revision surgery. However, because more younger people are having hip replacements, and wearing away of the joint surface becomes a problem after 15 to 20 years, revision surgery is becoming more common. Revision surgery is more difficult than first-time hip replacement surgery, and the outcome is generally not as good, so it is important to explore all available options before having additional surgery.

Doctors consider revision surgery for two reasons: if medication and lifestyle changes do not relieve pain and disability; or if x rays of the hip show that damage has occurred to the artificial hip that must be corrected before it is too late for a successful revision. This surgery is usually considered only when bone loss, wearing of the joint surfaces, or joint loosening shows up on an x ray. Other possible reasons for revision surgery include fracture, dislocation of the artificial parts, and infection.

## What Types of Exercise Are Most Suitable for Someone with a Total Hip Replacement?

Proper exercise can reduce joint pain and stiffness and increase flexibility and muscle strength. People who have an artificial hip should talk to their doctor or physical therapist about developing an appropriate exercise program. Most exercise programs begin with safe range-of-motion activities and muscle strengthening exercises. The doctor or therapist will decide when the patient can move on to more demanding activities. Many doctors recommend avoiding high-impact activities, such as basketball, jogging, and tennis. These activities can damage the new hip or cause loosening of its parts. Some recommended exercises are cross-country skiing, swimming, walking, and stationary bicycling. These exercises can increase muscle strength and cardiovascular fitness without injuring the new hip.

## What Hip Replacement Research Is Being Done?

To help avoid unsuccessful surgery, researchers are studying the types of patients most likely to benefit from a hip replacement. Researchers also are developing new surgical techniques, materials, and designs of prostheses, and studying ways to reduce the inflammatory response of the body to the prosthesis. Other areas of research address recovery and rehabilitation programs, such as home health and outpatient programs.

## Where Can People Find More Information about Hip Replacement Surgery?

*American Academy of Orthopaedic Surgeons*
6300 North River Road
Rosemont, IL 60018-4262
847-823-7186 or 800-346-AAOS
Fax: 847-823-8125
World Wide Web address: http://www.aaos.org

491

***The Hip Society***
951 Old County Road, #182
Belmont, CA 94002
650-596-6190
Fax: 650-508-2039
http://www.hipsoc.org

The Society maintains a list of physicians who are specialists in problems of the hip and provides physician referrals by geographic area.

## *Acknowledgments*

The NIAMS gratefully acknowledges the assistance of Charles A. Engh, M.D., of the Anderson Orthopaedic Research Institute, in Arlington, Virginia; James Panagis, M.D., M.P.H., of the National Institutes of Health; and Clement B. Sledge, M.D., of Brigham and Women's Hospital, in Boston, Massachusetts, in the review of this fact sheet. The National Arthritis and Musculoskeletal and Skin Diseases Information Clearinghouse (NAMSIC) is a public service sponsored by the NIAMS that provides health information and information sources. The NIAMS, a part of the National Institutes of Health (NIH), leads the Federal medical research effort in arthritis and musculoskeletal and skin diseases. The NIAMS sponsors research and research training throughout the United States as well as on the NIH campus in Bethesda, MD, and disseminates health and research information.

# Chapter 65

# *Coping with Chronic Pain*

Osteoporosis often causes painful fractures which can take many months to heal. In many cases, the pain tends to diminish as the fracture heals; however, vertebral fractures are an exception to this. When a vertebrae breaks, some people have no pain, while others have intense pain and muscle spasms that last long after the fracture has healed. Most new fractures heal in approximately three months. Pain that continues more than three months is generally considered to be chronic pain.

Pain is the body's way of responding to damaged tissue. When a bone breaks, nerves send pain messages through the spinal cord to the brain where they are interpreted. How a person responds to pain is determined by many factors, including her or his emotional outlook. For example, depression seems to increase a person's perception of pain and decreases her or his ability to cope with it. Often, treating the depression treats the pain as well.

Chronic pain is pain that lasts beyond the expected time for healing and interferes with normal life. The damaged tissues have healed, but the pain continues. The pain message may be triggered by muscle tension, stiffness, weakness, or spasms. Whatever the cause of chronic pain, feelings of frustration, anger, and fear make the pain more intense. Chronic pain can often diminish the quality of a person's life psychologically, socially, and physically.

Reprinted from *The Osteoporosis Report,* Winter 1996, © NOF, 1996. Reprinted with permission from the National Osteoporosis Foundation, Washington, D.C. 20037.

The following information will provide those suffering from chronic pain with an overview of different options for pain management. If you have chronic pain and need help managing it, you may wish to discuss these options with your doctor.

## Coping Strategies

### Physical Methods of Pain Management

*Heat and Ice*

Heat, in the form of warm showers or hot packs, can relieve chronic pain or stiff muscles. Cold packs or ice packs provide pain relief by numbing the pain-sensing nerves in the affected area. Cold also helps reduce swelling and inflammation. Depending on which feels better, apply heat or cold for 15 to 20 minutes at a time to the area where you feel the pain. To protect your skin, place a towel between your skin and the source for cold or heat.

- Warm towels or hot packs in the microwave for a quick source of heat
- Frozen juice cans or bags of frozen vegetables make instant cold packs
- Freezing a plastic, resealable bag filled with water makes a good ice bag

*Transcutaneous Electrical Nerve Stimulation (TENS)*

A TENS machine is a small machine that sends electrical impulses to certain parts of the body to block pain signals. Two electrodes are placed on the body where the person is experiencing the pain. The electrical current that is produced is very mild, but it can prevent pain messages from being transmitted to the brain. Pain relief can last for several hours. Some people may use a small, portable TENS unit that hooks on a belt for more continuous relief. TENS machines should be used under the supervision of a physician or physical therapist. They can be purchased or rented from hospital supply or surgical supply houses; however, a prescription is necessary for insurance reimbursement.

*Supports and Braces*

Spinal supports or braces reduce pain and inflammation by restricting movement. Following a vertebral fracture, a back brace or support will relieve pain and allow the person to resume normal activities while the fracture heals. However, continuous use of a back support can weaken back muscles. For this reason, exercises to strengthen the muscles in the back should be started as soon as possible.

*Exercise or Physical Therapy*

Prolonged inactivity increases weakness and causes loss of muscle mass and strength. Physical therapy and a regular exercise program can help a person regain strength, energy, and a more positive outlook on life. Because exercise raises the body's level of endorphins (natural pain killers produced by the brain), pain will diminish. Exercise also relieves tension, increases flexibility, strengthens muscles, and reduces fatigue. A physical therapist can help the person reorganize their home or work environment so that injuries can be avoided. Physical therapists also teach proper positioning, posture, and exercises to strengthen the back and abdominal muscles without injuring a weakened spine. Pool therapy is one of the best exercise techniques to gently improve back muscle strength and reduce pain.

*Acupuncture and Acupressure*

Acupuncture is the use of special needles which are inserted into the body at certain points. These needles stimulate nerve endings and cause the brain to release endorphins. It may take several acupuncture sessions before the pain is relieved. These techniques have been used in China especially to treat many types of pain and as an anesthetic.

Acupressure is direct pressure over trigger areas of the pain. This technique can be self-administered after training with an instructor.

*Massage Therapy*

Massage therapy can be a light, slow, circular motion with the fingertips or a deep and kneading motion that moves from the center of the body outward towards the fingers or toes. Massage relieves pain, relaxes stiff muscles, and smoothes out muscle knots by increasing the blood supply to the affected area and warming it. The person doing the massage uses oil or powder so that her/his hands slide smoothly over the skin. Massage can also include gentle pressure over affected areas or hard pressure over trigger points in muscle knots. However, deep muscle massage should not be done near the spine of a person who has spinal osteoporosis. Light, circular massage with fingers or the palm of the hand is best in this case.

## Psychological Methods of Pain Management

### Relaxation Training

Relaxation involves concentration and slow, deep breathing to release tension from muscles and relieve pain. Learning to relax takes a great deal of practice, but relaxation training can focus attention away from pain and release tension from all muscles.

Relaxation tapes are available to help achieve the desired effects.

### Biofeedback

Biofeedback is taught by a professional who uses special machines to help a person learn to control bodily functions such as heart rate and muscle tension. As the person learns to release muscle tension, the machine immediately indicates success. Biofeedback can be used to reinforce relaxation training. Once the technique is mastered, it can be practiced without the use of the machine.

### Visual Imagery or Distraction

Imagery involves concentrating on mental pictures of pleasant scenes or events or mentally repeating positive sayings to reduce pain. Tapes are also available to help visual imagery.

Distraction techniques focus the person's attention away from negative painful images to positive mental thoughts. This may include watching television or a favorite movie, reading a book or listening to a book on tape, listening to music, or talking to a friend.

### Hypnosis

Hypnosis can be used in two ways to reduce a person's perception of pain. Some people are hypnotized by a therapist and given a post-hypnotic suggestion that reduces the pain they feel; others are taught self-hypnosis and can hypnotize themselves when pain interrupts their ability to function. Self-hypnosis is a form of relaxation training.

### Individual or Family Therapy

A psychologist, psychiatrist, or psychiatric social worker can help people cope with the feelings of depression, frustration, and anger that often accompany chronic pain.

## Medications for Pain Management

### Over-the-Counter Pain Relievers

Aspirin, ibuprofen, naprosyn sodium, and acetaminophen can effectively relieve pain. While these medications are relatively safe, they can still cause side effects such as stomach upset. For this reason, these medications should be taken according to the manufacturer's directions. Before increasing the frequency of use or the dosage, the person should first check with her or his doctor or pharmacist.

### Non-Steroidal Anti-Inflammatory Medications (NSAIDs)

NSAIDs may be prescribed to treat mild to severe pain. These preparations block pain and treat inflammation. There are dozens of NSAIDs on the market, and a person may have to try several different brands to find the one that works best for her or his pain.

### Muscle Relaxants

Some patients also get relief from muscle spasms with well-tolerated muscle relaxants. These medications must be prescribed by the physician.

### Topical Pain Relievers

A variety of pain-relieving topical creams may also relieve pain when they are rubbed directly into the painful area. While some of these creams are available by prescription only, others may be purchased over-the-counter.

### Narcotic Pain Medications

Narcotics are powerful pain-relieving medications derived from opium or synthetic opium. Narcotics alter a person's perception of pain and also induce euphoria, mood changes, mental cloudiness, and deep sleep. These medications may be available in pill or skin patch form. The skin patch releases small amounts of the narcotic into the body through the skin. These drugs may also cause nausea, lethargy, and constipation. People with osteoporosis must be very careful when taking these medications. Narcotics can affect a person's balance and increase the chance of falling. After repeated and prolonged use people may become dependent or addicted to these medications. Narcotics are only available by prescription.

*Antidepressant Medications*

People who suffer from chronic pain frequently suffer from chronic depression as well. Several studies using antidepressant medications have noted that these medications may not only improve depression but may also relieve or reduce the amount of pain a person feels. Additional research is needed to determine whether antidepressants can treat the chronic pain of osteoporosis and which antidepressants give the best results.

*Nerve Block*

In some cases, a physician may perform a nerve block which involves the injection of pain-relieving medications into the tissues around an affected nerve. The block numbs the nerves and surrounding tissues so they can no longer sense pain. Pain relief may last for hours or months, depending on the medications used and the person's response to them.

All of these methods of pain management, alone and in combination, are used in hospitals and clinics across the country. People who are suffering from unrelieved chronic pain may wish to consult their physician for a referral to a physical therapist or a clinic specializing in pain management.

# Chapter 66

# *Behavioral and Relaxation Techniques for Chronic Pain and Insomnia*

## What Behavioral and Relaxation Approaches Are Used for Conditions Such as Chronic Pain and Insomnia?

### *Pain*

Pain is defined by the International Association for the Study of Pain as an unpleasant sensory experience associated with actual or potential tissue damage or described in terms of such damage. It is a complex, subjective, perceptual phenomenon with a number of contributing factors that are uniquely experienced by each individual. Pain is typically classified as acute, cancer-related, and chronic non-malignant. Acute pain is associated with a noxious event. Its severity is generally proportional to the degree of tissue injury and is expected to diminish with healing and time. Chronic non-malignant pain frequently develops following an injury but persists long after a reasonable period of healing. Its underlying causes are often not readily discernible, and the pain is disproportionate to demonstrable tissue damage. It is frequently accompanied by alteration of sleep, mood, sexual, vocational, and avocational function.

National Institutes of Health Consensus Development Program, *Integration of Behavioral and Relaxation Approaches into the Treatment of Chronic Pain and Insomnia,* NIH Techonology Assessment Statement Online, October 16-18, 1995 [cited August 2000], 1-34.

## *Insomnia*

Insomnia may be defined as a disturbance or perceived disturbance of the usual sleep pattern of the individual that has troublesome consequences. These consequences may include daytime fatigue and drowsiness, irritability, anxiety, depression, and somatic complaints. Categories of disturbed sleep are:

1. inability to fall asleep,
2. inability to maintain sleep, and
3. early awakening.

## *Selection Criteria*

A large variety of behavioral and relaxation approaches are used for conditions such as chronic pain and insomnia. The specific approaches that were addressed in this technology assessment conference represent three important selection criteria. First, somatically directed therapies with behavioral components (e.g., physical therapy, occupational therapy, acupuncture) were not considered. Second, the approaches were drawn from those reported in the scientific literature. Many commonly used behavioral approaches are not specifically incorporated into conventional medical care. For example, religious and spiritual approaches, which are the most commonly used health-related actions by the U.S. population, were not considered in this conference. Third, the approaches are a subset of those discussed in the literature and represent those selected by the conference organizers as most commonly used in clinical settings in the United States. Certain commonly used clinical interventions such as music, dance, recreational, and art therapies also were not addressed.

## *Relaxation Techniques*

Relaxation techniques are a group of behavioral therapeutic approaches that differ widely in their philosophical bases as well as in their methodologies and techniques. Their primary objective is the achievement of non-directed relaxation (rather than direct achievement of a specific therapeutic goal). They all share two basic components: (1) repetitive focus on a word, sound, prayer, phrase, body sensation, or muscular activity and(2) the adoption of a passive attitude toward intruding thoughts and a return to the focus. These techniques induce a common set of physiologic changes that result in decreased metabolic activity. Relaxation techniques may also be used in stress management (as self-regulatory techniques) and have been divided into deep and brief methods.

## Deep Methods

Deep methods include autogenic training, meditation, and progressive muscle relaxation (PMR). Autogenic training consists of imagining a peaceful environment and comforting bodily sensations. Six basic focusing techniques are used: heaviness in the limbs, warmth in the limbs, cardiac regulation, centering on breathing, warmth in the upper abdomen, and coolness in the forehead. Meditation is a self-directed practice for relaxing the body and calming the mind. A large variety of meditation techniques are commonly used; each has its own proponents. Meditation generally does not involve suggestion, auto-suggestion, or trance. The goal of mindfulness meditation is development of a non-judgmental awareness of bodily sensations and mental activities occurring in the present moment. Concentration meditation trains the person to passively attend to a bodily process, word, and/or a stimulus. Transcendental meditation focuses on a "suitable" sound or thought (the mantra) without attempting to actually concentrate on the sound or thought. There are also many movement meditations, such as yoga and walking meditation in Zen Buddhism. PMR focuses on reducing muscle tone in major muscle groups. Each of the 15 major muscle groups is tensed and then relaxed in sequence.

## Brief Methods

The brief methods, which include self-control relaxation, paced respiration, and deep breathing, generally require less time to acquire or practice and often represent abbreviated forms of a corresponding deep method. For example, self-control relaxation is an abbreviated form of PMR. Autogenic training may be abbreviated and converted to a self-control format. Paced respiration teaches patients to maintain slow breathing when anxiety threatens. Deep breathing involves taking several deep breaths, holding them for five seconds, and then exhaling slowly.

## Hypnotic Techniques

Hypnotic techniques induce states of selective attention focusing or diffusion combined with enhanced imagery. They are often used to induce relaxation and also may be a part of cognitive-behavioral techniques (CBT). The techniques have pre- and post-suggestion components. The pre-suggestion component involves attention focusing through the use of imagery, distraction, and/or relaxation. Subjects focus on relaxation and passively disregard intrusive thoughts. The pre-suggestion component of hypnosis has features that are similar to other relaxation techniques. The suggestion phase is characterized by introduction of specific goals, for example, analgesia may be specifically suggested. The post-suggestion component involves continued use of the new behavior following termination of hypnosis. Individuals vary widely in their hypnotic susceptibility and suggestibility, although the reasons for these differences are incompletely understood.

## Biofeedback Techniques

Biofeedback techniques are treatment methods that use monitoring instruments of varying degrees of sophistication to provide patients with physiologic information that allows them to reliably influence psycho-physiological responses of two kinds:

1.  responses not ordinarily under voluntary control and

2.  responses that ordinarily are easily regulated, but for which regulation has broken down.

Technologies that are commonly used include electromyography (EMG-BF), electroencephalography (EEG-BF), thermometers (thermal-BF), and galvanometry (electrodermal-BF). Biofeedback techniques often induce physiological responses similar to those of other relaxation techniques.

## Cognitive-Behavioral Techniques

Cognitive-Behavioral techniques (CBT) attempt to alter patterns of negative thoughts and dysfunctional attitudes in order to foster more healthy and adaptive thoughts, emotions, and actions. These interventions share four basic components: education, skills acquisition, cognitive and behavioral rehearsal, and generalization and maintenance. Relaxation techniques are frequently included as a behavioral component in CBT programs. The specific programs used to implement the four components can vary considerably. Each of the aforementioned therapeutic modalities may be practiced individually, or they may be combined as part of multimodal approaches to management of chronic pain or insomnia.

### *Relaxation and Behavioral Techniques for Insomnia*

Relaxation and behavioral techniques corresponding to those used for chronic pain may be employed for specific types of insomnia. Cognitive relaxation, various forms of biofeedback, and PMR may all be used in the treatment of insomnia. In addition, the following behavioral approaches are generally used in the management of insomnia.

- **Sleep hygiene**, which involves educating patients about behaviors that may interfere with the sleep process, with the hope that education about maladaptive behaviors will lead to behavioral modification.

- **Stimulus control therapy**, which seeks to create and protect conditioned association between the bedroom and sleep. Activities in the bedroom are restricted to sleep and sex.

- **Sleep restriction therapy**, in which patients provide a sleep log and are then asked to stay in bed only as long as they think they are currently sleeping. This usually leads to sleep deprivation and consolidation followed by a gradual increase in the length of time in bed.

- **Paradoxical intention** in which the patient is instructed not to fall asleep, with the expectation that efforts to avoid sleep will in fact induce it.

## *How Successful Are These Approaches?*

### *Pain*

A plethora of studies using a range of behavioral and relaxation approaches to treat chronic pain is reported in the literature. The measures of success reported in these studies depend on the rigor of the research design, the population studied, the length of follow-up, and the outcome measures identified. As the number of well-designed studies using a variety of behavioral and relaxation techniques grows, the use of meta-analysis as a means of demonstrating overall effectiveness increases.

One carefully analyzed review of studies on chronic pain, including cancer pain, was prepared under the auspices of the U.S. Agency for Health Care Policy and Research (AHCPR) in 1990. A great strength of the report was the careful categorization of the evidential basis of each intervention. The categorization was based on design of the studies and consistency of findings among the studies. These properties led to the development of a four-point scale that ranked the evidence as strong, moderate, fair, and weak; that scale is used in this panel report in evaluating both the AHCPR studies and additional data.

Evaluation of behavioral and relaxation interventions for chronic pain reduction in adults found the following:

**Relaxation.** The evidence is strong for the effectiveness of this class of techniques in reducing chronic pain in a variety of medical conditions.

**Hypnosis.** The evidence supporting the effectiveness of hypnosis in alleviating chronic pain associated with cancer is strong. In addition, the panel was presented with other data suggesting the effectiveness of hypnosis in other chronic pain conditions such as irritable bowel syndrome, oral mucositis, temporomandibular disorders, and tension headaches.

**Cognitive-Behavioral Techniques.** The evidence was moderate for the usefulness of cognitive-behavioral techniques (CBT) in chronic pain. In addition, a series of eight well-designed studies found CBT superior to placebo and to routine care for alleviating low back pain and rheumatoid arthritis and osteoarthritis, but inferior to hypnosis for oral mucositis, and, as mentioned, to EMG biofeedback for tension headache.

**Biofeedback.** The evidence is moderate for the effectiveness of biofeedback in relieving many types of chronic pain. Data were also reviewed showing EMG-BF to be more effective than psychological placebo for tension headache but equivalent in results to relaxation. For migraine headache biofeedback is equivalent to relaxation therapy and better than no treatment, but the superiority to psychological placebo is less clear.

**Multimodal Treatment.** Several meta-analyses address the effectiveness of pain clinic multimodal treatments. These studies indicate a consistent positive effect of the program of these centers on several categories of regional pain. Back and neck pain, dental or facial pain, joint pain, and migraine headaches have all shown a significant benefit.

Although there is relatively good evidence for the effectiveness of several behavioral and relaxation interventions in the treatment of chronic pain, there is insufficient data to conclude that one technique is more effective than another for a given condition. For any given individual patient, however, one approach may indeed be more appropriate than another.

## *Insomnia*

Behavioral treatments produce improvements in some aspects of sleep, the most pronounced of which are for sleep latency and time awake after sleep onset. Relaxation and biofeedback were both found to be effective in alleviating insomnia. Cognitive forms of relaxation such as meditation were slightly better than somatic forms of relaxation such as PMR. Sleep restriction, stimulus control, and multimodal treatment were the three most effective treatments in reducing insomnia. No data were presented or reviewed on the effectiveness of CBT or hypnosis. Improvements seen at treatment completion were maintained at follow-ups averaging six months in duration. Although these effects are statistically significant, it is questionable whether the magnitude of the improvements in sleep onset and total sleep time are clinically meaningful.

To adequately evaluate the relative success of different treatment modalities for insomnia a number of major issues need to be addressed.

First, valid objective measures of insomnia are needed. Some investigators rely on self-reports by patients, while others believe that insomnia must be documented electro-physiologically.

Second, what constitutes a therapeutic outcome should be determined. Some investigators use time until sleep onset, number of awakenings, and total sleep time as outcome measures, whereas others believe that impairment in daytime functioning is another important outcome measure. Both of these issues require resolution for research in the field to move forward.

## *Critique*

Although this literature offers substantial promise, the state of the art of the methodology in this field of behavioral and relaxation interventions indicates a need for thoughtful interpretation of these findings and prompt translation into programs of health care delivery. It should be noted that similar criticisms can be made of many conventional medical procedures.

Several cautions must be considered threats to the internal and external validity of the study results. The following problems exist regarding internal validity:

1.  The full and adequate comparability among treatment contrast groups may be absent;

2.  The sample sizes are sometimes small, lessening the ability to detect differences in efficacy;

3.  Complete blinding, which would be ideal, is compromised by patient and clinician awareness of the treatment;

4.  The treatments may not be well described and adequate procedures for standardization such as therapy manuals, therapist training, and reliable competency and integrity assessments have not always been carried out; and

5.  A potential publication bias in favor of authors dropping studies with small effects and negative results is a concern in a field characterized by studies with small numbers of patients.

With regard to the ability to generalize the findings of these investigations, the following considerations are important:

• The patients participating in these studies are usually not cognitively impaired. They must be capable not only of participating in the study treatments, but also of fulfilling all the requirements of participating in the study protocol.

• The therapists must be adequately trained to conduct the therapy competently.

• The cultural context in which the treatment is conducted may alter its acceptability and effectiveness.

In summary, this literature offers substantial promise and suggests a need for prompt translation into programs of health care delivery. At the same time, the state of the art of the methodology in the field of behavioral and relaxation interventions indicates a need for thoughtful interpretation of these findings. It should be noted that similar criticisms can be made of many conventional medical procedures.

## How Do These Approaches Work?

The mechanism of action of behavioral and relaxation approaches can be considered at two levels:

1. Determining how the procedure works to reduce cognitive and physiological arousal and to promote the most appropriate behavioral response and,

2. Identifying effects at more basic levels of functional anatomy, neuro-transmitter and other biochemical activity, and circadian rhythms. The exact biological actions are often unknown.

### *Pain*

There appear to be two pain transmission circuits. Some data suggest that a spinal cord-thalamic-frontal cortex-anterior cingulate pathway plays a role in the subjective psychological and physiological responses to pain, whereas a spinal cord-thalamic-somatosensory cortex pathway plays a role in pain sensation. A descending pathway involving the periaquaductal gray region modulates pain signals. This system can augment or inhibit pain transmission at the level of the dorsal spinal cord. Endogenous opioids are particularly concentrated in this pathway.

At the level of the spinal cord, serotonin and norepinephrine appear to play important roles. Relaxation techniques as a group generally alter sympathetic activity as indicated by decreases in oxygen consumption, respiratory and heart rate, and blood pressure. Increased slow wave activity on electroencephalography has also been reported. Although the mechanism for the decrease in sympathetic activity is unclear, one may infer decreased arousal (due to alterations in catecholamines or other neurochemical systems) plays a key role.

Hypnosis, in part because of its capacity for evoking intense relaxation, has been reported to reduce nausea associated with chemotherapy and has been shown to be helpful in reducing several types of pain, e.g., lower back and burn pain. Hypnosis does not appear to influence endorphin production, and its role in the production of catecholamines is not known. Hypnosis has been hypothesized to block pain from entering consciousness by activating the thalamic-frontal cortex-anterior cingulate pathway to inhibit impulse transmission from thalamic to cortical structures. Similarly, other CBTs may decrease transmission through this pathway. Moreover, the overlap in brain regions involved in pain modulation and anxiety suggest a possible role for CBT approaches affecting this area of function, although data are still evolving.

CBT also appears to exert a number of other effects that could alter pain intensity. Depression and anxiety increase subjective complaints of pain, and cognitive-behavioral approaches are well-documented for decreasing these affective states. In addition, these types of techniques may alter expectation, which also plays a key role in subjective experiences of pain intensity. They also may augment analgesic responses through behavioral conditioning. Finally, these techniques help patients feel empowered or less helpless and better able to deal with pain sensations.

## *Insomnia*

A cognitive-behavioral model for insomnia (see Figure 67.1) elucidates the interaction of insomnia with emotional, cognitive, and physiologic arousal: dysfunctional conditions, such as worry over sleep; and maladaptive habits (e.g., excessive time in bed and daytime napping) and the consequences of insomnia (e.g., fatigue and performance in impairment of activities).

In the treatment of insomnia, relaxation techniques have been used to reduce cognitive and physiological arousal and thus assist the induction of sleep as well as decrease awakenings during sleep.

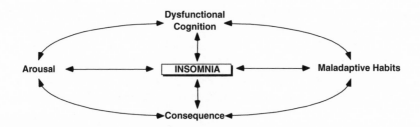

*Figure 66.1 MORIN CM (1993) Insomnia—The Guilford Press Adapted From Presentation by D. J. Buysse, M.D. at NIH Technology Conference 10-17-95.*

Relaxation is also likely to influence decreased activity in the entire sympathetic system, permitting a more rapid and effective "deafferentation" at sleep onset at the level of the thalamus. Relaxation may also enhance para-sympathetic activity in turn further decreasing autonomic tone. In addition, it has been suggested that alterations in cytokine activity (immune system) may play a role in insomnia or in response to treatment.

Cognitive approaches may decrease arousal and dysfunctional beliefs and thus improve sleep. Behavioral techniques including sleep restriction and stimulus control can be helpful in reducing physiologic arousal, reversing poor sleep habits, and shifting circadian rhythms. These effects appear to involve both cortical structures and deep nuclei (e.g., *locus ceruleus* and *suprachiasmatic nucleus*).

Knowing the mechanisms of action would reinforce and expand use of behavioral and relaxation techniques, but incorporation of these approaches into the treatment of chronic pain and insomnia can proceed on the basis of clinical efficacy, as has occurred with the discovery of other practices and products before their mode of action was completely delineated.

## Are There Barriers to the Appropriate Integration of These Approaches into Health Care?

One barrier to the integration of behavioral and relaxation techniques in standard medical care has been the emphasis on the biomedical model as the basis of medical education. The biomedical model defines disease in anatomic and patho-physiologic terms. Expansion to a bio-psychosocial model would increase emphasis on a patient's experience of disease and balance the anatomic/physiologic needs of patients with their psychosocial needs.

For example, of six factors identified to correlate with treatment failures of low back pain, all are psycho-social factors. The integration of behavioral and relaxation therapies with conventional medical procedures is necessary for the successful treatment of such conditions. Similarly, the importance of a comprehensive evaluation of a patient is emphasized in the field of insomnia where failure to identify a condition such as sleep apnea will result in inappropriate application of a behavioral therapy. Therapy should be matched to the illness and to the patient.

The integration of psycho-social issues with conventional medical approaches will necessitate the application of new methodologies to assess the success or failure of interventions. Therefore, additional barriers to integration include lack of standardization of outcome measures, lack of standardization or agreement on what constitutes successful outcome, and consensus on what constitutes appropriate follow-up. Methodologies appropriate for the evaluation of drugs may not be adequate for the evaluation of some psycho-social interventions, especially those involving patient experience and quality of life. Psycho-social research studies must maintain the high quality of those methods that have been painstakingly developed over the last few decades. Agreement needs to be reached for standards governing the demonstration of efficacy for psycho-social interventions.

Psychosocial interventions are often time intensive, creating potential blocks to provider and patient acceptance and compliance. Participation in biofeedback training typically includes up to 10 to 12 sessions of approximately 45 minutes to 1 hour each. Additionally home practice of these techniques is usually required. Thus, patient compliance and willingness to participate in these therapies will have to be addressed. Physicians will have to be educated on the efficacy of these techniques. They must also be willing to educate their patients about the importance and potential benefits of these interventions and to provide encouragement for the patient through the training processes.

Insurance companies provide a financial incentive or barrier to access of care depending upon their willingness to provide reimbursement. Traditionally, insurance companies have been reluctant to reimburse for some psycho-social interventions and reimburse others at rates below those for standard medical care. Psycho-social interventions should be reimbursed as part of comprehensive medical services at rates comparable to those for other medical care particularly in view of data supporting their effectiveness and data detailing the costs of failed medical and surgical interventions.

The evidence suggests that sleep disorders are significantly under-diagnosed. The prevalence and possible consequences of insomnia have begun to be documented. There are substantial disparities between patient reports of insomnia and the number of insomnia diagnoses, as well as between the number of prescriptions written for sleep medications and the number of recorded diagnoses of insomnia. Data indicate that insomnia is widespread, but the morbidity and mortality of this condition are not well understood. Without this information, it remains difficult for physicians to gauge how aggressive their intervention should be in the treatment of this disorder. Additionally, the efficacy of the behavioral approaches for treating this condition has not been adequately disseminated to the medical community.

Finally, who should be administering these therapies? Problems with credentialing and training have yet to be completely addressed in the field. Although the initial studies have been done by qualified and highly trained practitioners in each of these fields, the question remains as to how this will best translate into delivery of care in the community. Decisions will have to be made about which practitioners are best qualified and most cost-effective to provide these psycho-social interventions.

## What Are the Significant Issues for Future Research and Applications?

Research efforts on these therapies should include additional efficacy and effectiveness studies, cost-effectiveness studies, and efforts to replicate existing studies. Several specific issues should be addressed:

### *Outcomes*

- Outcome measures should be reliable, valid, and standardized for behavioral and relaxation interventions research in each area (chronic pain, insomnia) so that studies can be compared and combined.

- Qualitative research is needed to help determine patients' experiences with both insomnia and chronic pain and the impact of treatments.

- Future research should include examination of consequences/ outcomes of untreated chronic pain and insomnia; chronic pain and insomnia treated pharmacologically versus treated with behavioral and relaxation therapies; and combinations of pharmacologic and psycho-social treatments for chronic pain and insomnia.

### *Mechanism(s) of Action*

- Advances in the neuro-biological sciences and psycho-neuro-immunology are providing an improved scientific base for understanding mechanisms of action of behavioral and relaxation techniques, and need to be further investigated.

### *Covariates*

- Chronic pain and insomnia, as well as behavioral and relaxation therapies, involve factors such as values, beliefs, expectations, and behaviors, all of which are strongly culturally shaped. Research is needed to assess cross-cultural applicability, efficacy, and modifications of psycho-social therapeutic modalities.

• Research studies that examine the effectiveness of behavioral and relaxation approaches to insomnia and chronic pain should consider the influence of age, race, gender, religious belief, and socio-economic status on treatment effectiveness.

### Health Services

• The most effective timing of the introduction of behavioral interventions into the course of treatment should be studied.

• Research is needed to optimize the match between specific behavioral and relaxation techniques and specific patient groups and treatment settings.

### Integration into Clinical Care and Medical Education

• New and innovative methods of introducing psycho-social treatments into health care curricula and practice should be implemented.

## Conclusions

A number of well-defined behavioral and relaxation interventions are now available, some of which are commonly used to treat chronic pain and insomnia. Available data support the effectiveness of these interventions in relieving chronic pain and in achieving some reduction in insomnia. Data are currently insufficient to conclude with confidence that one technique is more effective than another for a given condition. For any given individual patient, however, one approach may indeed be more appropriate than another.

Behavioral and relaxation interventions clearly reduce arousal and hypnosis reduces pain perception. However, the exact biological underpinnings of these effects require further study, as is often the case with medical therapies. Although the literature demonstrates treatment effectiveness, the state of the art of the methodologies in this field indicates a need for thoughtful interpretation of the findings as well as an urgency to translate them into programs of health care delivery.

Although specific structural, bureaucratic, financial, and attitudinal barriers exist to the integration of these techniques, all are potentially surmountable with education and additional research, as patients shift from being passive participants in their treatment to becoming responsible, active partners in their rehabilitation.

The conference was co-sponsored by the National Institute of Mental Health, National Institute of Dental Research. National Heart, Lung, and Blood Institute, National Institute on Aging, National Cancer Institute, National Institute of Nursing Research, National Institute of Neurological Disorders and Stroke, and the National Institute of Arthritis and Musculoskeletal and Skin Diseases.

## More Information

This statement and the full text of other NIH statements are also available online through an electronic bulletin board system and through the Internet:

NIH Information Center BBS
1-800-NIH-BBS1 (644-2271)

Gopher
gopher://gopher.nih.gov/Health and Clinical Information

World Wide Web
http://text.nlm.nih.gov

ftp
ftp://public.nlm.nih.gov/hstat

## Publications Ordering Information

NIH Consensus Statements, NIH Technology Statements, and related materials are available be writing to the NIH Consensus Program Information Center, P.O. Box 2577, Kensington, Maryland 20891; by calling toll-free 1-888-NIH-CONSENSUS (1-888-644-2667); or by visiting the NIH consensus Development Program home page on the World Wide Web at http://consensus.nih.gov.

# Part Seven

# Additional Help and Information

# Chapter 67

# *Glossary of Important Terms*

## A

**Aerobic exercise:** Exercise that requires continuous, rhythmic motion of large muscle groups such as the quadriceps. Swimming, running, and walking are examples of aerobic exercise. Aerobic exercise also improves the ability to perform activities of daily living.

**Alendronate:** Alendronate is a medication used to treat and prevent osteoporosis. It is from a class of drugs called bisphosphonates, which inhibit bone breakdown. Alendronate has been shown to increase bone density and prevent fractures.

**Ankylosing spondylitis:** See Spondyloarthropathies.

**Antibody:** A special protein produced by the body's immune system that recognizes and helps fight infectious agents and other foreign substances that invade the body.

**Antinuclear antibody (ANA) test:** A blood test done to find out if the body is producing antinuclear antibodies.

---

This chapter contains definitions from the following National Institutes of Health (NIH) Web Publications, Office of Scientific and Health Communications [http://www.nih.gov/niams/healthinfo]: "Arthritis and Exercise Keywords," "Polymyalgia Rheumatica and Giant Cell Arteritis Glossary," "Psoriasis Glossary," and "Raynaud's Phenomenon Keywords." Some additional terms were extracted from the documents included in this volume.

**Antinuclear antibody:** Abnormal antibodies that are often present in people who have connective tissue diseases or other autoimmune disorders. These antibodies target material in the nucleus (the "command center") of healthy cells instead of fighting specific disease-causing agents.

**Arteries:** Large blood vessels that carry blood and oxygen from the heart to all parts of the body.

**Arterioles:** Small blood vessels that branch off from arteries and connect to capillaries.

**Artery:** Any tubular, branching vessel that carries blood from the heart throughout the body.

**Arthritis:** Literally means joint inflammation. It is a general term for more than 100 conditions known as rheumatic diseases. These diseases affect not only the joints but also other parts of the body, including important supporting structures such as muscles, tendons, and ligaments, as well as some internal organs. These diseases can cause pain, stiffness, and swelling in joints and may also affect other parts of the body.

**Atrophy:** Decrease in size or wasting away of a body part or tissue. When muscles are not used, they atrophy (get smaller and weaker).

**Autoantibodies:** Abnormal antibodies produced against the body's own tissues.

**Autoimmune disease:** A disease in which the immune system destroys or attacks a person's own tissues.

## B

**Benign:** A mild disease or condition that is not life threatening.

**Biofeedback:** A technique designed to help a person gain control over involuntary (independent of the will) body functions, such as heart rate, blood pressure, or skin temperature. A way to enhance a body signal so that one is aware of something that usually occurs at a level below consciousness. An electronic device provides information about a body function (such as heart rate) so that the person using biofeedback can learn to control that function. Biofeedback can help people with osteoporosis or arthritis learn to relax their muscles. In this case, an electronic device amplifies the sound of a muscle contracting, so the osteoporosis or arthritis patient knows that the muscle is not relaxed

**Biopsy:** The removal of tissue or cells from a person to examine them for signs of disease.

**Body mechanics:** Correct positioning of the body for a given task, such as lifting a heavy object or typing.

**Bone Density:** Bone density is expressed as grams of mineral per area or volume and in any given individual is determined by peak bone mass and amount of bone loss.

**Bone Density Test:** This safe, painless, and non-invasive test can determine your bone density, which is a measure of bone strength, and can predict your chances of sustaining a fracture in the future. It uses very low amounts of radiation and is much more sensitive than standard x-rays.

**Bone Formation:** Bone formation refers to the production of new bone tissue.

**Bone Mineral Density (BMD):** BMD measurements establish criteria for the diagnosis of osteoporosis. A T-score is defined as the number of standard deviations (SD) above or below the average BMD value for young healthy white women. This should be distinguished from a Z-score, which is defined as the number of SD above or below the average BMD for age- and gender-matched controls. According to the World Health Organization definition, osteoporosis is present when the T-score is at least minus 2.5 SD.

**Bone Quality:** Bone quality refers to bone architecture, turnover, damage accumulation (e.g., microfractures) and mineralization.

**Bone Resorption:** Bone resorption is the destruction of old bone tissue.

## C

**Calcitonin:** Calcitonin is a treatment option for postmenopausal women. Calcitonin is a hormone produced in the thyroid gland that is involved in calcium regulation and bone metabolism. This hormone has been shown to slow bone loss. It is available in nasal spray form or can be administered by injection.

**Capillaries:** Tiny blood vessels that carry blood between arterioles (the smallest arteries) and venules (the smallest veins). Capillaries form networks throughout the body's organs and tissues. They open and close in response to the organs' needs for oxygen and nutrients.

**Cardiovascular:** Involving the heart and the circulatory system.

**Cartilage:** A tough, stretchy tissue that covers the ends of bones to form a low-friction, shock-absorbing surface for joints.

**Collagen:** A fibrous protein that is one of the main building blocks of skin, tendon, bone, cartilage, and other connective tissues.

**Connective tissue disease:** A group of diseases that affect the body's connective tissues, including tissue in the joints, blood vessels, heart, skin, and other supporting structures. Some of these diseases are caused by a malfunctioning of the immune system. Connective tissue diseases are fairly common and include systemic lupus erythematosus, rheumatoid arthritis, scleroderma, polymyositis, and dermatomyositis.

**Connective tissue:** The supporting framework of the body and the internal organs—including bone, cartilage, and ligaments. The tissue that supports body structures and holds parts together. Some parts of the body, such as tendons and cartilage, are made up of connective tissue. Connective tissue is also the basic substance of bone and blood vessels.

**Cortical Bone:** Cortical bone is dense and compact. It forms the outer layer of the bones.

**Corticosteroids:** Potent anti-inflammatory hormones that are made naturally in the body or synthetically (man-made) for use as drugs. They also are called glucocorticoids. The most commonly prescribed drug of this type is prednisone.

**Cyanosis:** Bluish, grayish, or dark purple discoloration of the skin that occurs when blood cannot circulate freely and gives up all its oxygen.

**Cytokines:** Chemical messengers in the body that help direct and regulate response and are involved in cell-to-cell communication.

**D**

**Degenerative joint disease:** See Osteoarthritis (OA).

**Dermis:** The layer of skin beneath the epidermis.

## E

**Emollient:** A substance composed of fat or oil that soothes and softens the skin.

**Endorphin:** A substance produced in the brain or nervous system that stops pain naturally.

**Endurance:** The ability to continue a given task.

**Epidermis:** The outermost layer of skin.

**Erythrocyte sedimentation rate (ESR):** A blood test that determines how fast erythrocytes (red blood cells) settle out of unclotted blood and is used to detect inflammation in the body. Connective tissue diseases can change blood proteins, which changes how quickly red blood cells settle out of unclotted blood to the bottom of a test tube. Higher ESRs (indicating more rapid settling of red blood cells and the presence of inflammation) are found in all of the connective tissue diseases. Also referred to as the "sed rate" or ESR.

**Erythrodermic psoriasis:** A form of psoriasis characterized by widespread reddening and scaling of the skin often accompanied by itching or pain. Symptoms may be precipitated by severe sunburn, use of oral steroids, or a drug-related rash.

**Estrogen Replacement Therapy (ERT):** Estrogen replacement therapy (ERT) has been used to help prevent osteoporosis in women who no longer produce estrogen because of menopause or surgical removal of the ovaries. Estrogen replacement therapy (ERT) is medication that replaces or supplements the body's falling level of estrogen which results from menopause. ERT helps keep calcium in the bones and maintains bone density, thereby preventing osteoporosis. Recent research findings indicate that ERT also may protect against heart disease.

**Exercise:** Movement of the body designed to improve its physical condition. The goals of an osteoporosis or arthritis exercise program are to improve physical conditioning, muscle strength, flexibility, well-being, and function.

## F

**Fibromyalgia:** A chronic disorder characterized by widespread musculoskeletal pain, fatigue, and multiple tender points.

**Fibrous capsule:** A tough wrapping of tendons and ligaments that surrounds the joint.

**Flare:** A period of time in which disease symptoms reappear or become worse.

**Flexibility:** Ability to bend various joints and move freely.

## G

**Gangrene:** A condition that occurs when tissue dies. Tissue death is usually caused by a loss of blood supply. Gangrene may affect a small area, such as a finger or toe, or a large portion of a limb.

**Gene:** A unit of inheritance that contains the instructions, or code, that a cell uses to make a specific product, usually a protein. Genes are made of a substance called DNA. They govern every body function and determine inherited traits passed from parent to child.

**Genetics:** The science of understanding how diseases, conditions, and traits are inherited.

**Giant Cell Arteritis:** A disease causing inflammation of the temporal arteries and other arteries in the head and neck. Inflammation causes the arteries to narrow, reducing blood flow in the affected areas. The condition may cause persistent headaches and vision loss. It is also known as cranial arteritis, temporal arteritis, or Horton's disease.

**Gout:** A type of arthritis caused by the reaction of the body to needle-like crystals of uric acid that accumulate in joint spaces. This reaction causes inflammation, swelling, and pain in the affected joint, most commonly the big toe.

**Guttate psoriasis:** A form of psoriasis characterized by drop-like lesions on the trunk, limbs, and scalp. Symptoms may be triggered by viral respiratory infections or certain bacterial (streptococcal) infections.

## H

**Histologic examination:** The study of a tissue specimen by staining it and examining it under a microscope.

**Hydrotherapy:** Therapy that takes place in the water.

# I

**Idiopathic Juvenile Osteoporosis (IJO):** An onset of juvenile osteoporosis without apparent cause.

**Immune response:** The reactions of the immune system to foreign substances.

**Immune System:** A complex network of specialized cells and organs that work together to defend the body against attacks by "foreign" invaders such as bacteria and viruses. In some rheumatic conditions, it appears that the immune system does not function properly and may even work against the body.

**Incidence:** The number of new cases of a particular disease that occur in a population during a defined period of time, usually one year.

**Inflammation:** A characteristic reaction of tissues to injury or disease. It is marked by four signs: swelling, redness, heat, and pain.

**Internist:** A doctor who specializes in internal medicine (not requiring surgery).

**Inverse psoriasis:** A form of psoriasis characterized by large, dry, smooth, vividly red plaques in the folds of skin.

**Ischemic lesion:** A sore or other skin abnormality caused by an insufficient supply of blood to the tissue.

**Isometrics:** Isometric exercises are exercises that cause a muscle to contract and do work while joints do not move, for example, pushing against a wall.

# J

**Joint space:** The area enclosed within the fibrous capsule and synovium.

**Joint:** The place where two bones meet. Most joints are composed of cartilage, joint space, fibrous capsule, synovium, and ligaments.

**Juvenile Osteoporosis:** An early onset of osteoporosis. Osteoporosis is rare among children and adolescents. When it occurs, it is usually caused by an underlying medical disorder or by medications used to treat such disorders. This is called secondary osteoporosis. It may also be the result of a genetic disorder such as osteogenesis imperfecta.

Sometimes there is no identifiable cause of juvenile osteoporosis. This is known as idiopathic juvenile osteoporosis (IJO).

**Juvenile rheumatoid arthritis:** A chronic arthritis of childhood that causes pain, stiffness, swelling, and loss of function in the joints and may also affect other parts of the body.

## K

**Keratolytic:** A substance that promotes the softening and peeling of the epidermis.

## L

**Ligaments:** Stretchy bands of cord-like tissue that connect bone to bone.

## M

**Manipulation:** Trained professionals such as chiropractors or osteopaths use their hands to help restore normal movement to stiff joints.

**Methotrexate:** A drug often used to treat cancer that is also used in lower doses to treat some forms of arthritis.

**Microwaves:** Microwave therapy is a type of deep heat therapy. The electromagnetic waves pass between electrodes placed on the patient's skin. This creates heat that increases blood flow and relieves muscle and joint pain.

**Mobilization therapies:** A group of treatments that include traction, massage, and manipulation. When used by a trained professional, these methods can help control pain and increase joint and muscle motion.

**Muscle:** Tissue that can contract, producing movement or force. There are three types of muscle: striated muscle, attached to bones; smooth muscle, found in such tissues as the stomach and blood vessels; and cardiac muscle, which forms the walls of the heart. For striated muscle to function at its ideal level, the joint and surrounding structures must be in good condition.

## N

**Nailfold capillaroscopy:** A test used to identify the primary or secondary form of Raynaud's phenomenon. The examiner places a drop of oil on the nailfold (the skin at the cuticle or base of the nail) and uses a hand-held magnifying glass or microscope to look at the capillaries in the nailfold. Certain changes in theses capillaries can be characteristic of connective tissue diseases.

**Nonsteroidal anti-inflammatory drugs (NSAIDs):** A group of medications, including aspirin, ibuprofen, and related drugs, used to reduce inflammation that causes joint pain, stiffness, and swelling.

**NSAID:** An abbreviation for nonsteroidal anti-inflammatory drug. NSAIDs do not contain corticosteroids and are used to reduce pain and inflammation. Aspirin and ibuprofen are two types of NSAIDs.

## O

**Occult:** Disease or symptoms that are not readily detectable by physical examination or laboratory tests.

**Osteoblasts:** Osteoblasts are responsible for bone formation and completion of the bone remodeling cycle. Osteoblasts form new bone by secreting protein fibers into the cavities produced by the osteoclasts. Calcium salts harden these protein deposits, a process also controlled by osteoblasts.

**Osteoclasts:** Osteoclasts are responsible for bone resorption and initiation of the bone remodeling cycle. Osteoclasts destroy bone tissue by dissolving minerals. Other cells, macrophages, then digest the protein matrix.

**Osteoarthritis:** OA (also know as degenerative joint disease) primarily affects cartilage within the joints, causing it to fray, wear, ulcerate, and in extreme cases, to wear away entirely, leaving a bone-on-bone joint. At the edges of the joint, bony spurs may form. OA can cause joint pain, loss of function, reduced joint motion, and deformity. Disability results most often from disease in the spine and in the weight-bearing joints (knees and hips).

**Osteocytes:** Osteocytes are responsible for maintenance work within bone tissue. Osteocytes, former osteoblasts trapped by calcified tissue, perform maintenance work within the bone tissue and control local mineral exchange.

**Osteogenesis Imperfecta (OI):** Osteogenesis Imperfecta is a genetic disorder characterized by bones that break easily, often from little or no apparent cause. There are at least four distinct forms of the disorder, representing extreme variation in severity from one individual to another. For example, a person may have as few as ten or as many as several hundred fractures in a lifetime.

**Osteoporosis:** Osteoporosis is defined as a skeletal disorder characterized by compromised bone strength predisposing to an increased risk of fracture. Bone strength reflects the integration of two main features: bone density and bone quality. See primary and secondary osteoporosis and juvenile osteoporosis.

## P

**Phototherapy:** Use of natural or artificial light to treat a disease.

**Physiatrist:** A doctor who specializes in the diagnosis and management of injuries and diseases causing pain, loss of function, and disability. Treatment plans often include the use of exercise, massage, heat, electricity (TENS), relaxation techniques, splints and braces, and local injections to relieve pain.

**Plaques:** Patches of thickened and reddened skin that are covered by silvery scales.

**Polymyalgia Rheumatica:** A condition of unknown cause that affects the lining of joints, particularly in the shoulders and hips. Symptoms include pain and stiffness, typically in the neck, shoulders, and hips. It may be associated with giant cell arteritis.

**Polymyositis:** A rheumatic disease that causes weakness and inflammation of muscles.

**Predisposition:** A tendency to develop a certain disease.

**Prevalence:** The total number of people in a population with a certain disease at a given time.

**Primary Osteoporosis:** Primary osteoporosis can occur in both genders at all ages but often follows menopause in women and occurs later in life in men.

**Psoriasis vulgaris:** The most common form of psoriasis, characterized by reddened lesions covered by silvery scales.

**Psoriasis:** A chronic (long-lasting) skin disease characterized by scaling and inflammation. Scaling occurs when cells in the outer layer of skin reproduce faster than normal and pile up on the skin's surface. Possibly a disorder of the immune system.

**Psoriatic arthritis:** Joint inflammation that occurs in about 5 to 10 percent of people with psoriasis (a common skin disorder).

**PUVA:** A treatment sometimes used for extensive or severe psoriasis that combines oral or topical administration of a medicine called psoralen with exposure to ultraviolet A (UVA) light.

### R

**Raloxifene:** Raloxifene is a drug that was recently approved for the prevention of osteoporosis. It is from a new class of drugs called "Selective Estrogen Receptor Modulators" (SERMS) that appears to prevent bone loss throughout the body.

**Range of motion (ROM):** The ability of a joint to go through all its normal movements. A measurement of the extent to which a joint can go through all its normal spectrum of movements. Range-of-motion exercises help increase or maintain flexibility and movement in muscles, tendons, ligaments, and joints.

**Rehabilitation specialist:** See physiatrist.

**Relaxation therapy:** People with osteoporosis or arthritis use relaxation to release the tension in their muscles, which relieves pain.

**Rheumatoid Factor:** A special kind of antibody often found in people with rheumatoid arthritis.

**Rheumatoid arthritis:** An often chronic systemic disease that causes inflammatory changes in the synovium, or joint lining, that result in pain, stiffness, swelling, and loss of function in the joints. The disease can also affect other parts of the body.

**Rheumatologist:** A doctor who specializes in diagnosing and treating disorders that affect the joints, muscles, tendons, ligaments, and bones.

### S

**Secondary Osteoporosis:** Secondary osteoporosis is a result of medications, other conditions, or diseases. Examples include glucocorticoid-induced osteoporosis, hypogonadism, and celiac disease.

**Short waves:** These deliver deep heat to relieve pain. (Short waves are not used much currently because of problems in people with pacemakers.)

**Smooth muscle:** The muscles of the body that are not under a person's conscious control. Smooth muscle is found mainly in the internal organs, including the digestive tract, respiratory passages, urinary bladder, and walls of blood vessels.

**Spasm:** An involuntary, sudden muscle contraction. In Raynaud's phenomenon, involuntary contraction of the smooth muscle in the blood vessels decreases the flow of blood to the fingers or toes (which leads to color changes in the skin).

**Spondyloarthropathies:** A group of rheumatic diseases that affect the spine, such as Reiter's syndrome and ankylosing spondylitis.

**Strengthening exercises:** Exercises that build stronger muscles, for example, exercises that require movement against a force (weight lifting or isometric exercises).

**Synovial fluid:** Fluid released into movable joints by surrounding membranes. This fluid lubricates the joint and reduces friction.

**Synovitis:** Inflammation of the synovial membrane, the tissue that lines and protects the joint.

**Synovium:** A thin membrane that lines a joint and releases a fluid that allows the joint to move easily.

**Systemic lupus erythematosus:** Lupus is a type of immune system disorder known as an autoimmune disease, which causes the body to harm its own healthy cells and tissues. This leads to inflammation and damage of various body tissues. Lupus can affect many parts of the body, including the joints, skin, kidneys, heart, lungs, blood vessels, and brain.

**Systemic treatment:** A treatment, such as a pill, that is taken internally.

**Systemic:** Disease or symptoms that affect many different parts of the body.

# T

**T cell:** A type of white blood cell that is part of the immune system and normally helps protect the body against infection and disease. In psoriasis, it also can trigger inflammation and excessive skin cell reproduction.

**Temporal Arteries:** Vessels located over the temples on each side of the head, that supply blood to part of the head.

**Tendons:** Tough, fibrous cords of tissue that connect muscle to bone.

**TENS (transcutaneous electrical nerve stimulation):** Passes electricity to nerve cells through electrodes placed on the patient's skin. TENS is used to relieve pain.

**Topical agent:** A treatment, such as a cream, salve, or ointment, that is applied to the surface of the skin.

**Toxicity:** The potential of a drug or treatment to cause harmful side effects.

**Trabecular Bone:** Trabecular bone makes up the interior of bone, and has a spongy, honeycomb-like structure.

**Traction:** Gentle, steady pulling along the length of body structure, for example, the spine or neck.

**Transcutaneous:** Through the skin.

## U

**Ultrasound:** Sound waves that provide deep heat to relieve pain.

**UVB phototherapy:** An artificial light treatment used for mild psoriasis.

## V

**Vasodilator:** An agent, usually a drug, that widens blood vessels and allows more blood to reach the tissues.

**Vasospasm or Vasoconstriction:** A sudden muscle contraction that narrows the blood vessels, reducing blood flow to a part of the body.

# Chapter 68

# *Directory of Resources*

**American Academy of Orthopaedic Surgeons**
6300 North River Road
Rosemont, IL 60018-4262
847-823-7186
800-346-AAOS
Fax-on Demand: 800/999-2939
E-mail: custserv@aaos.org
http://www.aaos.org

**American Anorexia and Bulimia Association, Inc.**
165W. 46th St. #1108
New York, NY 10036
212-575-6200
Fax: 212-278-0698
E-mail: info@aabainc.org
http://www.aabainc.org

**American Association of Retired Persons (AARP) Women's Initiative** has a fact sheet, *Hormone Replacement Therapy: Facts to Help You Decide*. To obtain a copy, write:
AARP
601 E Street, N.W.
Washington, D.C. 20049
800-424-3410
E-mail: member@aarp.org
http://www.aarp.org

**American College of Obstetricians and Gynecologists (ACOG)**
offers the following pamphlets, *Hormone Replacement Therapy, Preventing Osteoporosis, and The Menopause Years*. To obtain copies, send a self-addressed envelope to:
ACOG
409 12th Street, S.W.
P.O. Box 96920
Washington, D.C. 20024-2188
E-mail: resources@acog.org
http://www.acog.org

**American College of Sports Medicine**
401 W. Michigan St.
Indianapolis, IN 46202
317-637-9200
Fax: 317-634-7817
E-mail: mkeckhaver@acsm.org
http://www.acsm.org

**American Speech-Language-Hearing Association (ASHA)**
10801 Rockville Pike
Rockville, MD 20852
ASHA Line: 888-321-ASHA
ASHA Action Center: 800-498-2071
TTY: 301-571-0457
Fax-on-Demand: 877-541-5035
E-mail: actioncenter@asha.org
http://www.asha.org

ASHA is the national professional, scientific, and credentialing association for speech-language pathologists and audiologists. Part of its mission is to ensure that individuals with hearing disorders have access to high quality services to help them communicate more effectively. A toll-free HELPLINE is available for those seeking information. ASHA can also provide a list of certified audiologists.

## American Academy of Otolaryngology—Head and Neck Surgery (AAO-HNS)
1 Prince Street
Alexandria, VA 22314-3357
703-836-4444; TTY: 703-519-1585
Fax: 703-519-1587
E-mail: entinfo@aol.com
http://www.entnet.org

The AAO-HNS is the not-for-profit professional, educational, and research association for ear, nose, and throat specialists. They have fact sheets on hearing loss and can also provide patients with a list of specialists.

## American Dietetic Association Nutrition Resources
216 W. Jackson Blvd
Chicago, IL 6060-6995
312-899-0040
E-mail: cdr@eatright.org
http://www.eatright.org

## American Society for Bone and Mineral Research
2025 M Street, NW, Suite 800
Washington, D.C. 20036-3309
202-367-1161
Fax: 262-367-2161
E-mail: asbmrc@dc.sba.com
http://wwwasbmr.org/

## Anorexia Nervosa and Related Eating Disorders
PO Box 5102
Eugene, OR 97405
503-344-1144
E-mail: jarinor@rio.com
www.anred.com

## Children's Brittle Bone Foundation (CBBF)
7701 95th St.
Pleasant Prairie, WI 53158
847-433-4981
Fax: 262-947-0724
e-mail info@cbbf.org
http://www.cbbf.org

**Dairy Council of California**
1101 National Drive, Suite B
Sacramento, CA 95834
In California: 888-868-3133
Outside California: 888-868-3083
http://www.dairycouncilofca.org

**ERIC Clearinghouse on Disabilities and Gifted Education**
**Council for Exceptional Children**
1920 Association Drive
Reston, VA 20191-1589
800-328-0272
E-mail: ericec@cec.sped.org
http://ericec.org/index.html

**HEATH Resource Center** (National Clearinghouse on
Postsecondary Education for Individuals with Disabilities)
One Dupont Circle, NW, Suite 800
Washington, D.C. 20036-1193
800-544-3284, 202-939-9320
E-mail: health@ace.nche.edu
http://www.acenet.edu/about/programs/Access&Equity/HEALTH/
home.html

**Hip Society**
951 Old County Road, #182
Belmont, CA 94002
650-596-6190
Fax: 650-508-2039
http://www,hipsoc.org

**International Bone and Mineral Society**
2025 M Street, NW, Suite 800
Washington, D.C. 20036-3309
202-367-1121
Fax: 202-367-2121
E-mail: IBMS@dc.sba.com
http://www.IBMSonline.org

## International Osteoporosis Foundation
71, cours Albert-Thomas
69447 Lyon Cedex 03
France
Tel: +33 472 91 41 77
Fax: +33 472 36 90 52
E-mail: info@ioflyon.org
http://www.osteofound.org

## International Society for Clinical Densitometry
2025 Main Stree, NW, Suite 800
Washington, D.C. 20036-2422
202-367-1132; Fax: 202-367-2132
E-mail: iscd@dc.sba.com
http://www.iscd.org

## MAGIC Foundation
1327 N. Harlem Avenue
Oak Park, IL 60303
708-383-0808; Fax: 708-383-0899
E-mail: mary@magicfoundation.org
http://magicfoundation.org

## National Association of Anorexia Nervosa and Associated Disorders
Box 7
Highland Park, IL 60035
National Hotline: 847-831-3438
Fax: 847-433-4632
E-mail: info@anad.org
http://www.anad.org

**National Cancer Institute (NCI),** part of NIH, funds cancer research and offers information for health professionals and the public. For more information about cancer risks and other related issues, call: 1-800-4-CANCER
NCI Public Inquiries Office
Building 31, Room 10A03
31 Center Drive, MSC 2580
Bethesda, MD 20892-2580
301-435-3848
http://www.nci.noh.gov

**The National Collegiate Athletic Association**
700 W. Washington Ave.
P.O. Box 6222
Indiana, IN 46206-6222
317-917-6222
Fax: 317-917-6888
E-mail: wrenfro@ncaa.org
http://www.ncaa.org

**National Eating Disorders Organization**
6655 S. Yale Ave.
Tulsa, OK 74136
918-481-4044
Fax: 918-481-4076
http://www.kidsource.com/nedo/nedointro.html

**National Gaucher Foundation**
11140 Rockville Pike, Ste 350
Rockville, MD 20852-3106
301-816-1515
800-925-8885 or 800-GAUCHER
E-mail: ngf@gaucherdisease.org

**National Heart, Lung, and Blood Institute,** part of NIH, carries out research and provides educational information on heart disease, stroke, and other related topics. For more information call: 301-251-1222
E-mail: nhlbiinfo@rover.nhlbi.nih.gov
http://www.nhlbi.nih.gov

**National Institute of Health (NIH)**
Bethesda, MD, 20892
E-mail: nihinfo@od.hin.gov
http://www.nih.gov

**National Institute of Arthritis and Musculoskeletal and Skin Diseases (NIAMS)**
9000 Rockville Pike, Building 31, Room 4C32
Bethesda MD 20894
301-496-8190
TTY: 301-565-2966
Fax: 301-480-2814
http://www.nih.gov/niams

**National Institute on Aging Information Center** has information on menopause, osteoporosis, and a variety of other topics related to health and aging. Contact:
Building 31, Room 5C27
31 Center Drive, MSC 2292
Bethesda, MD 20892
301-496-1752
800-222-2225
800-222-4225 (TTY)
http://www.nih.gov/nia

**National Institute on Deafness and Other Communication Disorders (NIDCD) Clearinghouse**
National Institutes of Health
31 Center Drive, MSC 2320
Bethesda, MD 20892-2320
301-496-7343
TTY: 301-402-0252
Fax: 301-402-0018
http://www.nih.gov/nidcd

The NIDCD Clearinghouse is a national resource center for information about the normal and disordered mechanisms of hearing, balance, smell, taste, voice, speech, and language. It provides an information service to respond to professional and public inquiries; develops and distributes publications such as fact sheets, bibliographies, information packets, and organization directories; and maintains a database of references to journal articles, books, audiovisual materials, brochures, facts sheets, and other educational materials.

**National Organization for Rare Disorders (NORD)**
P.O. Box 8923
(100 Route 37)
Fairfield CT 06812-8923
orphan@rarediseases.org
Tel: 203-746-6518
800-999-NORD (-6673)
Fax: 203-746-6481
http://www.pcnet.com/~orphan

**National Osteoporosis Foundation (NOF)** has information for health professionals and the public. Contact:
NOF
1232 22nd Street, N.W.
Washington, D.C. 20036-4603
202-223-2226
E-mail: communications@nof.org
http://www.nof.org

**National Tay-Sachs and Allied Diseases Association**
2001 Beacon Street
Suite 204
Brighton MA 02146
NTSAD-boston@worldnet.att.net
617-277-4463; 800-90-NTSAD (906-8723)
Fax: 617-277-0134
http://www.nstad.org

**National Women's Health Network** distributes educational materials on a variety of women's health topics. Contact:
National Women's Health Network
514 10th Street, N.W.
Washington, D.C. 20004
202-347-1140; Fax: 202-347-1168
http://www.aoa.dhhs.gov/aoa/dir/203.html

**National Information Center for Children and Youth with Disabilities**
P.O. Box
1492 Washington, D.C. 20013
800-695-0285 (Voice/TTY)
202-884-8200 (Voice/TTY)
Fax: 202-884-8441
E-mail: nichcy@aed.org
http://www.nechcy.org

**North American Menopause Society (NAMS)** answers written requests for information. Write: NAMS
P.O. Box 94527
Cleveland, Ohio 44105-4527
440-442-7550
http://www.menopause.org

**Older Women's League (OWL)** educates the public about problems and issues of concern to middle age and older women. Contact:
666 11th Street, N.W., Suite 700
Washington, D.C. 20001
202-783-6686 or 800-825-3695
Fax: 202-638-2356
E-mail: owlinfo@owl-national.org
http://www.owl-national.org

**Osteoporosis and Related Bone Diseases—National Resource Center (ORBD)**
1232 22nd St., NW,
Washington, D.C. 20037-1292
202-223-0344 or 800-624-BONE
TTY (202) 466-4315
Fax: 202-293-2356
E-mail orbdnrc@nof.org
http://www.osteo.org

National Resource Center on Osteoporosis and Related Bone Diseases is a national clearinghouse with information on the risks, prevention, and treatment of osteoporosis. For more information call: 1-800-624-BONE

**Osteogenesis Imperfecta Foundation (OI)**
840 West Diamond Ave.
Suite 210
Gaithersburg, MD 20878
301-947-0083 or 800-981-2663
Fax: 301-947-0456
e-mail bonelink@oif.org
http://www.oif.org

**Paget Foundation for Paget's Disease of Bone and Related Disorders**
120 Wall St., Suite 1602
New York, NY 10005-4001
212-509-5335
Fax: 202-509-8492
E-mail: pagetfdn@aol.com
http://www.paget.org

## Self-Help for Hard of Hearing People, Inc. (SHHH)
7910 Woodmont Avenue, Suite 1200
Bethesda, MD 20814
301-657-2248
TTY: 301-657-2249
Fax: 301-913-9413
E-mail: national@shhh.org
http://www.shhh.org

SHHH is a national self-help organization for those who are hard of hearing. SHHH can help with information on coping with hearing loss.

## Sports, Cardiovascular, and Wellness Nutritionists (SCAN)
A practice group of the American Dietetic Assocration
90 S. Cascade Ave., Suite 1190
Colorado Springs, CO 80903
719-475-7751
www.nutrifit.org

## State Department of Education
Division of Special Education
State Capital
http://ericps.ed.uic.edu/eece/statlink.html

## The Bones Page
http://www.geocities.com/CapeCanaveral/Lab/3608/

## U.S. National Library of Medicine (NLM)
8600 Rockville Pike
Bethesda, MD 20894
888-346-3656 or 301-594-5983
E-mail: custserv@nlm.nih.gov
http://www.nlm.nih.gov

## *Support Groups*

National Osteoporosis Foundation
**Building Strength Together**
515 N. State ST.
Chicago, IL 60610
312-464-5110
Fax: 312-464-5863
email supgroup@nof.org

## Osteogenesis Imperfecta Foundation

**Support Groups:** OI Foundation has support groups across the country that are run by volunteers. When asked what they derive from the support groups, members say that they are looking for information on OI, that they derive a sense of comfort through hearing from others who have had similar experiences, and it is a place where they can go to seek advice. Older persons with OI believe that they can share their experiences with younger people, thus helping them to cope. And, at all levels, there is the desire for friendship.

If you are interested in joining a support group, contact the OI Foundation listed below. Please note that each group is a regional support group that may include several states:

| | | | |
|---|---|---|---|
| Alaska | 907-457-2841 | Missouri | 636-931-4746 |
| Arizona | 602-833-2112 | New Jersey | 201-797-1914 |
| | | | 201-489-9232 |
| Central | | | |
| California | 559-439-4823 | Ohio | 937-833-5933 |
| | | | 513-753-3062 |
| Northern | 408-554-1747 | | |
| California | 510-228-0488 | Oklahoma | 580-228-2933 |
| Southern | | Oregon | 503-926-3869 |
| California | 310-796-4923 | | |
| | | Texas | |
| Delaware | 717-361-7266 | (Houston area) | 409-321-4031 |
| Georgia | 404-315-7217 | Texas | |
| Illinois | 708-452-0997 | (Central) | 512-388-5887 |
| | | Texas | |
| Indiana | 317-873-0549 | (San Antonio) | 210-521-2989 |
| Iowa | 515-684-7080 | Utah | 801-536-3570 |
| Kentucky | 606-744-7203 | Virginia | 804-379-6798 |
| Kansas | 816-650-6344 | Washington | 206-285-8002 |
| Massachu- | | Wisconsin | 608-226-9339 |
| setts | 781-982-0101 | | |

**One-on-One Support:** The Foundation also has staff and local volunteers who can provide support and information by telephone or e-mail.

Contact the Foundation to request assistance and the name of a support volunteer whom you can call.

**Mentoring Program:** For young people with OI (teens and young adults), the OI Foundation offers the PASS IT ON! Mentoring Program. The mission of the PASS IT ON! program is to create a network of mentors who can share their experiences of living with OI by providing advice, guidance, and coping skills to others with OI. All PASS IT ON! mentors complete a screening process, including an interview, references, and a background check.

Are you a young person with OI who is interested in getting to know an adult with OI who can offer support and guidance? Maybe you have specific concerns about school, dating, accessibility, driving, travel or getting a job. Or perhaps you would just like to get to know an older person with OI to learn how he or she has managed OI. We currently have volunteers who are eager to work with young people in the following parts of the country: Northern California, Central Florida, Southern Ohio, Northern Virginia, and Western and Southeastern Michigan. We will try to match interested young people with a mentor based on interests, type/severity of OI, type of support requested, and geographic location.

If you are interested in participating (whether you live in one of these areas or elsewhere), contact volunteer Jamie Kendall (wunjo1871 @aol.com), who is coordinating the program, or the OI Foundation.

**KeyPals Program:** Young people age 9 to 17 who have OI and are interested in having a pen pal are invited to join the OI Foundation's KeyPals Program. While most participants correspond by e-mail, "snail mail" users can also be accommodated. To request an application, contact the OI Foundation.

### *Suggested Readings—Consumer Articles*

Anderson, W., Chitwood, S., & Hayden, D. (in press). *Negotiating the special education maze: A guide for parents and teachers* (3rd ed.). Bethesda, MD: Woodbine.

Bilezikian, John P. et al. *The Parathyroids: Basic and Clinical Concepts.* New York: Raven Press, 1994.

National Institutes of Health. "Diagnosis and Management of Asymptomatic Primary Hyperparathyroidism: Consensus Development Conference Statement," *Annals of Internal Medicine*

Vol. 114, No. 7, April 1, 1991. 593-596. Reprints are also available from the Office of Medical Applications of Research (OMAR) Consensus Program Clearinghouse, P.O. Box 2577, Kensington, MD 20891 1-800-NIH-OMAR.

NICHCY (1997, Feb.). Parenting a child with special needs: A guide to reading and resources. 2nd ed., NICHCY News Digest.

Parisien, May, et al. "Bone Disease in Primary Hyperparathyroidism," *Endocrinology and Metabolism Clinics of North America.* Vol. 19, No. 1, March, 1990.

Potts, John T., Jr. "Management of Asymptomatic Hyperparathyroidism," *Journal of Endocrinology and Metabolism*

## Suggested Readings—Research Articles

Appendicular bone density and age predict hip fracture in women. The Study of Osteoporotic Fractures Research Group: [http://www.medmedia.com:80/ lib0/55.htm]

Intermittent cyclical etidronate treatment of postmenopausal osteoporosis: [http://www.medmedia.com:80/lib0/103.htm]

A prospective study to evaluate the dose of vitamin D required to correct low 25-hydroxyvitamin D levels, calcium, and alkaline phosphatase in patients at risk of developing antiepileptic drug-induced osteomalacia: [http://www.medmedia.com:80/lib1/44.htm]

Hypothalamic osteopenia—body weight and skeletal mass in the premenopausal woman: [http://www.medmedia.com:80/lib1/95.htm]

The coexistence and characteristics of osteoarthritis and osteoporosis: [http://www.medmedia.com:80/lib3/210.htm]

Effect of intense physical activity on the bone-mineral content in the lower limbs of young adults. [http://www.medmedia.com:80/lib3/210.htm]

Assessment of the risk of vertebral fracture in menopausal women: [http://www.medmedia.com:80/lib4/44.htm]

Proximal femoral fractures: [http://www.medmedia.com:80/lib9/44htm]

Age- and sex-specific incidence of femoral neck and trochanteric fractures. An analysis based on 20,538 fractures in Stockholm

County, Sweden, 1972-1981: [http://www.medmedia.com:80/lib9/133.htm]

Osteoporosis and proximal femoral fractures in the female elderly of Jerusalem: [http://www.medmedia.com:80/lib9/194.htm]

A controlled trial of the effect of calcium supplementation on bone density in postmenopausal women: [http://www.medmedia.com:80/18/122.htm]

Intermittent cyclical etidronate treatment of postmenopausal osteoporosis: [http://www.medmedia.com:80/18/23.htm]

Effect of intermittent cyclical etidronate therapy on bone mass and fracture rate in women with postmenopausal osteoporosis: [http://www.medmedia.com:80/18/24.htm]

Treatment of postmenopausal osteoporosis with calcitriol or calcium: [http://www.medmedia.com:80/j1/75.htm]

Original Articles: Prevention Of Postmenopausal Osteoporosis — A Comparative Study of Exercise, Calcium Supplementation, and Hormone-Replacement Therapy: [http://www.medmedia.com:80/j4/114.htm]

Effect of calcium supplementation on bone loss in postmenopausal women: [http://www.medmedia.com:80/j7/75.htm]

Vitamin D3 and calcium to prevent hip fractures in the elderly women: [http://www.medmedia.com:80/j7/77.htm]

Total body bone density in amenorrheic runners: [http://www.medmedia.com:80/a3/20.htm]

Effect of calcium supplementation on bone loss in postmenopausal women: [http://www.medmedia.com:80/a5/135/htm]

The effect of postmenopausal estrogen therapy on bone density in elderly women: [http://www.medmedia.com:80/a5/61.htm]

Bone density at various sites for prediction of hip fractures: SR Cummings et al. *Lancet*. Vol 341. 1993. p 72-75.

Menstrual irregularity and stress fractures in collegiate female distance runners: Barrow G, Saha S: *Am J Sports Med* 1988;16:209-216.

Osteoporosis: current modes of prevention and treatment: JM Lane and M. Nydick MD. *AOS*. Vol 7. No 1. Jan/Feb. 1999 p 19.

# *Index*

# *Index*

Page numbers followed by 'n' indicate a footnote. Page numbers in *italics* indicate a table or illustration.

## A

AAO-HNS *see* American Academy of Otolaryngology-Head and Neck Surgery

AARP *see* American Association of Retired Persons

"Accessing Programs for Infants, Toddlers, and Preschoolers with Disabilities" 144

ACOG *see* American College of Obstetricians and Gynecologists

activities of daily living (ADL), osteoporotic fractures 6

Actonel (risedronate) 16, 88

acupressure, pain management 128, 495

acupuncture, pain management 128, 495

Addison's disease, amenorrhea 244

Administration on Aging (AoA) 323n

adolescents
  amenorrhea 249
  bone basics 44–47, 313–14
  bone mass 69

adolescents, continued
  female athlete triad 277
  osteogenesis imperfecta 137–38
  osteoporosis 9–10, 37–42, 92–93, 523–24

aerobic exercise, defined 517

Aerobics and Fitness Association of America 91n

African Americans
  bone density 7
  fracture risks statistics 5
  osteoporosis 97–100

"After the Vertebral Fracture" 445n

"Age- and sex-specific incidence of femoral neck and trochanteric fractures" 543

age factor
  bone basics 57–60
  bone density 30
  calcium requirements 33
  osteoporosis 29, 57, 385–88, 428–29

Agency for Health Care Policy and Research (AHCPR) 503–4

Agency for Healthcare Research and Quality, Consensus Development Conference on Osteoporosis Prevention 4

Albertson, Ann 317

547

Committee on Special Education
(CSE), special education services 144
"Concise review for primary-care physicians: Treatment options"
(Khosla) 443
connective tissue, defined 520
connective tissue disease, defined 520
"A controlled trial of the effect of calcium supplementation" 544
Copyright Clearinghouse Center, contact information 254
cortical bone, defined 520
corticosteroids *38*, 76
defined 520
osteoporosis risk 87, 305–9
cortisone 29, *35*
Council for Exceptional Children 534
counseling
nutrition 239, 250–54, 279
pain management 129, 496
Crohn's disease 215
CSE *see* Committee on Special Education
Cummings, Nancy 75
Cummings, S. R. 66, 544
Cushing's syndrome 29, 35, *38*
amenorrhea 244
cyanosis, defined 520
Cybermedical, Inc., bone density
215n
cyclophosphamide 76
cytokines 185, 216
defined 520

**D**

Dairy Council of California, contact
information 319, 534
Dargent-Molina, P. 443
Dawson-Hughes, Bess 295, 296, 372,
374, 460
degenerative joint disease *see* osteoarthritis
Delmas, P. D. 443
deoxypyridinolines 14
Depo-Provera (medroxyprogesterone
acetate) 239, 240, 245, 246, 247–50,
254–55

depression 78, 95
bone loss 303–4
fractures 237–38
dermis, defined 520
DEXA scan *see* dual energy photon
absorptiometry
DHHS *see* US Department of Health
and Human Services
diabetes mellitus *38*
"Diagnosis and Management of
Asymptomatic Primary Hyperparathyroidism" 119, 542
dialysis, hypercalcemia 203
Didronel (etidronate disodium) 16,
167, 200–201, *436*
diet and nutrition *38*, 441
bone development 10–11, 45–46,
48–49, 314–15
calcium 318–19
osteoporosis 98–99
distraction, pain management 129, 496
diuretics, hypercalcemia 197–98
dowager's hump 27
Drinkwater, Barbara L. 91, 94
dual energy photon absorptiometry
(DEXA scan) 312, 408, 457, 459–60,
463–64
*see also* bone scans
dual x-ray absorptiometry 77, 111
Dunne and Associates 234
Dunstan, Colin R. 62, 63, 64
Durie, B. G. M. 164

**E**

ear
depicted *172*
described 171
eating disorders
amenorrhea 244–45
bone health 316
female athletes 276
*see also* anorexia nervosa; bulimia;
diet and nutrition; nutrition
counseling
education
hypercalcemia 205
osteogenesis imperfecta 142–47

# Health Reference Series

## COMPLETE CATALOG

## AIDS Sourcebook, 1st Edition

*Basic Information about AIDS and HIV Infection, Featuring Historical and Statistical Data, Current Research, Prevention, and Other Special Topics of Interest for Persons Living with AIDS*

*Along with Source Listings for Further Assistance*

Edited by Karen Bellenir and Peter D. Dresser. 831 pages. 1995. 0-7808-0031-1. $78.

"One strength of this book is its practical emphasis. The intended audience is the lay reader . . . useful as an educational tool for health care providers who work with AIDS patients. Recommended for public libraries as well as hospital or academic libraries that collect consumer materials."
— *Bulletin of the Medical Library Association, Jan '96*

"This is the most comprehensive volume of its kind on an important medical topic. Highly recommended for all libraries." — *Reference Book Review, '96*

"Very useful reference for all libraries."
— *Choice, Association of College and Research Libraries, Oct '95*

"There is a wealth of information here that can provide much educational assistance. It is a must book for all libraries and should be on the desk of each and every congressional leader. Highly recommended."
— *AIDS Book Review Journal, Aug '95*

"Recommended for most collections."
— *Library Journal, Jul '95*

■

## AIDS Sourcebook, 2nd Edition

*Basic Consumer Health Information about Acquired Immune Deficiency Syndrome (AIDS) and Human Immunodeficiency Virus (HIV) Infection, Featuring Updated Statistical Data, Reports on Recent Research and Prevention Initiatives, and Other Special Topics of Interest for Persons Living with AIDS, Including New Antiretroviral Treatment Options, Strategies for Combating Opportunistic Infections, Information about Clinical Trials, and More*

*Along with a Glossary of Important Terms and Resource Listings for Further Help and Information*

Edited by Karen Bellenir. 751 pages. 1999. 0-7808-0225-X. $78.

"Highly recommended."
— *American Reference Books Annual, 2000*

"Excellent sourcebook. This continues to be a highly recommended book. There is no other book that provides as much information as this book provides."
— *AIDS Book Review Journal, Dec-Jan 2000*

"Recommended reference source."
— *Booklist, American Library Association, Dec '99*

"A solid text for college-level health libraries."
— *The Bookwatch, Aug '99*

Cited in *Reference Sources for Small and Medium-Sized Libraries, American Library Association, 1999*

■

## Alcoholism Sourcebook

*Basic Consumer Health Information about the Physical and Mental Consequences of Alcohol Abuse, Including Liver Disease, Pancreatitis, Wernicke-Korsakoff Syndrome (Alcoholic Dementia), Fetal Alcohol Syndrome, Heart Disease, Kidney Disorders, Gastrointestinal Problems, and Immune System Compromise and Featuring Facts about Addiction, Detoxification, Alcohol Withdrawal, Recovery, and the Maintenance of Sobriety*

*Along with a Glossary and Directories of Resources for Further Help and Information*

Edited by Karen Bellenir. 613 pages. 2000. 0-7808-0325-6. $78.

"Recommended reference source."
— *Booklist, American Library Association, Dec '00*

"Presents a wealth of information on alcohol use and abuse and its effects on the body and mind, treatment, and prevention." — *SciTech Book News, Dec '00*

"Important new health guide which packs in the latest consumer information about the problems of alcoholism." — *Reviewer's Bookwatch, Nov '00*

*SEE ALSO Drug Abuse Sourcebook, Substance Abuse Sourcebook*

■

## Allergies Sourcebook

*Basic Information about Major Forms and Mechanisms of Common Allergic Reactions, Sensitivities, and Intolerances, Including Anaphylaxis, Asthma, Hives and Other Dermatologic Symptoms, Rhinitis, and Sinusitis*

*Along with Their Usual Triggers Like Animal Fur, Chemicals, Drugs, Dust, Foods, Insects, Latex, Pollen, and Poison Ivy, Oak, and Sumac; Plus Information on Prevention, Identification, and Treatment*

Edited by Allan R. Cook. 611 pages. 1997. 0-7808-0036-2. $78.

■

## Alternative Medicine Sourcebook

*Basic Consumer Health Information about Alternatives to Conventional Medicine, Including Acupressure, Acupuncture, Aromatherapy, Ayurveda, Bioelectromagnetics, Environmental Medicine, Essence*

Therapy, Food and Nutrition Therapy, Herbal Therapy, Homeopathy, Imaging, Massage, Naturopathy, Reflexology, Relaxation and Meditation, Sound Therapy, Vitamin and Mineral Therapy, and Yoga, and More

Edited by Allan R. Cook. 737 pages. 1999. 0-7808-0200-4. $78.

**"Recommended reference source."**
—*Booklist, American Library Association, Feb '00*

**"A great addition to the reference collection of every type of library."** —*American Reference Books Annual, 2000*

■

# Alzheimer's, Stroke & 29 Other Neurological Disorders Sourcebook, 1st Edition

*Basic Information for the Layperson on 31 Diseases or Disorders Affecting the Brain and Nervous System, First Describing the Illness, Then Listing Symptoms, Diagnostic Methods, and Treatment Options, and Including Statistics on Incidences and Causes*

Edited by Frank E. Bair. 579 pages. 1993. 1-55888-748-2. $78.

**"Nontechnical reference book that provides reader-friendly information."**
—*Family Caregiver Alliance Update, Winter '96*

**"Should be included in any library's patient education section."** —*American Reference Books Annual, 1994*

**"Written in an approachable and accessible style. Recommended for patient education and consumer health collections in health science center and public libraries."** —*Academic Library Book Review, Dec '93*

**"It is very handy to have information on more than thirty neurological disorders under one cover, and there is no recent source like it."** —*Reference Quarterly, American Library Association, Fall '93*

**SEE ALSO** *Brain Disorders Sourcebook*

■

# Alzheimer's Disease Sourcebook, 2nd Edition

*Basic Consumer Health Information about Alzheimer's Disease, Related Disorders, and Other Dementias, Including Multi-Infarct Dementia, AIDS-Related Dementia, Alcoholic Dementia, Huntington's Disease, Delirium, and Confusional States*

*Along with Reports Detailing Current Research Efforts in Prevention and Treatment, Long-Term Care Issues, and Listings of Sources for Additional Help and Information*

Edited by Karen Bellenir. 524 pages. 1999. 0-7808-0223-3. $78.

**"Provides a wealth of useful information not otherwise available in one place. This resource is recommended for all types of libraries."**
—*American Reference Books Annual, 2000*

**"Recommended reference source."**
—*Booklist, American Library Association, Oct '99*

# Arthritis Sourcebook

*Basic Consumer Health Information about Specific Forms of Arthritis and Related Disorders, Including Rheumatoid Arthritis, Osteoarthritis, Gout, Polymyalgia Rheumatica, Psoriatic Arthritis, Spondyloarthropathies, Juvenile Rheumatoid Arthritis, and Juvenile Ankylosing Spondylitis*

*Along with Information about Medical, Surgical, and Alternative Treatment Options, and Including Strategies for Coping with Pain, Fatigue, and Stress*

Edited by Allan R. Cook. 550 pages. 1998. 0-7808-0201-2. $78.

**". . . accessible to the layperson."**
—*Reference and Research Book News, Feb '99*

■

# Asthma Sourcebook

*Basic Consumer Health Information about Asthma, Including Symptoms, Traditional and Nontraditional Remedies, Treatment Advances, Quality-of-Life Aids, Medical Research Updates, and the Role of Allergies, Exercise, Age, the Environment, and Genetics in the Development of Asthma*

*Along with Statistical Data, a Glossary, and Directories of Support Groups, and Other Resources for Further Information*

Edited by Annemarie S. Muth. 628 pages. 2000. 0-7808-0381-7. $78.

**"Highly recommended."** —*The Bookwatch, Jan '01*

■

# Back & Neck Disorders Sourcebook

*Basic Information about Disorders and Injuries of the Spinal Cord and Vertebrae, Including Facts on Chiropractic Treatment, Surgical Interventions, Paralysis, and Rehabilitation*

*Along with Advice for Preventing Back Trouble*

Edited by Karen Bellenir. 548 pages. 1997. 0-7808-0202-0. $78.

**"The strength of this work is its basic, easy-to-read format. Recommended."**
—*Reference and User Services Quarterly, American Library Association, Winter '97*

■

# Blood & Circulatory Disorders Sourcebook

*Basic Information about Blood and Its Components, Anemias, Leukemias, Bleeding Disorders, and Circulatory Disorders, Including Aplastic Anemia, Thalassemia, Sickle-Cell Disease, Hemochromatosis, Hemophilia, Von Willebrand Disease, and Vascular Diseases*

*Along with a Special Section on Blood Transfusions and Blood Supply Safety, a Glossary, and Source Listings for Further Help and Information*

Edited by Karen Bellenir and Linda M. Shin. 554 pages. 1998. 0-7808-0203-9. $78.

"Recommended reference source."
—*Booklist, American Library Association, Feb '99*

"An important reference sourcebook written in simple language for everyday, non-technical users. "
—*Reviewer's Bookwatch, Jan '99*

■

# Brain Disorders Sourcebook

*Basic Consumer Health Information about Strokes, Epilepsy, Amyotrophic Lateral Sclerosis (ALS/Lou Gehrig's Disease), Parkinson's Disease, Brain Tumors, Cerebral Palsy, Headache, Tourette Syndrome, and More*

*Along with Statistical Data, Treatment and Rehabilitation Options, Coping Strategies, Reports on Current Research Initiatives, a Glossary, and Resource Listings for Additional Help and Information*

Edited by Karen Bellenir. 481 pages. 1999. 0-7808-0229-2. $78.

"Belongs on the shelves of any library with a consumer health collection."        —*E-Streams, Mar '00*

"Recommended reference source."
—*Booklist, American Library Association, Oct '99*

**SEE ALSO** *Alzheimer's, Stroke & 29 Other Neurological Disorders Sourcebook, 1st Edition*

■

# Breast Cancer Sourcebook

*Basic Consumer Health Information about Breast Cancer, Including Diagnostic Methods, Treatment Options, Alternative Therapies, Self-Help Information, Related Health Concerns, Statistical and Demographic Data, and Facts for Men with Breast Cancer*

*Along with Reports on Current Research Initiatives, a Glossary of Related Medical Terms, and a Directory of Sources for Further Help and Information*

Edited by Edward J. Prucha and Karen Bellenir. 600 pages. 2001. 0-7808-0244-6. $78.

**SEE ALSO** *Cancer Sourcebook for Women, 1st and 2nd Editions, Women's Health Concerns Sourcebook*

■

# Burns Sourcebook

*Basic Consumer Health Information about Various Types of Burns and Scalds, Including Flame, Heat, Cold, Electrical, Chemical, and Sun Burns*

*Along with Information on Short-Term and Long-Term Treatments, Tissue Reconstruction, Plastic Surgery, Prevention Suggestions, and First Aid*

Edited by Allan R. Cook. 604 pages. 1999. 0-7808-0204-7. $78.

"This key reference guide is an invaluable addition to all health care and public libraries in confronting this ongoing health issue."
—*American Reference Books Annual, 2000*

"This is an exceptional addition to the series and is highly recommended for all consumer health collections, hospital libraries, and academic medical centers."        —*E-Streams, Mar '00*

"Recommended reference source."
—*Booklist, American Library Association, Dec '99*

**SEE ALSO** *Skin Disorders Sourcebook*

■

# Cancer Sourcebook, 1st Edition

*Basic Information on Cancer Types, Symptoms, Diagnostic Methods, and Treatments, Including Statistics on Cancer Occurrences Worldwide and the Risks Associated with Known Carcinogens and Activities*

Edited by Frank E. Bair. 932 pages. 1990. 1-55888-888-8. $78.

**Cited in** *Reference Sources for Small and Medium-Sized Libraries, American Library Association, 1999*

"Written in nontechnical language. Useful for patients, their families, medical professionals, and librarians."
—*Guide to Reference Books, 1996*

"Designed with the non-medical professional in mind. Libraries and medical facilities interested in patient education should certainly consider adding the *Cancer Sourcebook* to their holdings. This compact collection of reliable information . . . is an invaluable tool for helping patients and patients' families and friends to take the first steps in coping with the many difficulties of cancer."
—*Medical Reference Services Quarterly, Winter '91*

"Specifically created for the nontechnical reader . . . an important resource for the general reader trying to understand the complexities of cancer."
—*American Reference Books Annual, 1991*

"This publication's nontechnical nature and very comprehensive format make it useful for both the general public and undergraduate students."
—*Choice, Association of College and Research Libraries, Oct '90*

■

# New Cancer Sourcebook, 2nd Edition

*Basic Information about Major Forms and Stages of Cancer, Featuring Facts about Primary and Secondary Tumors of the Respiratory, Nervous, Lymphatic, Circulatory, Skeletal, and Gastrointestinal Systems, and Specific Organs; Statistical and Demographic Data; Treatment Options; and Strategies for Coping*

Edited by Allan R. Cook. 1,313 pages. 1996. 0-7808-0041-9. $78.

"An excellent resource for patients with newly diagnosed cancer and their families. The dialogue is simple, direct, and comprehensive. Highly recommended for patients and families to aid in their understanding of cancer and its treatment."
—*Booklist Health Sciences Supplement, American Library Association, Oct '97*

"The amount of factual and useful information is extensive. The writing is very clear, geared to general readers. Recommended for all levels."
— *Choice, Association of College and Research Libraries, Jan '97*

## Cancer Sourcebook, 3rd Edition

*Basic Consumer Health Information about Major Forms and Stages of Cancer, Featuring Facts about Primary and Secondary Tumors of the Respiratory, Nervous, Lymphatic, Circulatory, Skeletal, and Gastrointestinal Systems, and Specific Organs*

*Along with Statistical and Demographic Data, Treatment Options, Strategies for Coping, a Glossary, and a Directory of Sources for Additional Help and Information*

Edited by Edward J. Prucha. 1,069 pages. 2000. 0-7808-0227-6. $78.

"Recommended reference source."
— *Booklist, American Library Association, Dec '00*

## Cancer Sourcebook for Women, 1st Edition

*Basic Information about Specific Forms of Cancer That Affect Women, Featuring Facts about Breast Cancer, Cervical Cancer, Ovarian Cancer, Cancer of the Uterus and Uterine Sarcoma, Cancer of the Vagina, and Cancer of the Vulva; Statistical and Demographic Data; Treatments, Self-Help Management Suggestions, and Current Research Initiatives*

Edited by Allan R. Cook and Peter D. Dresser. 524 pages. 1996. 0-7808-0076-1. $78.

". . . written in easily understandable, non-technical language. Recommended for public libraries or hospital and academic libraries that collect patient education or consumer health materials."
— *Medical Reference Services Quarterly, Spring '97*

"Would be of value in a consumer health library. . . . written with the health care consumer in mind. Medical jargon is at a minimum, and medical terms are explained in clear, understandable sentences."
— *Bulletin of the Medical Library Association, Oct '96*

"The availability under one cover of all these pertinent publications, grouped under cohesive headings, makes this certainly a most useful sourcebook."
— *Choice, Association of College and Research Libraries, Jun '96*

"Presents a comprehensive knowledge base for general readers. Men and women both benefit from the gold mine of information nestled between the two covers of this book. Recommended."
— *Academic Library Book Review, Summer '96*

"This timely book is highly recommended for consumer health and patient education collections in all libraries."
— *Library Journal, Apr '96*

**SEE ALSO** *Breast Cancer Sourcebook, Women's Health Concerns Sourcebook*

## Cancer Sourcebook for Women, 2nd Edition

*Basic Consumer Health Information about Specific Forms of Cancer That Affect Women, Including Cervical Cancer, Ovarian Cancer, Endometrial Cancer, Uterine Sarcoma, Vaginal Cancer, Vulvar Cancer, and Gestational Trophoblastic Tumor; and Featuring Statistical Information, Facts about Tests and Treatments, a Glossary of Cancer Terms, and an Extensive List of Additional Resources*

Edited by Karen Bellenir. 600 pages. 2001. 0-7808-0226-8. $78.

**SEE ALSO** *Breast Cancer Sourcebook, Women's Health Concerns Sourcebook*

## Cardiovascular Diseases & Disorders Sourcebook, 1st Edition

*Basic Information about Cardiovascular Diseases and Disorders, Featuring Facts about the Cardiovascular System, Demographic and Statistical Data, Descriptions of Pharmacological and Surgical Interventions, Lifestyle Modifications, and a Special Section Focusing on Heart Disorders in Children*

Edited by Karen Bellenir and Peter D. Dresser. 683 pages. 1995. 0-7808-0032-X. $78.

". . . comprehensive format provides an extensive overview on this subject."
— *Choice, Association of College and Research Libraries, Jun '96*

". . . an easily understood, complete, up-to-date resource. This well executed public health tool will make valuable information available to those that need it most, patients and their families. The typeface, sturdy non-reflective paper, and library binding add a feel of quality found wanting in other publications. Highly recommended for academic and general libraries. "
— *Academic Library Book Review, Summer '96*

**SEE ALSO** *Healthy Heart Sourcebook for Women, Heart Diseases & Disorders Sourcebook, 2nd Edition*

## Caregiving Sourcebook

*Basic Consumer Health Information for Caregivers, Including a Profile of Caregivers, Caregiving Responsibilities, Tips for Specific Conditions, Care Environments, and the Effects of Caregiving*

*Along with Legal Issues, Financial Concerns, Future Planning, a Glossary, and a Listing of Additional Resources*

Edited by Joyce Brennfleck Shannon. 550 pages. 2001. 0-7808-0331-0. $78.

# Colds, Flu & Other Common Ailments Sourcebook

*Basic Consumer Health Information about Common Ailments and Injuries, Including Colds, Coughs, the Flu, Sinus Problems, Headaches, Fever, Nausea and Vomiting, Menstrual Cramps, Diarrhea, Constipation, Hemorrhoids, Back Pain, Dandruff, Dry and Itchy Skin, Cuts, Scrapes, Sprains, Bruises, and More*

*Along with Information about Prevention, Self-Care, Choosing a Doctor, Over-the-Counter Medications, Folk Remedies, and Alternative Therapies, and Including a Glossary of Important Terms and a Directory of Resources for Further Help and Information*

Edited by Chad T. Kimball. 600 pages. 2001. 0-7808-0435-X. $78.

■

# Communication Disorders Sourcebook

*Basic Information about Deafness and Hearing Loss, Speech and Language Disorders, Voice Disorders, Balance and Vestibular Disorders, and Disorders of Smell, Taste, and Touch*

Edited by Linda M. Ross. 533 pages. 1996. 0-7808-0077-X. $78.

**"This is skillfully edited and is a welcome resource for the layperson. It should be found in every public and medical library."** *— Booklist Health Sciences Supplement, American Library Association, Oct '97*

■

# Congenital Disorders Sourcebook

*Basic Information about Disorders Acquired during Gestation, Including Spina Bifida, Hydrocephalus, Cerebral Palsy, Heart Defects, Craniofacial Abnormalities, Fetal Alcohol Syndrome, and More*

*Along with Current Treatment Options and Statistical Data*

Edited by Karen Bellenir. 607 pages. 1997. 0-7808-0205-5. $78.

**"Recommended reference source."** *— Booklist, American Library Association, Oct '97*

**SEE ALSO** *Pregnancy & Birth Sourcebook*

■

# Consumer Issues in Health Care Sourcebook

*Basic Information about Health Care Fundamentals and Related Consumer Issues, Including Exams and Screening Tests, Physician Specialties, Choosing a Doctor, Using Prescription and Over-the-Counter Medications Safely, Avoiding Health Scams, Managing Common Health Risks in the Home, Care Options for Chronically or Terminally Ill Patients, and a List of Resources for Obtaining Help and Further Information*

Edited by Karen Bellenir. 618 pages. 1998. 0-7808-0221-7. $78.

**"Both public and academic libraries will want to have a copy in their collection for readers who are interested in self-education on health issues."** *—American Reference Books Annual, 2000*

**"The editor has researched the literature from government agencies and others, saving readers the time and effort of having to do the research themselves. Recommended for public libraries."** *—Reference and User Services Quarterly, American Library Association, Spring '99*

**"Recommended reference source."** *—Booklist, American Library Association, Dec '98*

■

# Contagious & Non-Contagious Infectious Diseases Sourcebook

*Basic Information about Contagious Diseases like Measles, Polio, Hepatitis B, and Infectious Mononucleosis, and Non-Contagious Infectious Diseases like Tetanus and Toxic Shock Syndrome, and Diseases Occurring as Secondary Infections Such as Shingles and Reye Syndrome*

*Along with Vaccination, Prevention, and Treatment Information, and a Section Describing Emerging Infectious Disease Threats*

Edited by Karen Bellenir and Peter D. Dresser. 566 pages. 1996. 0-7808-0075-3. $78.

■

# Death & Dying Sourcebook

*Basic Consumer Health Information for the Layperson about End-of-Life Care and Related Ethical and Legal Issues, Including Chief Causes of Death, Autopsies, Pain Management for the Terminally Ill, Life Support Systems, Insurance, Euthanasia, Assisted Suicide, Hospice Programs, Living Wills, Funeral Planning, Counseling, Mourning, Organ Donation, and Physician Training*

*Along with Statistical Data, a Glossary, and Listings of Sources for Further Help and Information*

Edited by Annemarie S. Muth. 641 pages. 1999. 0-7808-0230-6. $78.

**"Recommended reference source."** *—Booklist, American Library Association, Aug '00*

**"This book is a definite must for all those involved in end-of-life care."** *— Doody's Review Service, 2000*

■

# Diabetes Sourcebook, 1st Edition

*Basic Information about Insulin-Dependent and Non-insulin-Dependent Diabetes Mellitus, Gestational Diabetes, and Diabetic Complications, Symptoms, Treatment, and Research Results, Including Statistics on Prevalence, Morbidity, and Mortality*

*Along with Source Listings for Further Help and Information*

Edited by Karen Bellenir and Peter D. Dresser. 827 pages. 1994. 1-55888-751-2. $78.

"... very informative and understandable for the layperson without being simplistic. It provides a comprehensive overview for laypersons who want a general understanding of the disease or who want to focus on various aspects of the disease."
— *Bulletin of the Medical Library Association, Jan '96*

■

# Diabetes Sourcebook, 2nd Edition

*Basic Consumer Health Information about Type 1 Diabetes (Insulin-Dependent or Juvenile-Onset Diabetes), Type 2 (Noninsulin-Dependent or Adult-Onset Diabetes), Gestational Diabetes, and Related Disorders, Including Diabetes Prevalence Data, Management Issues, the Role of Diet and Exercise in Controlling Diabetes, Insulin and Other Diabetes Medicines, and Complications of Diabetes Such as Eye Diseases, Periodontal Disease, Amputation, and End-Stage Renal Disease*

*Along with Reports on Current Research Initiatives, a Glossary, and Resource Listings for Further Help and Information*

Edited by Karen Bellenir. 688 pages. 1998. 0-7808-0224-1. $78.

"This comprehensive book is an excellent addition for high school, academic, medical, and public libraries. This volume is highly recommended."
—*American Reference Books Annual, 2000*

"An invaluable reference." — *Library Journal, May '00*

Selected as one of the 250 "Best Health Sciences Books of 1999." — *Doody's Rating Service, Mar-Apr 2000*

"Recommended reference source."
— *Booklist, American Library Association, Feb '99*

"... provides reliable mainstream medical information ... belongs on the shelves of any library with a consumer health collection." — *E-Streams, Sep '99*

"Provides useful information for the general public."
— *Healthlines, University of Michigan Health Management Research Center, Sep/Oct '99*

■

# Diet & Nutrition Sourcebook, 1st Edition

*Basic Information about Nutrition, Including the Dietary Guidelines for Americans, the Food Guide Pyramid, and Their Applications in Daily Diet, Nutritional Advice for Specific Age Groups, Current Nutritional Issues and Controversies, the New Food Label and How to Use It to Promote Healthy Eating, and Recent Developments in Nutritional Research*

Edited by Dan R. Harris. 662 pages. 1996. 0-7808-0084-2. $78.

"Useful reference as a food and nutrition sourcebook for the general consumer." — *Booklist Health Sciences Supplement, American Library Association, Oct '97*

"Recommended for public libraries and medical libraries that receive general information requests on nutrition. It is readable and will appeal to those interested in learning more about healthy dietary practices."
— *Medical Reference Services Quarterly, Fall '97*

"An abundance of medical and social statistics is translated into readable information geared toward the general reader." — *Bookwatch, Mar '97*

"With dozens of questionable diet books on the market, it is so refreshing to find a reliable and factual reference book. Recommended to aspiring professionals, librarians, and others seeking and giving reliable dietary advice. An excellent compilation." — *Choice, Association of College and Research Libraries, Feb '97*

SEE ALSO *Digestive Diseases & Disorders Sourcebook, Gastrointestinal Diseases & Disorders Sourcebook*

■

# Diet & Nutrition Sourcebook, 2nd Edition

*Basic Consumer Health Information about Dietary Guidelines, Recommended Daily Intake Values, Vitamins, Minerals, Fiber, Fat, Weight Control, Dietary Supplements, and Food Additives*

*Along with Special Sections on Nutrition Needs throughout Life and Nutrition for People with Such Specific Medical Concerns as Allergies, High Blood Cholesterol, Hypertension, Diabetes, Celiac Disease, Seizure Disorders, Phenylketonuria (PKU), Cancer, and Eating Disorders, and Including Reports on Current Nutrition Research and Source Listings for Additional Help and Information*

Edited by Karen Bellenir. 650 pages. 1999. 0-7808-0228-4. $78.

"This book is an excellent source of basic diet and nutrition information." — *Booklist Health Sciences Supplement, American Library Association, Dec '00*

"This reference document should be in any public library, but it would be a very good guide for beginning students in the health sciences. If the other books in this publisher's series are as good as this, they should all be in the health sciences collections."
—*American Reference Books Annual, 2000*

"This book is an excellent general nutrition reference for consumers who desire to take an active role in their health care for prevention. Consumers of all ages who select this book can feel confident they are receiving current and accurate information."
— *Journal of Nutrition for the Elderly, Vol. 19, No. 4, '00*

"Recommended reference source."
—*Booklist, American Library Association, Dec '99*

SEE ALSO *Digestive Diseases & Disorders Sourcebook, Gastrointestinal Diseases & Disorders Sourcebook*

■

# Digestive Diseases & Disorders Sourcebook

*Basic Consumer Health Information about Diseases and Disorders that Impact the Upper and Lower Digestive System, Including Celiac Disease, Constipation, Crohn's Disease, Cyclic Vomiting Syndrome, Diarrhea, Diverticulosis and Diverticulitis, Gallstones, Heart-*

burn, Hemorrhoids, Hernias, Indigestion (Dyspepsia), Irritable Bowel Syndrome, Lactose Intolerance, Ulcers, and More

Along with Information about Medications and Other Treatments, Tips for Maintaining a Healthy Digestive Tract, a Glossary, and Directory of Digestive Diseases Organizations

Edited by Karen Bellenir. 335 pages. 1999. 0-7808-0327-2. $48.

"This title is recommended for public, hospital, and health sciences libraries with consumer health collections." — *E-Streams, Jul-Aug '00*

"Recommended reference source."
— *Booklist, American Library Association, May '00*

*SEE ALSO* Diet & Nutrition Sourcebook, 1st and 2nd Editions, Gastrointestinal Diseases & Disorders Sourcebook

■

# Disabilities Sourcebook

Basic Consumer Health Information about Physical and Psychiatric Disabilities, Including Descriptions of Major Causes of Disability, Assistive and Adaptive Aids, Workplace Issues, and Accessibility Concerns

Along with Information about the Americans with Disabilities Act, a Glossary, and Resources for Additional Help and Information

Edited by Dawn D. Matthews. 616 pages. 2000. 0-7808-0389-2. $78.

"An excellent source book in easy-to-read format covering many current topics; highly recommended for all libraries." — *Choice, Association of College and Research Libraries, Jan '01*

"Recommended reference source."
— *Booklist, American Library Association, Jul '00*

"An involving, invaluable handbook."
— *The Bookwatch, May '00*

■

# Domestic Violence & Child Abuse Sourcebook

Basic Consumer Health Information about Spousal/Partner, Child, Sibling, Parent, and Elder Abuse, Covering Physical, Emotional, and Sexual Abuse, Teen Dating Violence, and Stalking; Includes Information about Hotlines, Safe Houses, Safety Plans, and Other Resources for Support and Assistance, Community Initiatives, and Reports on Current Directions in Research and Treatment

Along with a Glossary, Sources for Further Reading, and Governmental and Non-Governmental Organizations Contact Information

Edited by Helene Henderson. 1,064 pages. 2000. 0-7808-0235-7. $78.

# Drug Abuse Sourcebook

Basic Consumer Health Information about Illicit Substances of Abuse and the Diversion of Prescription Medications, Including Depressants, Hallucinogens, Inhalants, Marijuana, Narcotics, Stimulants, and Anabolic Steroids

Along with Facts about Related Health Risks, Treatment Issues, and Substance Abuse Prevention Programs, a Glossary of Terms, Statistical Data, and Directories of Hotline Services, Self-Help Groups, and Organizations Able to Provide Further Information

Edited by Karen Bellenir. 629 pages. 2000. 0-7808-0242-X. $78.

"Highly recommended." — *The Bookwatch, Jan '01*

*SEE ALSO* Alcoholism Sourcebook, Substance Abuse Sourcebook

■

# Ear, Nose & Throat Disorders Sourcebook

Basic Information about Disorders of the Ears, Nose, Sinus Cavities, Pharynx, and Larynx, Including Ear Infections, Tinnitus, Vestibular Disorders, Allergic and Non-Allergic Rhinitis, Sore Throats, Tonsillitis, and Cancers That Affect the Ears, Nose, Sinuses, and Throat

Along with Reports on Current Research Initiatives, a Glossary of Related Medical Terms, and a Directory of Sources for Further Help and Information

Edited by Karen Bellenir and Linda M. Shin. 576 pages. 1998. 0-7808-0206-3. $78.

"Overall, this sourcebook is helpful for the consumer seeking information on ENT issues. It is recommended for public libraries."
— *American Reference Books Annual, 1999*

"Recommended reference source."
— *Booklist, American Library Association, Dec '98*

■

# Endocrine & Metabolic Disorders Sourcebook

Basic Information for the Layperson about Pancreatic and Insulin-Related Disorders Such as Pancreatitis, Diabetes, and Hypoglycemia; Adrenal Gland Disorders Such as Cushing's Syndrome, Addison's Disease, and Congenital Adrenal Hyperplasia; Pituitary Gland Disorders Such as Growth Hormone Deficiency, Acromegaly, and Pituitary Tumors; Thyroid Disorders Such as Hypothyroidism, Graves' Disease, Hashimoto's Disease, and Goiter; Hyperparathyroidism; and Other Diseases and Syndromes of Hormone Imbalance or Metabolic Dysfunction

Along with Reports on Current Research Initiatives

Edited by Linda M. Shin. 574 pages. 1998. 0-7808-0207-1. $78.

"Omnigraphics has produced another needed resource for health information consumers."
— *American Reference Books Annual, 2000*

"Recommended reference source."
— *Booklist, American Library Association, Dec '98*

## Environmentally Induced Disorders Sourcebook

*Basic Information about Diseases and Syndromes Linked to Exposure to Pollutants and Other Substances in Outdoor and Indoor Environments Such as Lead, Asbestos, Formaldehyde, Mercury, Emissions, Noise, and More*

Edited by Allan R. Cook. 620 pages. 1997. 0-7808-0083-4. $78.

**"Recommended reference source."**
— *Booklist, American Library Association, Sep '98*

**"This book will be a useful addition to anyone's library."** — *Choice Health Sciences Supplement, Association of College and Research Libraries, May '98*

**". . . a good survey of numerous environmentally induced physical disorders . . . a useful addition to anyone's library."**
— *Doody's Health Sciences Book Reviews, Jan '98*

**". . . provide[s] introductory information from the best authorities around. Since this volume covers topics that potentially affect everyone, it will surely be one of the most frequently consulted volumes in the *Health Reference Series*."** — *Rettig on Reference, Nov '97*

■

## Ethnic Diseases Sourcebook

*Basic Consumer Health Information for Ethnic and Racial Minority Groups in the United States, Including General Health Indicators and Behaviors, Ethnic Diseases, Genetic Testing, the Impact of Chronic Diseases, Women's Health, Mental Health Issues, and Preventive Health Care Services*

*Along with a Glossary and a Listing of Additional Resources*

Edited by Joyce Brennfleck Shannon. 600 pages. 2001. 0-7808-0336-1. $78.

■

## Family Planning Sourcebook

*Basic Consumer Health Information about Planning for Pregnancy and Contraception, Including Traditional Methods, Barrier Methods, Hormonal Methods, Permanent Methods, Future Methods, Emergency Contraception, and Birth Control Choices for Women at Each Stage of Life*

*Along with Statistics, a Glossary, and Sources of Additional Information*

Edited by Amy Marcaccio Keyzer. 520 pages. 2001. 0-7808-0379-5. $78.

**SEE ALSO** *Pregnancy & Birth Sourcebook*

## Fitness & Exercise Sourcebook, 1st Edition

*Basic Information on Fitness and Exercise, Including Fitness Activities for Specific Age Groups, Exercise for People with Specific Medical Conditions, How to Begin a Fitness Program in Running, Walking, Swimming, Cycling, and Other Athletic Activities, and Recent Research in Fitness and Exercise*

Edited by Dan R. Harris. 663 pages. 1996. 0-7808-0186-5. $78.

**"A good resource for general readers."**
— *Choice, Association of College and Research Libraries, Nov '97*

**"The perennial popularity of the topic . . . make this an appealing selection for public libraries."**
— *Rettig on Reference, Jun/Jul '97*

■

## Fitness & Exercise Sourcebook, 2nd Edition

*Basic Consumer Health Information about the Fundamentals of Fitness and Exercise, Including How to Begin and Maintain a Fitness Program, Fitness as a Lifestyle, the Link between Fitness and Diet, Advice for Specific Groups of People, Exercise as It Relates to Specific Medical Conditions, and Recent Research in Fitness and Exercise*

*Along with a Glossary of Important Terms and Resources for Additional Help and Information*

Edited by Kristen M. Gledhill. 600 pages. 2001. 0-7808-0334-5. $78.

■

## Food & Animal Borne Diseases Sourcebook

*Basic Information about Diseases That Can Be Spread to Humans through the Ingestion of Contaminated Food or Water or by Contact with Infected Animals and Insects, Such as Botulism, E. Coli, Hepatitis A, Trichinosis, Lyme Disease, and Rabies*

*Along with Information Regarding Prevention and Treatment Methods, and Including a Special Section for International Travelers Describing Diseases Such as Cholera, Malaria, Travelers' Diarrhea, and Yellow Fever, and Offering Recommendations for Avoiding Illness*

Edited by Karen Bellenir and Peter D. Dresser. 535 pages. 1995. 0-7808-0033-8. $78.

**"Targeting general readers and providing them with a single, comprehensive source of information on selected topics, this book continues, with the excellent caliber of its predecessors, to catalog topical information on health matters of general interest. Readable and thorough, this valuable resource is highly recommended for all libraries."**
— *Academic Library Book Review, Summer '96*

**"A comprehensive collection of authoritative information."** — *Emergency Medical Services, Oct '95*

# Food Safety Sourcebook

*Basic Consumer Health Information about the Safe Handling of Meat, Poultry, Seafood, Eggs, Fruit Juices, and Other Food Items, and Facts about Pesticides, Drinking Water, Food Safety Overseas, and the Onset, Duration, and Symptoms of Foodborne Illnesses, Including Types of Pathogenic Bacteria, Parasitic Protozoa, Worms, Viruses, and Natural Toxins*

*Along with the Role of the Consumer, the Food Handler, and the Government in Food Safety; a Glossary, and Resources for Additional Help and Information*

Edited by Dawn D. Matthews. 339 pages. 1999. 0-7808-0326-4. $48.

"This book is recommended for public libraries and universities with home economic and food science programs." —*E-Streams, Nov '00*

"This book takes the complex issues of food safety and foodborne pathogens and presents them in an easily understood manner. [It does] an excellent job of covering a large and often confusing topic."
—*American Reference Books Annual, 2000*

"Recommended reference source."
—*Booklist, American Library Association, May '00*

■

# Forensic Medicine Sourcebook

*Basic Consumer Information for the Layperson about Forensic Medicine, Including Crime Scene Investigation, Evidence Collection and Analysis, Expert Testimony, Computer-Aided Criminal Identification, Digital Imaging in the Courtroom, DNA Profiling, Accident Reconstruction, Autopsies, Ballistics, Drugs and Explosives Detection, Latent Fingerprints, Product Tampering, and Questioned Document Examination*

*Along with Statistical Data, a Glossary of Forensics Terminology, and Listings of Sources for Further Help and Information*

Edited by Annemarie S. Muth. 574 pages. 1999. 0-7808-0232-2. $78.

"There are several items that make this book attractive to consumers who are seeking certain forensic data.... This is a useful current source for those seeking general forensic medical answers."
—*American Reference Books Annual, 2000*

"Recommended for public libraries."
—*Reference & User Services Quarterly, American Library Association, Spring 2000*

"Recommended reference source."
—*Booklist, American Library Association, Feb '00*

"A wealth of information, useful statistics, references are up-to-date and extremely complete. This wonderful collection of data will help students who are interested in a career in any type of forensic field. It is a great resource for attorneys who need information about types of expert witnesses needed in a particular case. It also offers useful information for fiction and nonfiction writers whose work involves a crime. A fascinating compilation. All levels." —*Choice, Association of College and Research Libraries, Jan 2000*

# Gastrointestinal Diseases & Disorders Sourcebook

*Basic Information about Gastroesophageal Reflux Disease (Heartburn), Ulcers, Diverticulosis, Irritable Bowel Syndrome, Crohn's Disease, Ulcerative Colitis, Diarrhea, Constipation, Lactose Intolerance, Hemorrhoids, Hepatitis, Cirrhosis, and Other Digestive Problems, Featuring Statistics, Descriptions of Symptoms, and Current Treatment Methods of Interest for Persons Living with Upper and Lower Gastrointestinal Maladies*

Edited by Linda M. Ross. 413 pages. 1996. 0-7808-0078-8. $78.

". . . very readable form. The successful editorial work that brought this material together into a useful and understandable reference makes accessible to all readers information that can help them more effectively understand and obtain help for digestive tract problems."
—*Choice, Association of College and Research Libraries, Feb '97*

*SEE ALSO Diet & Nutrition Sourcebook, 1st and 2nd Editions, Digestive Diseases & Disorders Sourcebook*

■

# Genetic Disorders Sourcebook, 1st Edition

*Basic Information about Heritable Diseases and Disorders Such as Down Syndrome, PKU, Hemophilia, Von Willebrand Disease, Gaucher Disease, Tay-Sachs Disease, and Sickle-Cell Disease, Along with Information about Genetic Screening, Gene Therapy, Home Care, and Including Source Listings for Further Help and Information on More Than 300 Disorders*

Edited by Karen Bellenir. 642 pages. 1996. 0-7808-0034-6. $78.

"Recommended for undergraduate libraries or libraries that serve the public."
—*Science & Technology Libraries, Vol. 18, No. 1, '99*

"Provides essential medical information to both the general public and those diagnosed with a serious or fatal genetic disease or disorder."
—*Choice, Association of College and Research Libraries, Jan '97*

"Geared toward the lay public. It would be well placed in all public libraries and in those hospital and medical libraries in which access to genetic references is limited." —*Doody's Health Sciences Book Review, Oct '96*

■

# Genetic Disorders Sourcebook, 2nd Edition

*Basic Consumer Health Information about Hereditary Diseases and Disorders, Including Cystic Fibrosis, Down Syndrome, Hemophilia, Huntington's Disease, Sickle Cell Anemia, and More; Facts about Genes, Gene Research and Therapy, Genetic Screening, Ethics of Gene Testing, Genetic Counseling, and Advice on Coping and Caring*

*Along with a Glossary of Genetic Terminology and a Resource List for Help, Support, and Further Information*

Edited by Kathy Massimini. 768 pages. 2001. 0-7808-0241-1. $78.

■

# Head Trauma Sourcebook

*Basic Information for the Layperson about Open-Head and Closed-Head Injuries, Treatment Advances, Recovery, and Rehabilitation*

*Along with Reports on Current Research Initiatives*

Edited by Karen Bellenir. 414 pages. 1997. 0-7808-0208-X. $78.

■

# Health Insurance Sourcebook

*Basic Information about Managed Care Organizations, Traditional Fee-for-Service Insurance, Insurance Portability and Pre-Existing Conditions Clauses, Medicare, Medicaid, Social Security, and Military Health Care*

*Along with Information about Insurance Fraud*

Edited by Wendy Wilcox. 530 pages. 1997. 0-7808-0222-5. $78.

"Particularly useful because it brings much of this information together in one volume. This book will be a handy reference source in the health sciences library, hospital library, college and university library, and medium to large public library."
—*Medical Reference Services Quarterly, Fall '98*

Awarded "Books of the Year Award"
—*American Journal of Nursing, 1997*

"The layout of the book is particularly helpful as it provides easy access to reference material. A most useful addition to the vast amount of information about health insurance. The use of data from U.S. government agencies is most commendable. Useful in a library or learning center for healthcare professional students."
—*Doody's Health Sciences Book Reviews, Nov '97*

■

# Healthy Aging Sourcebook

*Basic Consumer Health Information about Maintaining Health through the Aging Process, Including Advice on Nutrition, Exercise, and Sleep, Help in Making Decisions about Midlife Issues and Retirement, and Guidance Concerning Practical and Informed Choices in Health Consumerism*

*Along with Data Concerning the Theories of Aging, Different Experiences in Aging by Minority Groups, and Facts about Aging Now and Aging in the Future; and Featuring a Glossary, a Guide to Consumer Help, Additional Suggested Reading, and Practical Resource Directory*

Edited by Jenifer Swanson. 536 pages. 1999. 0-7808-0390-6. $78.

"Recommended reference source."
—*Booklist, American Library Association, Feb '00*

***SEE ALSO*** *Physical & Mental Issues in Aging Sourcebook*

# Healthy Heart Sourcebook for Women

*Basic Consumer Health Information about Cardiac Issues Specific to Women, Including Facts about Major Risk Factors and Prevention, Treatment and Control Strategies, and Important Dietary Issues*

*Along with a Special Section Regarding the Pros and Cons of Hormone Replacement Therapy and Its Impact on Heart Health, and Additional Help, Including Recipes, a Glossary, and a Directory of Resources*

Edited by Dawn D. Matthews. 336 pages. 2000. 0-7808-0329-9. $48.

"Contains very important information about coronary artery disease that all women should know. The information is current and presented in an easy-to-read format. The book will make a good addition to any library."
—*American Medical Writers Association Journal, Summer '00*

"Important, basic reference."
—*Reviewer's Bookwatch, Jul '00*

***SEE ALSO*** *Cardiovascular Diseases & Disorders Sourcebook, 1st Edition, Heart Diseases & Disorders Sourcebook, 2nd Edition, Women's Health Concerns Sourcebook*

■

# Heart Diseases & Disorders Sourcebook, 2nd Edition

*Basic Consumer Health Information about Heart Attacks, Angina, Rhythm Disorders, Heart Failure, Valve Disease, Congenital Heart Disorders, and More, Including Descriptions of Surgical Procedures and Other Interventions, Medications, Cardiac Rehabilitation, Risk Identification, and Prevention Tips*

*Along with Statistical Data, Reports on Current Research Initiatives, a Glossary of Cardiovascular Terms, and Resource Directory*

Edited by Karen Bellenir. 612 pages. 2000. 0-7808-0238-1. $78.

"Recommended reference source."
—*Booklist, American Library Association, Dec '00*

"Provides comprehensive coverage of matters related to the heart. This title is recommended for health sciences and public libraries with consumer health collections."
—*E-Streams, Oct '00*

***SEE ALSO*** *Cardiovascular Diseases & Disorders Sourcebook, 1st Edition, Healthy Heart Sourcebook for Women*

■

# Immune System Disorders Sourcebook

*Basic Information about Lupus, Multiple Sclerosis, Guillain-Barré Syndrome, Chronic Granulomatous Disease, and More*

*Along with Statistical and Demographic Data and Reports on Current Research Initiatives*

Edited by Allan R. Cook. 608 pages. 1997. 0-7808-0209-8. $78.

## Infant & Toddler Health Sourcebook

*Basic Consumer Health Information about the Physical and Mental Development of Newborns, Infants, and Toddlers, Including Neonatal Concerns, Nutrition Recommendations, Immunization Schedules, Common Pediatric Disorders, Assessments and Milestones, Safety Tips, and Advice for Parents and Other Caregivers*

*Along with a Glossary of Terms and Resource Listings for Additional Help*

Edited by Jenifer Swanson. 585 pages. 2000. 0-7808-0246-2. $78.

## Kidney & Urinary Tract Diseases & Disorders Sourcebook

*Basic Information about Kidney Stones, Urinary Incontinence, Bladder Disease, End Stage Renal Disease, Dialysis, and More*

*Along with Statistical and Demographic Data and Reports on Current Research Initiatives*

Edited by Linda M. Ross. 602 pages. 1997. 0-7808-0079-6. $78.

## Learning Disabilities Sourcebook

*Basic Information about Disorders Such as Dyslexia, Visual and Auditory Processing Deficits, Attention Deficit/Hyperactivity Disorder, and Autism*

*Along with Statistical and Demographic Data, Reports on Current Research Initiatives, an Explanation of the Assessment Process, and a Special Section for Adults with Learning Disabilities*

Edited by Linda M. Shin. 579 pages. 1998. 0-7808-0210-1. $78.

**Named "Outstanding Reference Book of 1999."**
— *New York Public Library, Feb 2000*

**"An excellent candidate for inclusion in a public library reference section. It's a great source of information. Teachers will also find the book useful. Definitely worth reading."**
— *Journal of Adolescent & Adult Literacy, Feb 2000*

**"Readable . . . provides a solid base of information regarding successful techniques used with individuals who have learning disabilities, as well as practical suggestions for educators and family members. Clear language, concise descriptions, and pertinent information for contacting multiple resources add to the strength of this book as a useful tool."**
— *Choice, Association of College and Research Libraries, Feb '99*

**"Recommended reference source."**
— *Booklist, American Library Association, Sep '98*

**"This is a useful resource for libraries and for those who don't have the time to identify and locate the individual publications."**
— *Disability Resources Monthly, Sep '98*

## Liver Disorders Sourcebook

*Basic Consumer Health Information about the Liver and How It Works; Liver Diseases, Including Cancer, Cirrhosis, Hepatitis, and Toxic and Drug Related Diseases; Tips for Maintaining a Healthy Liver; Laboratory Tests, Radiology Tests, and Facts about Liver Transplantation*

*Along with a Section on Support Groups, a Glossary, and Resource Listings*

Edited by Joyce Brennfleck Shannon. 591 pages. 2000. 0-7808-0383-3. $78.

**"This title is recommended for health sciences and public libraries with consumer health collections."**
— *E-Streams, Oct '00*

**"Recommended reference source."**
— *Booklist, American Library Association, Jun '00*

## Medical Tests Sourcebook

*Basic Consumer Health Information about Medical Tests, Including Periodic Health Exams, General Screening Tests, Tests You Can Do at Home, Findings of the U.S. Preventive Services Task Force, X-ray and Radiology Tests, Electrical Tests, Tests of Blood and Other Body Fluids and Tissues, Scope Tests, Lung Tests, Genetic Tests, Pregnancy Tests, Newborn Screening Tests, Sexually Transmitted Disease Tests, and Computer Aided Diagnoses*

*Along with a Section on Paying for Medical Tests, a Glossary, and Resource Listings*

Edited by Joyce Brennfleck Shannon. 691 pages. 1999. 0-7808-0243-8. $78.

**"A valuable reference guide."**
— *American Reference Books Annual, 2000*

**"Recommended for hospital and health sciences libraries with consumer health collections."**
— *E-Streams, Mar '00*

**"This is an overall excellent reference with a wealth of general knowledge that may aid those who are reluctant to get vital tests performed."**
— *Today's Librarian, Jan 2000*

## Men's Health Concerns Sourcebook

*Basic Information about Health Issues That Affect Men, Featuring Facts about the Top Causes of Death in Men, Including Heart Disease, Stroke, Cancers, Prostate Disorders, Chronic Obstructive Pulmonary Disease, Pneumonia and Influenza, Human Immunodeficiency Virus and Acquired Immune Deficiency Syndrome, Diabetes Mellitus, Stress, Suicide, Accidents and Homicides; and Facts about Common Concerns for Men, Including Impotence, Contraception, Circumcision, Sleep Disorders, Snoring, Hair Loss, Diet, Nutrition, Exercise, Kidney and Urological Disorders, and Backaches*

Edited by Allan R. Cook. 738 pages. 1998. 0-7808-0212-8. $78.

"This comprehensive resource and the series are highly recommended."
—*American Reference Books Annual, 2000*

"Recommended reference source."
—*Booklist, American Library Association, Dec '98*

■

# Mental Health Disorders Sourcebook, 1st Edition

*Basic Information about Schizophrenia, Depression, Bipolar Disorder, Panic Disorder, Obsessive-Compulsive Disorder, Phobias and Other Anxiety Disorders, Paranoia and Other Personality Disorders, Eating Disorders, and Sleep Disorders*

*Along with Information about Treatment and Therapies*

Edited by Karen Bellenir. 548 pages. 1995. 0-7808-0040-0. $78.

"This is an excellent new book . . . written in easy-to-understand language."    —*Booklist Health Sciences Supplement, American Library Association, Oct '97*

". . . useful for public and academic libraries and consumer health collections."
—*Medical Reference Services Quarterly, Spring '97*

"The great strengths of the book are its readability and its inclusion of places to find more information. Especially recommended."    —*Reference Quarterly, American Library Association, Winter '96*

". . . a good resource for a consumer health library."
—*Bulletin of the Medical Library Association, Oct '96*

"The information is data-based and couched in brief, concise language that avoids jargon. . . . a useful reference source."    —*Readings, Sep '96*

"The text is well organized and adequately written for its target audience."    —*Choice, Association of College and Research Libraries, Jun '96*

". . . provides information on a wide range of mental disorders, presented in nontechnical language."
—*Exceptional Child Education Resources, Spring '96*

"Recommended for public and academic libraries."
—*Reference Book Review, 1996*

■

# Mental Health Disorders Sourcebook, 2nd Edition

*Basic Consumer Health Information about Anxiety Disorders, Depression and Other Mood Disorders, Eating Disorders, Personality Disorders, Schizophrenia, and More, Including Disease Descriptions, Treatment Options, and Reports on Current Research Initiatives*

*Along with Statistical Data, Tips for Maintaining Mental Health, a Glossary, and Directory of Sources for Additional Help and Information*

Edited by Karen Bellenir. 605 pages. 2000. 0-7808-0240-3. $78.

"Recommended reference source."
—*Booklist, American Library Association, Jun '00*

# Mental Retardation Sourcebook

*Basic Consumer Health Information about Mental Retardation and Its Causes, Including Down Syndrome, Fetal Alcohol Syndrome, Fragile X Syndrome, Genetic Conditions, Injury, and Environmental Sources*

*Along with Preventive Strategies, Parenting Issues, Educational Implications, Health Care Needs, Employment and Economic Matters, Legal Issues, a Glossary, and a Resource Listing for Additional Help and Information*

Edited by Joyce Brennfleck Shannon. 642 pages. 2000. 0-7808-0377-9. $78.

"The strength of this work is that it compiles many basic fact sheets and addresses for further information in one volume. It is intended and suitable for the general public. The sourcebook is relevant to any collection providing health information to the general public."
—*E-Streams, Nov '00*

"From preventing retardation to parenting and family challenges, this covers health, social and legal issues and will prove an invaluable overview."
—*Reviewer's Bookwatch, Jul '00*

■

# Obesity Sourcebook

*Basic Consumer Health Information about Diseases and Other Problems Associated with Obesity, and Including Facts about Risk Factors, Prevention Issues, and Management Approaches*

*Along with Statistical and Demographic Data, Information about Special Populations, Research Updates, a Glossary, and Source Listings for Further Help and Information*

Edited by Wilma Caldwell and Chad T. Kimball. 376 pages. 2001. 0-7808-0333-7. $48.

■

# Ophthalmic Disorders Sourcebook

*Basic Information about Glaucoma, Cataracts, Macular Degeneration, Strabismus, Refractive Disorders, and More*

*Along with Statistical and Demographic Data and Reports on Current Research Initiatives*

Edited by Linda M. Ross. 631 pages. 1996. 0-7808-0081-8. $78.

■

# Oral Health Sourcebook

*Basic Information about Diseases and Conditions Affecting Oral Health, Including Cavities, Gum Disease, Dry Mouth, Oral Cancers, Fever Blisters, Canker Sores, Oral Thrush, Bad Breath, Temporomandibular Disorders, and other Craniofacial Syndromes*

*Along with Statistical Data on the Oral Health of Americans, Oral Hygiene, Emergency First Aid, Information on Treatment Procedures and Methods of Replacing Lost Teeth*

Edited by Allan R. Cook. 558 pages. 1997. 0-7808-0082-6. $78.

"Unique source which will fill a gap in dental sources for patients and the lay public. A valuable reference tool even in a library with thousands of books on dentistry. Comprehensive, clear, inexpensive, and easy to read and use. It fills an enormous gap in the health care literature." —Reference and User Services Quarterly, American Library Association, Summer '98

"Recommended reference source." —Booklist, American Library Association, Dec '97

# Osteoporosis Sourcebook

Basic Consumer Health Information about Primary and Secondary Osteoporosis and Juvenile Osteoporosis and Related Conditions, Including Fibrous Dysplasia, Gaucher Disease, Hyperthyroidism, Hypophosphatasia, Myeloma, Osteopetrosis, Osteogenesis Imperfecta, and Paget's Disease

Along with Information about Risk Factors, Treatments, Traditional and Non-Traditional Pain Management, a Glossary of Related Terms, and a Directory of Resources

Edited by Allan R. Cook. 584 pages. 2001. 0-7808-0239-X. $78.

SEE ALSO Women's Health Concerns Sourcebook

# Pain Sourcebook

Basic Information about Specific Forms of Acute and Chronic Pain, Including Headaches, Back Pain, Muscular Pain, Neuralgia, Surgical Pain, and Cancer Pain

Along with Pain Relief Options Such as Analgesics, Narcotics, Nerve Blocks, Transcutaneous Nerve Stimulation, and Alternative Forms of Pain Control, Including Biofeedback, Imaging, Behavior Modification, and Relaxation Techniques

Edited by Allan R. Cook. 667 pages. 1997. 0-7808-0213-6. $78.

"The text is readable, easily understood, and well indexed. This excellent volume belongs in all patient education libraries, consumer health sections of public libraries, and many personal collections." —American Reference Books Annual, 1999

"A beneficial reference." —Booklist Health Sciences Supplement, American Library Association, Oct '98

"The information is basic in terms of scholarship and is appropriate for general readers. Written in journalistic style ... intended for non-professionals. Quite thorough in its coverage of different pain conditions and summarizes the latest clinical information regarding pain treatment." —Choice, Association of College and Research Libraries, Jun '98

"Recommended reference source." —Booklist, American Library Association, Mar '98

# Pediatric Cancer Sourcebook

Basic Consumer Health Information about Leukemias, Brain Tumors, Sarcomas, Lymphomas, and Other Cancers in Infants, Children, and Adolescents, Including Descriptions of Cancers, Treatments, and Coping Strategies

Along with Suggestions for Parents, Caregivers, and Concerned Relatives, a Glossary of Cancer Terms, and Resource Listings

Edited by Edward J. Prucha. 587 pages. 1999. 0-7808-0245-4. $78.

"A valuable addition to all libraries specializing in health services and many public libraries." —American Reference Books Annual, 2000

"Recommended reference source." —Booklist, American Library Association, Feb '00

"An excellent source of information. Recommended for public, hospital, and health science libraries with consumer health collections." —E-Streams, Jun '00

# Physical & Mental Issues in Aging Sourcebook

Basic Consumer Health Information on Physical and Mental Disorders Associated with the Aging Process, Including Concerns about Cardiovascular Disease, Pulmonary Disease, Oral Health, Digestive Disorders, Musculoskeletal and Skin Disorders, Metabolic Changes, Sexual and Reproductive Issues, and Changes in Vision, Hearing, and Other Senses

Along with Data about Longevity and Causes of Death, Information on Acute and Chronic Pain, Descriptions of Mental Concerns, a Glossary of Terms, and Resource Listings for Additional Help

Edited by Jenifer Swanson. 660 pages. 1999. 0-7808-0233-0. $78.

"Recommended for public libraries." —American Reference Books Annual, 2000

"This is a treasure of health information for the layperson." —Choice Health Sciences Supplement, Association of College & Research Libraries, May 2000

"Recommended reference source." —Booklist, American Library Association, Oct '99

SEE ALSO Healthy Aging Sourcebook

# Podiatry Sourcebook

Basic Consumer Health Information about Foot Conditions, Diseases, and Injuries, Including Bunions, Corns, Calluses, Athlete's Foot, Plantar Warts, Hammertoes and Clawtoes, Club Foot, Heel Pain, Gout, and More

Along with Facts about Foot Care, Disease Prevention, Foot Safety, Choosing a Foot Care Specialist, a Glossary of Terms, and Resource Listings for Additional Information

Edited by M. Lisa Weatherford. 600 pages. 2001. 0-7808-0215-2. $78.

# Pregnancy & Birth Sourcebook

*Basic Information about Planning for Pregnancy, Maternal Health, Fetal Growth and Development, Labor and Delivery, Postpartum and Perinatal Care, Pregnancy in Mothers with Special Concerns, and Disorders of Pregnancy, Including Genetic Counseling, Nutrition and Exercise, Obstetrical Tests, Pregnancy Discomfort, Multiple Births, Cesarean Sections, Medical Testing of Newborns, Breastfeeding, Gestational Diabetes, and Ectopic Pregnancy*

Edited by Heather E. Aldred. 737 pages. 1997. 0-7808-0216-0. $78.

**"A well-organized handbook. Recommended."**
— *Choice, Association of College and Research Libraries, Apr '98*

**"Recommended reference source."**
— *Booklist, American Library Association, Mar '98*

**"Recommended for public libraries."**
— *American Reference Books Annual, 1998*

***SEE ALSO*** *Congenital Disorders Sourcebook, Family Planning Sourcebook*

■

# Public Health Sourcebook

*Basic Information about Government Health Agencies, Including National Health Statistics and Trends, Healthy People 2000 Program Goals and Objectives, the Centers for Disease Control and Prevention, the Food and Drug Administration, and the National Institutes of Health*

*Along with Full Contact Information for Each Agency*

Edited by Wendy Wilcox. 698 pages. 1998. 0-7808-0220-9. $78.

**"Recommended reference source."**
— *Booklist, American Library Association, Sep '98*

**"This consumer guide provides welcome assistance in navigating the maze of federal health agencies and their data on public health concerns."**
— *SciTech Book News, Sep '98*

■

# Reconstructive & Cosmetic Surgery Sourcebook

*Basic Consumer Health Information on Cosmetic and Reconstructive Plastic Surgery, Including Statistical Information about Different Surgical Procedures, Things to Consider Prior to Surgery, Plastic Surgery Techniques and Tools, Emotional and Psychological Considerations, and Procedure-Specific Information*

*Along with a Glossary of Terms and a Listing of Resources for Additional Help and Information*

Edited by M. Lisa Weatherford. 374 pages. 2001. 0-7808-0214-4. $48.

# Rehabilitation Sourcebook

*Basic Consumer Health Information about Rehabilitation for People Recovering from Heart Surgery, Spinal Cord Injury, Stroke, Orthopedic Impairments, Amputation, Pulmonary Impairments, Traumatic Injury, and More, Including Physical Therapy, Occupational Therapy, Speech/ Language Therapy, Massage Therapy, Dance Therapy, Art Therapy, and Recreational Therapy*

*Along with Information on Assistive and Adaptive Devices, a Glossary, and Resources for Additional Help and Information*

Edited by Dawn D. Matthews. 531 pages. 1999. 0-7808-0236-5. $78.

**"Recommended reference source."**
— *Booklist, American Library Association, May '00*

■

# Respiratory Diseases & Disorders Sourcebook

*Basic Information about Respiratory Diseases and Disorders, Including Asthma, Cystic Fibrosis, Pneumonia, the Common Cold, Influenza, and Others, Featuring Facts about the Respiratory System, Statistical and Demographic Data, Treatments, Self-Help Management Suggestions, and Current Research Initiatives*

Edited by Allan R. Cook and Peter D. Dresser. 771 pages. 1995. 0-7808-0037-0. $78.

**"Designed for the layperson and for patients and their families coping with respiratory illness. . . . an extensive array of information on diagnosis, treatment, management, and prevention of respiratory illnesses for the general reader."** — *Choice, Association of College and Research Libraries, Jun '96*

**"A highly recommended text for all collections. It is a comforting reminder of the power of knowledge that good books carry between their covers."**
— *Academic Library Book Review, Spring '96*

**"A comprehensive collection of authoritative information presented in a nontechnical, humanitarian style for patients, families, and caregivers."**
— *Association of Operating Room Nurses, Sep/Oct '95*

■

# Sexually Transmitted Diseases Sourcebook, 1st Edition

*Basic Information about Herpes, Chlamydia, Gonorrhea, Hepatitis, Nongonoccocal Urethritis, Pelvic Inflammatory Disease, Syphilis, AIDS, and More*

*Along with Current Data on Treatments and Preventions*

Edited by Linda M. Ross. 550 pages. 1997. 0-7808-0217-9. $78.

# Sexually Transmitted Diseases Sourcebook, 2nd Edition

*Basic Consumer Health Information about Sexually Transmitted Diseases, Including Information on the Diagnosis and Treatment of Chlamydia, Gonorrhea, Hepatitis, Herpes, HIV, Mononucleosis, Syphilis, and Others*

*Along with Information on Prevention, Such as Condom Use, Vaccines, and STD Education; And Featuring a Section on Issues Related to Youth and Adolescents, a Glossary, and Resources for Additional Help and Information*

Edited by Dawn D. Matthews. 538 pages. 2001. 0-7808-0249-7. $78.

# Skin Disorders Sourcebook

*Basic Information about Common Skin and Scalp Conditions Caused by Aging, Allergies, Immune Reactions, Sun Exposure, Infectious Organisms, Parasites, Cosmetics, and Skin Traumas, Including Abrasions, Cuts, and Pressure Sores*

*Along with Information on Prevention and Treatment*

Edited by Allan R. Cook. 647 pages. 1997. 0-7808-0080-X. $78.

". . . comprehensive, easily read reference book."
— *Doody's Health Sciences Book Reviews, Oct '97*

**SEE ALSO** *Burns Sourcebook*

# Sleep Disorders Sourcebook

*Basic Consumer Health Information about Sleep and Its Disorders, Including Insomnia, Sleepwalking, Sleep Apnea, Restless Leg Syndrome, and Narcolepsy*

*Along with Data about Shiftwork and Its Effects, Information on the Societal Costs of Sleep Deprivation, Descriptions of Treatment Options, a Glossary of Terms, and Resource Listings for Additional Help*

Edited by Jenifer Swanson. 439 pages. 1998. 0-7808-0234-9. $78.

"This text will complement any home or medical library. It is user-friendly and ideal for the adult reader."
— *American Reference Books Annual, 2000*

"Recommended reference source."
— *Booklist, American Library Association, Feb '99*

"A useful resource that provides accurate, relevant, and accessible information on sleep to the general public. Health care providers who deal with sleep disorders patients may also find it helpful in being prepared to answer some of the questions patients ask."
— *Respiratory Care, Jul '99*

# Sports Injuries Sourcebook

*Basic Consumer Health Information about Common Sports Injuries, Prevention of Injury in Specific Sports, Tips for Training, and Rehabilitation from Injury*

*Along with Information about Special Concerns for Children, Young Girls in Athletic Training Programs, Senior Athletes, and Women Athletes, and a Directory of Resources for Further Help and Information*

Edited by Heather E. Aldred. 624 pages. 1999. 0-7808-0218-7. $78.

"Public libraries and undergraduate academic libraries will find this book useful for its nontechnical language." — *American Reference Books Annual, 2000*

"While this easy-to-read book is recommended for all libraries, it should prove to be especially useful for public, high school, and academic libraries; certainly it should be on the bookshelf of every school gymnasium." — *E-Streams, Mar '00*

# Substance Abuse Sourcebook

*Basic Health-Related Information about the Abuse of Legal and Illegal Substances Such as Alcohol, Tobacco, Prescription Drugs, Marijuana, Cocaine, and Heroin; and Including Facts about Substance Abuse Prevention Strategies, Intervention Methods, Treatment and Recovery Programs, and a Section Addressing the Special Problems Related to Substance Abuse during Pregnancy*

Edited by Karen Bellenir. 573 pages. 1996. 0-7808-0038-9. $78.

"A valuable addition to any health reference section. Highly recommended."
— *The Book Report, Mar/Apr '97*

". . . a comprehensive collection of substance abuse information that's both highly readable and compact. Families and caregivers of substance abusers will find the information enlightening and helpful, while teachers, social workers and journalists should benefit from the concise format. Recommended."
— *Drug Abuse Update, Winter '96/'97*

**SEE ALSO** *Alcoholism Sourcebook, Drug Abuse Sourcebook*

# Traveler's Health Sourcebook

*Basic Consumer Health Information for Travelers, Including Physical and Medical Preparations, Transportation Health and Safety, Essential Information about Food and Water, Sun Exposure, Insect and Snake Bites, Camping and Wilderness Medicine, and Travel with Physical or Medical Disabilities*

*Along with International Travel Tips, Vaccination Recommendations, Geographical Health Issues, Disease Risks, a Glossary, and a Listing of Additional Resources*

Edited by Joyce Brennfleck Shannon. 613 pages. 2000. 0-7808-0384-1. $78.

## Women's Health Concerns Sourcebook

*Basic Information about Health Issues That Affect Women, Featuring Facts about Menstruation and Other Gynecological Concerns, Including Endometriosis, Fibroids, Menopause, and Vaginitis; Reproductive Concerns, Including Birth Control, Infertility, and Abortion; and Facts about Additional Physical, Emotional, and Mental Health Concerns Prevalent among Women Such as Osteoporosis, Urinary Tract Disorders, Eating Disorders, and Depression*

*Along with Tips for Maintaining a Healthy Lifestyle*

Edited by Heather E. Aldred. 567 pages. 1997. 0-7808-0219-5. $78.

**"Handy compilation. There is an impressive range of diseases, devices, disorders, procedures, and other physical and emotional issues covered . . . well organized, illustrated, and indexed."** — *Choice, Association of College and Research Libraries, Jan '98*

**SEE ALSO** *Breast Cancer Sourcebook, Cancer Sourcebook for Women, 1st and 2nd Editions, Healthy Heart Sourcebook for Women, Osteoporosis Sourcebook*

■

## Workplace Health & Safety Sourcebook

*Basic Consumer Health Information about Workplace Health and Safety, Including the Effect of Workplace Hazards on the Lungs, Skin, Heart, Ears, Eyes, Brain, Reproductive Organs, Musculoskeletal System, and Other Organs and Body Parts*

*Along with Information about Occupational Cancer, Personal Protective Equipment, Toxic and Hazardous Chemicals, Child Labor, Stress, and Workplace Violence*

Edited by Chad T. Kimball. 626 pages. 2000. 0-7808-0231-4. $78.

**"Highly recommended."** — *The Bookwatch, Jan '01*

■

## Worldwide Health Sourcebook

*Basic Information about Global Health Issues, Including Malnutrition, Reproductive Health, Disease Dispersion and Prevention, Emerging Diseases, Risky Health Behaviors, and the Leading Causes of Death*

*Along with Global Health Concerns for Children, Women, and the Elderly, Mental Health Issues, Research and Technology Advancements, and Economic, Environmental, and Political Health Implications, a Glossary, and a Resource Listing for Additional Help and Information*

Edited by Joyce Brennfleck Shannon. 500 pages. 2001. 0-7808-0330-2. $78.

## Health Reference Series Cumulative Index 1999

*A Comprehensive Index to the Individual Volumes of the Health Reference Series, Including a Subject Index, Name Index, Organization Index, and Publication Index*

*Along with a Master List of Acronyms and Abbreviations*

Edited by Edward J. Prucha, Anne Holmes, and Robert Rudnick. 990 pages. 2000. 0-7808-0382-5. $78.

**"Essential for collections that hold any of the numerous *Health Reference Series* titles."**
— *Choice, Association of College and Research Libraries, Nov '00*